I0066224

Encyclopedia of Ovarian Cancer

Encyclopedia of Ovarian Cancer

Edited by **Lester Price**

hayle
medical

New York

Published by Hayle Medical,
30 West, 37th Street, Suite 612,
New York, NY 10018, USA
www.haylemedical.com

Encyclopedia of Ovarian Cancer
Edited by Lester Price

International Standard Book Number: 978-1-63241-188-4 (Hardback)

Printed in the United States of America.

Contents

Preface

Over the recent decade, advancements and applications have progressed exponentially. This has led to the increased interest in this field and projects are being conducted to enhance knowledge. The main objective of this book is to present some of the critical challenges and provide insights into possible solutions. This book will answer the varied questions that arise in the field and also provide an increased scope for furthering studies.

Research-focused detailed information regarding ovarian cancer has been illustrated in this descriptive book. Ovarian cancer accounts for more deaths across the world than the rest of the gynecologic diseases put together. Researchers and scientists from across the globe have reviewed the essential biological and basic science aspects associated with ovarian cancer. This book elucidates the molecular biological characteristics of the disease and also highlights molecular biology methodologies for the purpose of comprehending this cancer. These techniques have been formulated with the purpose of characterizing the tumor genetics, expression and protein function and describing the genetic mechanisms for optimization of immunotherapies. The book also discusses clinical and therapeutic perspectives associated with ovarian cancer and describes an overview of present research on aspects of malignant transformation, metastasis, and growth control. The aim of this book is to serve as a handy source of information for researchers, practitioners as well as students interested in acquiring advanced knowledge about this disease.

I hope that this book, with its visionary approach, will be a valuable addition and will promote interest among readers. Each of the authors has provided their extraordinary competence in their specific fields by providing different perspectives as they come from diverse nations and regions. I thank them for their contributions.

Editor

1

Ovarian Cancer Incidence: Current and Comprehensive Statistics

Sherri L. Stewart
Division of Cancer Prevention and Control, Centers for Disease Control and Prevention
USA

1. Introduction

Ovarian cancer is a commonly diagnosed and particularly deadly gynecologic malignancy worldwide. It ranks among the top ten diagnosed cancers and top five deadliest cancers in most countries (Ferlay et al., 2010). Several cancer incidence data sources have been used to measure ovarian cancer burden across the world; however, the statistics presented are often not population-based, which can lead to misrepresentation of the burden due to incomplete or inaccurate data. An accurate assessment of ovarian cancer burden is essential as incidence data are used for many purposes including to generate hypotheses regarding etiology, allocate resources and funding toward new treatment discovery and clinical trials, and determine which populations of women may benefit from more education or greater surveillance for the disease. The purpose of this chapter is to present global comprehensive ovarian cancer incidence data. Data collected are from several resources, and every effort is made to present only high-quality data from population-based data sources. Because of changing age structures of populations and differences in data quality and coverage of various data sources over time, only the most recent data are presented. This will aid in preventing misinterpretation of temporal trends.

2. Data sources and interpretation

Data on the incidence of ovarian cancer (the number of new cases per year) is collected by population-based cancer registries; however, only certain countries have national registries that collect this information. In the United States, a law passed in 1992 established nationwide cancer surveillance. This law resulted in the establishment of the National Program of Cancer Registries (NPCR), which is administered by the Centers for Disease Control and Prevention (CDC), and provides cancer incidence data for 96% of the U.S. population (U.S.Cancer Statistics Working Group, 2010). When combined with data from the existing Surveillance, Epidemiology, and End Results (SEER) program, administered by the National Cancer Institute (NCI), 100% of the U.S. population is accounted for. Several other countries including Canada, Singapore, Denmark, Finland, Iceland, Norway, and Sweden have nationwide registry systems (Thun et al., 2011). Many other countries base their incidence on cancers collected in certain regions or groups of regions, and therefore these results vary in quality (Thun et al., 2011). Cancer registries typically require a period of one to two years to collect all required information on cancer diagnoses in the geographic areas covered. For that reason, most incidence data reported is two to three years behind the current calendar year.

Incidence rates take into account the number of new cases of cancer (numerator), and also the population at risk for the cancer (denominator). Most incidence rates are age-adjusted or standardized in order to allow comparisons across populations with differing age structures. Several age distributions are available for standardization. In international data, which is compiled from population-based registries by the International Agency for Research on Cancer (IARC), the 1960 world standard population is used (Ferlay et al., 2010). Within specific countries, such as the United States, the 2000 U.S. standard population is used (Thun et al., 2011; U.S.Cancer Statistics Working Group, 2010). Differences in age standardization methodology can result in a variance of rates reported from the same country. Age-specific rates for certain age poulations (e.g., children) are often reported; these rates are often not age-adjusted or standardized. Most rates are expressed per 100,000 persons, and in the case of ovarian cancer per 100,000 women.

In this chapter, data are presented from a variety of sources, including monographs and peer-reviewed literature. Data are presented from the IARC public-use monograph (GLOBOCAN 2008) on case counts and rates for countries around the world (Ferlay et al., 2010). Since the United States also produces a comprehensive monograph annually, data are also presented for this country from the public-use *United States Cancer Statistics* (*USCS*) website (U.S.Cancer Statistics Working Group, 2010). Overall case and rate data from peer-reviewed articles are also included for countries (including the United States) that have published ovarian cancer incidence information from population-based registries. These articles may be a better source of data for some countries than monographs, as they may contain more complete or up-to-date information. Demographic- and clinical factor-specific data, and temporal trends are presented from monographs when available, and are supplemented with data from the most recent peer-reviewed publications for all countries available. Clinical factor data and temporal trends especially (histology, stage, laterality) are most often contained in peer-reviewed publications as opposed to monogaphs. To prevent misinterpretation, only data from the most recent publications (monograph or peer-reviewed publication) are presented. Table 1 lists data sources, years and population covered for each.

3. Global ovarian cancer incidence

A total of 224,747 new cases of ovarian cancer were reported worldwide in 2008, with 99,521 cases being diagnosed in more developed regions, and 125,226 being diagnosed in less developed regions (Ferlay et al., 2010). Ovarian cancer was the seventh most common cancer diagnosis among women in the world overall, and fifth most common cancer diagnosis among women in more developed regions (Ferlay et al., 2010). The world rate is estimated to be 6.3 per 100,000, and is higher in developed countries and regions (9.3) compared to others (Ferlay et al., 2010). Incidence rates for selected regions, continents and countries are shown in Table 2. Rates range from 3.8 in the Southern and Western African regions to 11.8 in the region of Northern Europe. Continental rates are highest in Europe (10.1), followed by North America (8.7), Australia (including New Zealand, 7.8), South America (6.2), Asia (5.1), and Africa (4.2).

Figure 1 displays a categorization of ovarian cancer incidence rates around the world. Rates for individual countries range from 1.8 in Samoa to 14.6 in Latvia (Ferlay et al., 2010).

Author and publication year	Data year(s)	Population*
Ferlay et al., 2010	2008	World
U.S. Cancer Statistics Working Group, 2010	2007	United States (99.1%)
Koper et al., 1996	1989-1991	Netherlands
Ioka et al., 2003	1975-1998	Osaka, Japan
Mahdy et al., 1999	1988-1997	Alexandria, Egypt
Zambon et al., 2004	1986-1997	Several regions in Italy
Kohler et al., 2011	Rates: 2003-2007; Trends: 1998-2007	United States (93%)
Tamakoshi et al., 2001	1975-1993	Several regions in Japan
Jin et al.,1993	1979-1989	Shanghai, China
Dey et al., 2010	1999-2002	Tanta, Egypt
Minelli et al., 2007	1998-2002	Umbria, Italy
Goodman & Howe, 2003	1992-1997	United States (52%)
Goodman et al., 2003	1992-1997	United States (52%)
Boger-Megiddo & Weiss, 2005	1992-2000	United States (26%)
Stiller, 2007	NR	World
Brookfield et al., 2009	1973-2005	United States (9%)
Poynter et al., 2010	1975-2006	United States (9%)
Smith et al., 2006	1973-2002	United States (9%)
Goodman and Shvetsov, 2009	1995-2004	United States (64%)
Jaaback et al., 2006	1993-2003	Royal United Hospital, UK
Stewart et al, 2007	1998-2003	United States (83.1%)
Riska et al., 2003	1953-1997	Finland
Pfeiffer et al., 1989	1978-1983	Denmark

Table 1. Data years and populations covered for monographs and articles cited throughout this chapter. *The population coverage for a particular country or region is provided when available from reports. NR=not reported.

In the United States, 20,749 ovarian cases were diagnosed in 2007 (the most recent year for which data are available), for an incidence rate of 12.2 per 100,000 women (U.S.Cancer Statistics Working Group, 2010). Koper et al. reported a rate of 14.9 in the Netherlands, similar to that found in the United States (Koper et al., 1996). In Osaka, Japan the overall rate reported was 5.4 (Ioka et al., 2003), and in Alexandria, Egypt, the rate was 3.16 (Mahdy et al., 1999). An Italian network of cancer registries reported 7,690 cases of ovarian cancer from 1986 through 1997 (Zambon et al., 2004). Few countries publish trends in ovarian cancer incidence over time. This may be due to differing methods of data collection and data quality issues, especially for countries that do not have a national registry. In the United States, a recent report estimates that ovarian cancer incidence has been decreasing since 1998, with a significant decline of 2.3% per year from 2003-2007 (Kohler et al., 2011). The reasons for this decrease are unclear, but are likely not artefactual due to the long-standing high-quality data available for the United States. A Japanese analysis based on data from several regional cancer registries reported a 1.5 fold increase in ovarian cancer rates from 1975 to 1993 (Tamakoshi et al., 2001). The Chinese Shanghai Cancer Registry also reported an increase in ovarian cancer incidence from 1979-1989 (Jin et al., 1993). Some of these increases may be due to increases in population coverage or completeness of data within the registry; however, the Chinese increase is thought to be a birth cohort effect in women born between 1925-1935 (Jin et al., 1993).

Region	Case count	Rate
World	224747	6.3
More developed regions	99521	9.3
Less developed regions	125226	5.0
Africa	13976	4.2
Sub-Saharan Africa	9961	4.0
Eastern Africa	3840	4.0
Middle Africa	1728	4.3
Northern Africa	4015	4.8
Southern Africa	893	3.8
Western Africa	3500	3.8
Latin America and Caribbean	16981	5.9
Caribbean	1005	4.3
Central America	3571	5.2
South America	12405	6.2
Northern America	23895	8.7
Asia	102408	5.1
Eastern Asia	40831	4.3
South-Eastern Asia	18580	6.6
South-Central Asia	38797	5.5
Western Asia	4200	4.8
Europe	65697	10.1
Central and Eastern Europe	27071	11.0
Northern Europe	10256	11.8
Southern Europe	11751	8.4
Western Europe	16619	8.9
Oceania	1790	7.6
Australia/New Zealand	1601	7.8
Melanesia	161	5.1
Micronesia/Polynesia	28	5.5
Micronesia	15	6.1
Polynesia	13	5.0

Table 2. Ovarian cancer incidence counts and rates for selected regions and continents worldwide. Rates are per 100,000 women and age-standardized to the 1960 world standard population. Source: Ferlay et al., 2011.

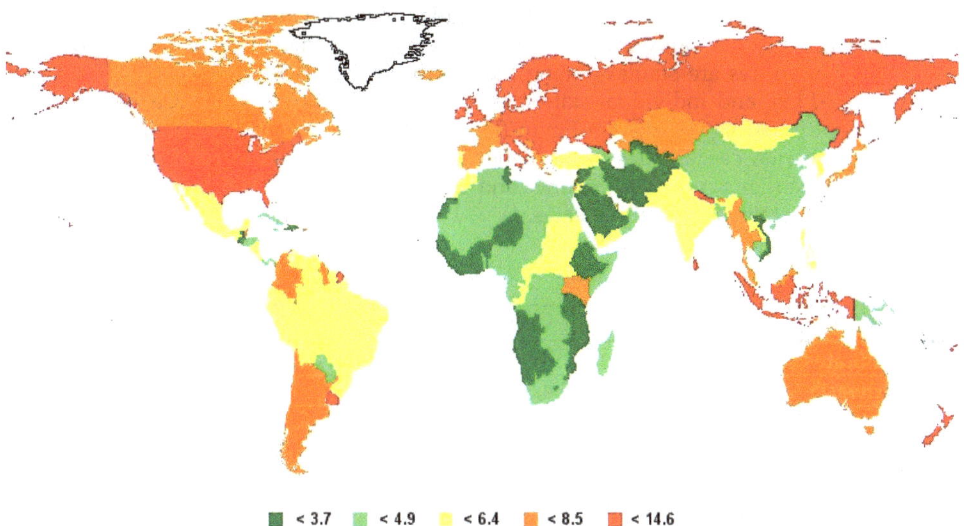

Fig. 1. Map of ovarian cancer rates worldwide. Rates are per 100,000 women and are age-standardized to the 1960 world standard population. Data were not included for white areas on the map. Source: Ferlay et al., 2011.

Incidence patterns stratified by region can assist with assessment of environmental or cultural factors that may increase risk. Regional variation in ovarian cancer rates exists, and this variation can sometimes be substantial. Percentages of ovarian cancer cases in World Health Organization regions are shown in Figure 2, these percentages range from 4.4% in the Eastern Mediterranean region (EMRO) to 31.0% in the European region (EURO) (Ferlay et al., 2010).

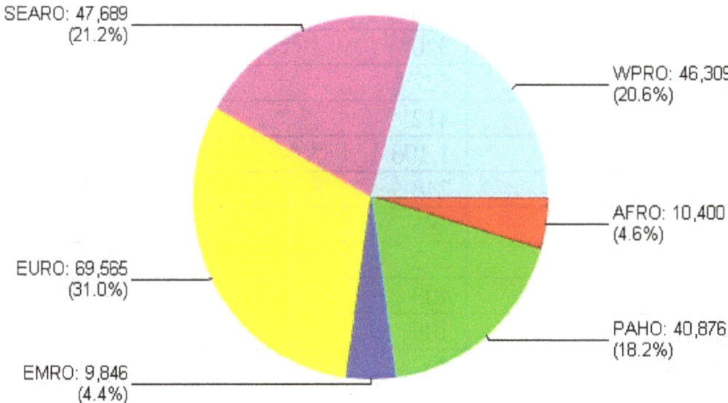

Fig. 2. Percentage of ovarian cancer cases by World Health Organization (WHO) health organization region. SEARO=Southeast Asia Regional Office, EURO=European Regional Office; EMRO=Eastern Mediterranean Regional Office; WPRO=Western Pacific Regional Office; AFRO=Africa Regional Office; PAHO=Pan American Health Organization. Source: Ferlay et al., 2011.

These numbers do not take into account the population, and may likely be reflective of the population coverage of cancer registration in these areas. In the United States, ovarian cancer incidence rates are similar among the Northeast, Midwest, and South U.S. Census regions (11.7-12.9), and individual state rates range from 7.3 to 15.4 (U.S.Cancer Statistics Working Group, 2010). Studies in Egypt (Dey et al., 2010) and Italy (Minelli et al., 2007) have found ovarian cancer rates to be higher in urban compared to rural areas. Table 3 displays the ovarian cancer case counts and incidence rates by U.S. census region and division, and by state in the United States.

Geographic Area	Case count	Rate
United States	**20,749**	**12.2**
Northeast	**4,375**	**12.9**
New England	**1,057**	**11.9**
Connecticut	268	12.1
Maine	98	11.8
Massachusetts	473	11.8
New Hampshire	99	12.5
Rhode Island	77	11.8
Vermont	42	10.8
Middle Atlantic	3,318	13.3
New Jersey	696	13.3
New York	1,516	13
Pennsylvania	1,106	13.7
Midwest	**4,724**	**12.3**
East North Central	3,318	12.4
Illinois	896	12.6
Indiana	428	11.7
Michigan	755	13.1
Detroit	320	13.7
Ohio	827	12
Wisconsin	412	12.7
West North Central	1,406	12.1
Iowa	248	13.7
Kansas	196	12.6
Minnesota	352	12.1
Missouri	403	11.5
Nebraska	108	10.4
North Dakota	46	12.9
South Dakota	53	11.4
South	**7,298**	**11.7**
South Atlantic	**4,045**	**11.9**
Delaware	78	15.4
District of Columbia	31	9.4
Florida	1,391	11.8

Geographic Area	Case count	Rate
Georgia	638	13.2
Atlanta	191	12.1
Maryland	367	11.2
North Carolina	612	12
South Carolina	295	11.4
Virginia	491	11.3
West Virginia	142	11.9
East South Central	**1,187**	**11.2**
Alabama	312	11.1
Kentucky	278	11.3
Mississippi	173	10.3
Tennessee	424	11.8
West South Central	**2,066**	**11.6**
Arkansas	188	11
Louisiana*	237	9.6
Oklahoma	272	13
Texas	1,369	11.8
West	**NR**	**NR**
Mountain	**NR**	**NR**
Arizona	397	11.6
Colorado	334	13.3
Idaho	119	15
Montana	65	11
Nevada	NR	NR
New Mexico	129	11.9
Utah	103	9.1
Wyoming	22	7.3
Pacific	**3,183**	**12.4**
Alaska	37	13.1
California	2,319	12.3
San Francisco-Oakland	317	12.8
San Jose-Monterey	158	12.8
Los Angeles	626	12.6
Hawaii	92	12.2
Oregon	280	12.7
Washington	455	12.5
Seattle-Puget Sound	332	13.2

Table 3. Ovarian cancer incidence counts and rates for the United States, U.S. Census regions and divisions and individual states. Rates are per 100,000 women and age-adjusted to the 2000 U.S. standard. Data presented cover 99.1% of the U.S. population. *Indicates that data differ from that presented by the Louisiana Tumor Registry and the SEER Program. NR=not reported. Source: (U.S.Cancer Statistics Working Group, 2010).

3.1 Clinical factors (histology, stage, laterality) and ovarian cancer incidence

Ovarian cancers are classified into three main histologic groups: epithelial tumors, sex cord-stromal tumors, and germ cell tumors (Cannistra et al., 2011). Epithelial tumors are believed to originate from the surface epithelium of the ovary (Chen et al., 2003). There are four main subtypes of epithelial tumors: serous, mucinous, endometrioid, and clear cell adenocarcinomas (Chen et al., 2003). Sex cord-stromal tumors originate in granulosa or thecal cells, or other stromal cells. Germ cell tumors are formed by cells that are believed to be derived from primordial germ cells, and they include the subtypes dysgerminomas, teratomas, and yolk sac tumors, among other subtypes (Chen et al., 2003). Several histologic-specific ovarian cancer incidence studies are published in the peer-reviewed literature, and most are based on populations in the United States. In a 2003 publication, Goodman et al. reported that 91.9% of ovarian tumors were epithelial, 1.2% were sex cord-stromal, and 1.9% were germ cell (Goodman & Howe, 2003). Serous adenocarcinoma was the most incident epithelial subtype, accounting for 37.7% of all ovarian tumors (Goodman & Howe, 2003). These U.S. data are consistent with those from the Netherlands, where 89% of all ovarian cancer diagnoses were reported to be epithelial tumors (Koper et al., 1996).

Effective early detection methods for ovarian cancer do not currently exist, and symptoms for ovarian cancer can be vague and gastrointestinal (as opposed to gynecologic) in nature. Because of this, many ovarian tumors are diagnosed at advanced stages. In the United States, studies show that about 20% of all ovarian cancer cases are localized stage at diagnosis, about 13% are regional stage, and the majority are distant stage (58%) (Goodman et al., 2003). This distribution differs by histologic type. Sex cord-stromal and germ cell tumors are more often diagnosed at localized stages (>50%) compared to epithelial tumors (19%) (Goodman et al., 2003). In the Netherlands, two thirds of all ovarian cancers were found to be extended to the pelvis or beyond at diagnosis (Koper et al., 1996).

There is a paucity of analyses on laterality. In a U.S. population, serous adenocarcinomas were were found to be bilateral at diagnoses in 57.5% of cases, and other epithelial tumors ranged in bilaterality from 13.3% to 35.6% (Boger-Megiddo & Weiss, 2005).

3.2 Demographic factors (age and race/ethnicity) and ovarian cancer incidence

Age is commonly reported in most ovarian cancer incidence publications. Globally, ovarian cancer incidence rates increase with advancing age and range from 0.2 among those aged 0-14 to 29.2 among those aged 75 years and older (Ferlay et al., 2010). A similar pattern is seen in more developed countries; however, the incidence rates are higher and range from 0.3 to 42.6 (Ferlay et al., 2010). In the United States, ovarian cancer incidence rates range from 0.3 in those aged 5-9 years to 44.2 in women aged 85 and older (U.S.Cancer Statistics Working Group, 2010). The peak ovarian cancer incidence rate of 50.6 is found among women aged 80-84 in the United States (U.S.Cancer Statistics Working Group, 2010). In developing countries, ovarian cancer occurs in younger women. In Ghana, the mean age of ovarian cases seen in a teaching hospital was 46.4 years (Nkyekyer, 2000), and in Kyrgyzstan, the average age of ovarian cancer patients was 37.9, with the highest incidence rate (11.2 per 60,0000 women) observed among those aged 40-49 (Igisinov & Umaralieva, 2008).

Several published studies limit their age-specific ovarian cancer analyses to children and adolescents, and many of these specifically report on ovarian germ cell tumors, which are diagnosed in high numbers among children and adolescents (Young et al., 2003). In an international study of cancer among adolescents, ovarian germ cell tumors were found in the highest rates among those aged 15-19 (Stiller, 2007). A study from the United States reported an overall ovarian cancer incidence rate of 0.102 for girls aged 9 years and younger, and 1.072 for girls aged 10-19 years (Brookfield et al., 2009). Other studies in the United States comparing germ cell tumor rates concluded that the incidence of ovarian germ cell tumors was significantly higher in Hispanic compared to non-Hispanic girls aged 10-19 (Poynter et al., 2010; Smith et al., 2006), and Asian/Pacific Islanders (0.059) compared to other ethnicities (Smith et al., 2006). Consistent with international studies, girls aged 15-19 years had the highest germ cell rates in the United States and it was reported that these rates are increasing (Smith et al., 2006).

Most reports examining ovarian cancer by race and/or ethnicity are in the United States population. This is likely due to the diversity in the racial and ethnic make-up of the United States. In 2007, it was reported that ovarian cancer incidence rates were highest among U.S. white women (12.6), followed by black (9.1), Asian/Pacific Islander (A/PI) (9.0), and American Indian/Alaska Native (AI/AN) women (8.0) (U.S.Cancer Statistics Working Group, 2010). Rates were lower in Hispanic women (10.2) compared to non-Hispanic women (11.3) (U.S.Cancer Statistics Working Group, 2010). Some U.S. studies have used enhanced population denominator data to probe race-specific rates further in an attempt to provide more accurate or meaningful rates. Studies using denominator data adjusted for Indian Health Service delivery regions in the United States (Espey et al., 2007; Kohler et al., 2011) report ovarian cancer incidence rates of 11.3 (Kohler et al., 2011) among AI/AN women. The most recent report examining trends concluded that ovarian cancer incidence rates have been decreasing at about 1.0% per year since 1998 among most racial and ethnic groups in the United States, with the exception of A/PI women (Kohler et al., 2011).

4. Primary peritoneal and primary fallopian tube cancers

Primary peritoneal cancer (PPC) and primary fallopian tube cancer (PFTC) are rare malignancies, but share many similarities to ovarian cancer. These three cancers are clinically managed in a similar manner (Cannistra et al., 2011). Due to their rarity, these cancers are generally not reported as a distinct or separate category in statistical monographs; reports of their incidence are limited to relatively few peer-reviewed publications. In the United States, the incidence rate of PPC is estimated to be 0.678 (Goodman & Shvetsov, 2009a). PPCs were diagnosed at later ages (mean age 67 years) and more advanced stages (85% regional/distant diagnoses) than ovarian cancer (mean age 63, 75% regional/distant diagnoses) in this same population (Goodman & Shvetsov, 2009a). In contrast, a study from a UK cancer center examining PPC found that age and tumor characteristics (stage and grade) were similar among ovarian and primary peritoneal tumors (Jaaback et al., 2006). The U.S. incidence rate of PFTC is 0.41 (Stewart et al., 2007). The vast majority of PFTCs (89%) are unilateral at diagnosis, and about 30% are diagnosed at each localized, regional and distant stages (Stewart et al., 2007). U.S. PFTC rates are similar to those reported from Finland (0.3) (Riska et al., 2003) and Denmark (0.5) (Pfeiffer et al., 1989). U.S. studies have suggested that the rates of both PPC (Goodman & Shvetsov, 2009a; Howe et al., 2001) and PFTC (Goodman & Shvetsov, 2009a; Stewart et al., 2007) are increasing. It is thought that some of this increase may be due to reduction in the misclassification of PPC and PFTC as ovarian cancer (Stewart et al., 2007, Goodman & Shvetsov, 2009b).

5. Discussion

Ovarian cancer incidence rates reported from countries with nationwide cancer registration and those from more developed countries are generally similar to each other. In less developed countries and regions, ovarian cancer rates are relatively lower, and this is likely due in part to the lack of quality data from large portions of the population in these countries. Additionally, cancers that are related to infectious agents (i.e. not ovarian cancer), are some of the most incident cancers in developing countries (Thun et al., 2011). It should be noted; however, that while cancer overall has typically been more incident in industrialized and comparatively wealthy nations, it is suggested that cancer incidence is increasing in low and medium resource countries (Thun et al., 2009). This increase may be a result of an increased lifespan due to advances in medical treatment in these countries, as well as the adoption of Western patterns of diet, physical activity, and tobacco use (Thun et al., 2011).

Several factors, including genetic, reproductive, hormonal and behavioral factors have been suggested to increase risk for ovarian cancer. Genetic factors perhaps have the strongest and most consistent association with increased risk for ovarian cancer. At least 10% of all epithelial ovarian cancers are reported to be hereditary, with the majority (about 90%) of these related to mutations in BRCA genes and 10% related to mutations associated with Lynch syndrome (Prat et al., 2005). Hereditary ovarian cancers have distinct patterns from sporadic ovarian cancers. Many are diagnosed at younger ages and less advanced stages than sporadic ovarian cancers (Prat et al., 2005). Regarding reproductive factors, studies over several years have consistently associated nulliparity with increased risk of ovarian cancer (Modan et al., 2001; Risch et al, 1994; Vachon et al., 2002). It is estimated that nulliparity may increase risk only slighty in the average-risk population (relative risk [RR]=1.4, 95% confidence interval [CI] 1.9-2.4), but may have a more substantial effect in women with a family history of ovarian cancer (Vachon et al., 2002). Hysterectomy and tubal ligation have been consistently associated with conferring a decreased risk for ovarian cancer. Tubal ligation has been estimated to decrease risk substantially (RR= 0.33, 95% CI 0.16 to 0.64), while hysterectomy may have a weaker, but still protective association (RR= 0.67, 95% CI 0.45 to 1.00) (Hankinson et al., 1993). Oral contraceptive use has been suggested to decrease risk for ovarian cancer, while post-menopausal hormone replacement therapy use is suggested to increase risk for ovarian cancer. However, conclusions from hormonal studies have generally been less consistent and more difficult to interpret than genetic and reproductive factor studies. Although some studies have shown a protective effect of oral contraceptives on ovarian cancer (Beral et al., 2008), IARC classifies estrogen, combined estrogen-progesterone oral contraceptives, and combined estrogen-progesterone hormone replacement therapy as class one carcinogens, concluding there is sufficient evidence for their carcinogenicity in humans (IARC 2007). The relationship between behavioral factors, such as tobacco use, physical activity, and obesity and ovarian cancer has been less reported compared to the other factors mentioned. Available results are generally inconclusive. Some studies have suggested a modest increased risk of ovarian cancer in obese women (Leitzmann, et al., 2009); however, others have found no relationship between body mass index and ovarian cancer (Fairfield et al., 2002). Similarly with physical activity, one study concluded there was a modest inverse association of physical activity and ovarian cancer risk (Biesma et al., 2006), while another concluded there was no association (Hannan et al., 2004). Smoking has been shown to increase risk for the epithelial subtype mucinous adenocarcinoma, but does not increase risk for other more incident subtypes (Jordan et al., 2006).

6. Conclusion

Although ovarian cancer patterns vary widely around the world, incidence rates are high in several regions. The etiology and natural history of ovarian cancer are poorly understood, and much more research is needed to elucidate factors that may increase or decrease risk for ovarian cancer. The analysis of incidence patterns both within and between populations is essential to revealing potential causes of and risk factors for ovarian cancer. Incidence rates from countries with high-quality data should continue to be analyzed with respect to histology and stage variation, as these types of analyses may provide clues to the pathogenesis of the disease. Currently, a major goal of ovarian cancer research is to develop an effective test that can detect the disease at its earliest stages, which would ultimately result in decreased mortality. Increased knowledge of ovarian cancer etiology and pathogenesis would greatly enhance the development of this tool. Expansions in ovarian cancer incidence registration and analyses will be very valuable in this endeavor.

7. Acknowledgement

The author gratefully acknowledges Sun Hee Rim, MPH and Troy D. Querec, PhD for their expert assistance with this chapter. Additionally, the author is especially grateful to Cheryll C. Thomas, MSPH for her critical review and thoughtful comments regarding this chapter. The findings and conclusions of this report are those of the author and do not represent the official position of the Centers for Disease Control and Prevention.

8. References

Beral, V.; Doll, R.; Hermon, C.; Peto, R. & Reeves, G. (2008). Ovarian cancer and oral contraceptives: collaborative: reanalysis of data from 45 epidemiological studies including 23, 257 women with ovarian cancer and 87, 303 controls.*Lancet,* Vol. 371, No. 9609, (2008), pp. (303-14)

Biesma, R.G.; Schouten, L.J.; Dirx, M.J.; Goldbohm, R.A. & van den Brandt, P.A.(2006) Physical activity and risk of ovarian cancer: results from the Netherlands Cohort Study (The Netherlands). *Cancer Causes Contro,* Vol 17, No. 1 (2006), pp. (109-15)

Boger-Megiddo, I. & Weiss, N.S. (2005). Histologic subtypes and laterality of primary epithelial ovarian tumors. *Gynecol.Oncol.,* Vol 97, No. 1 (April 2005), pp. (80-83)

Brookfield, K.F.; Cheung, M.C.; Koniaris, L.G.; Sola, J.E. & Fischer, A.C. (2009). A population-based analysis of 1037 malignant ovarian tumors in the pediatric population. *J.Surg.Res.,* Vol. 156, No. 1, (September 2009), pp. (45-49)

Cannistra, S.A.; Gershenson, D.M.; & Recht, A.(2011). Ovarian cancer, fallopian tube carcinoma, and peritoneal carcinoma. In: *DeVita, Hellman, and Rosenberg's Cancer: Principles and Practice of Oncology, 9th Edition.,* DeVita, V.T.; Lawrence, T.S. &

Rosenberg, S.A.pp. (1368-1391) Lippincott, Williams, & Wilkins, ISBN 978-1-4511-0545-2, Philadelphia, PA, USA

Chen, V.W.; Ruiz, B.; Killeen, J.L.; Cote, T.R.; Wu, X.C. & Correa, C.N.(2003) Pathology and classification of ovarian tumors. *Cancer,* Vol 97, No. 10 Suppl., (May 2003), pp. (2631-2642)

Dey, S.; Hablas, A.; Seifeldin, I.A; Ismail, K.; . Ramadan, M.; El-Hamzawy, H.; Wilson, M.L.; Banerjee, M.; Boffetta, P.; Harford, J.; Merajver, S.D.; & Soliman, A.S.E et al. (2010). Urban-rural differences of gynaecological malignancies in Egypt (1999-2002). *BJOG.*, Vol. 117, No. 3, (February 2010), pp. (348-355)..

Espey, D.K.; Wu, X.C.; Swan, J.; Wiggins, C.; Jim, M.A.; Ward, E.; Wingo, P.A.; Howe, H.L.; Ries, L.A.; Miller, B.A.; Jemal, A.; Ahmed, F.; Cobb, N.; Kaur, J.S. & Edwards, B.K.. (2007). Annual report to the nation on the status of cancer, 1975-2004, featuring cancer in American Indians and Alaska Natives. *Cancer,* Vol. 110, No. 10, (November 2007), pp., (2119-2152)

Fairfield, K.M.; Willett, W.C.; Rosner, B.A.; Manson, J.E.; Speizer, F.E.; & Hankinson, S.E. (2002). Obesity, Weight Gain, and Ovarian Cancer. *Obstetrics & Gynecology* Vol 100, No. 2, (pp. 288–296)

Ferlay J.; Shin H.R.; Bray F.; Forman, D., Mathers, C. & Parkin, D.M. (2008) GLOBOCAN 2008 v1.2, Cancer Incidence and Mortality Worldwide: IARC CancerBase No. 10 [Internet]. Lyon, France: International Agency for Research on Cancer; 2010. Available from: http://globocan.iarc.fr, accessed on 21/07/2011.

Goodman, M.T.; Correa, C.N.; Tung, K.H.; Roffers, S.D.; Cheng, Wu, X; Young, J.L., Jr.; Wilkens, L.R.; Carney, M.E.; & Howe, H.L. (2003). Stage at diagnosis of ovarian cancer in the United States, 1992-1997. *Cancer,* Vol 97, No. 10 Suppl., (May 2003), pp. (2648-2659).

Goodman, M. T. & Howe, H. L. (2003). Descriptive epidemiology of ovarian cancer in the United States, 1992-1997. *Cancer,* Vol 97, No. 10 Suppl., (May 2003), pp (2615-2630).

Goodman, M.T. & Shvetsov, Y.B.. (2009) Rapidly increasing incidence of papillary serous carcinoma of the peritoneum in the United States: fact or artifact? *Int J Cancer,* Vol 124, No. 9, (May 2009), pp. (2231-2235)

Goodman, M. T. & Shvetsov, Y. B. (2009). Incidence of ovarian, peritoneal, and fallopian tube carcinomas in the United States, 1995-2004. *Cancer Epidemiol.Biomarkers Prev., 18,* 132-139.

Hankinson, S.E.; Hunter, D.J.; Colditz, G.A.; Willett, W.C.; Stampfer, M.J.; Rosner, B.; Hennekens, C.H. & Speizer, F.E. (2003) Tubal ligation, hysterectomy, and risk of ovarian cancer. A prospective study. *JAMA,* Vol. 270, No. 23, (December 2003), pp.(2813-2818).

Hannan, L.M.; Leitzmann, M.F.; Lacey, J.V. Jr; Colbert, L.H.; Albanes, D.; Schatzkin, A.; & Schairer, C. (2004) Physical activity and risk of ovarian cancer: a prospective cohort study in the United States. *Cancer Epidemiol Biomarkers Prev.,* Vol 13, No. 5, pp (765-70).

Howe, H.L.; Wingo, P.A.; Thun, M.J.; Ries, L.A.; Rosenberg, H.M.; Feigal, E.G. & Edwards, B.K. (2001). Annual report to the nation on the status of cancer (1973 through 1998), featuring cancers with recent increasing trends. *J.Natl.Cancer Inst.,* Vol 93, No. 11, (May 2001), pp. (824-842).

IARC (2007). IARC Monographs on the Evaluation of Carcinogenic Risks to Humans. Combined Estrogen-Progestogen Contraceptives and Combined Estrogen-Progestogen Menopausal Therapy. Vol 91. ISBN 9789283212911

Igisinov, N. & Umaralieva, G. (2008). Epidemiology of ovarian cancer in Kyrgyzstan women of reproductive age. *Asian Pac.J.Cancer Prev.*, Vol. 9, No. 2, (April 2008), pp. (331-334).

Ioka, A; Tsukuma, H.; Ajiki, W. & Oshima, A. (2003). Ovarian cancer incidence and survival by histologic type in Osaka, Japan. *Cancer Sci.*, Vol. 94, No. 3 (March 2003), pp. (292-296).

Jaaback, K.S.; Ludeman, L.; Clayton, N.L.; & Hirschowitz, L. (2006). Primary peritoneal carcinoma in a UK cancer center: comparison with advanced ovarian carcinoma over a 5-year period. *Int.J.Gynecol.Cancer., Vol 16 Suppl, (January 2006), pp. (* 123-128).

Jin, F.; Shu, X.O.; Devesa, S.S.; Zheng, W.; Blot, W. J. & Gao, Y.T. (1993). Incidence trends for cancers of the breast, ovary, and corpus uteri in urban Shanghai, 1972-89. *Cancer Causes Control.*, Vol 4, No. 4(July 1993), pp. (355-360).

Jordan, S.J.; Whiteman, D.C.; Purdie, D.M.; Green, A.C. & Webb, P.M. (2006) Does smoking increase risk of ovarian cancer? A systematic review. Gynecol Oncol., Vol. 103, No. 3, (December 2006), pp. (1122-9).

Kohler, B.A.; Ward, E.; McCarthy, B.J.; Schymura, M.J.; Ries, L.A.; Eheman, C.; Jemal, A.; Anderson, R.N.; Ajani, U.A. & Edwards, B.K. (2011). Annual report to the nation on the status of cancer, 1975-2007, featuring tumors of the brain and other nervous system. *J.Natl.Cancer Inst.*, Vol. 103, No. 9, (May 2011), pp. (714-736).

Koper, N.P.; Kiemeney, L.A.; Massuger, L.F.; Thomas, C.M.; Schijf, C.P. & Verbeek, A.L. (1996). Ovarian cancer incidence (1989-1991) and mortality (1954-1993) in The Netherlands. *Obstet.Gynecol., Vol. 88, No. 3* (September 1996), pp. (387-393).

Leitzmann, M. F.; Koebnick, C.; Danforth, K.N.; Brinton, L.A.; Moore, S.C.; Hollenbeck, A.R.; Schatzkin, A. & Lacey, J. V. (2009), Body mass index and risk of ovarian cancer. *Cancer*, Vol. 115, pp (812–822).

Mahdy, N.H.; Abdel-Fattah, M. & Ghanem, H. (1999). Ovarian cancer in Alexandria from 1988 to 1997: trends and survival. *East Mediterr.Health J.*, Vol. 5, No. 4(July 1999), pp. (727-739).

Minelli, L.; Stracci, F.; Cassetti, T.; Canosa, A.; Scheibel, M.; Sapia, I.E.; Romagnoli, C. & La, Rosa F. (2007). Urban-rural differences in gynaecological cancer occurrence in a central region of Italy: 1978-1982 and 1998-2002. *Eur.J.Gynaecol.Oncol.*, Vol. 28, No. 6, pp. (468-472).

Nkyekyer, K. (2000). Pattern of gynaecological cancers in Ghana. *East Afr.Med.J.*, Vol. 77, No. 10, (October 2000), pp. (534-538).

Pfeiffer P.; Mogensen, H.; Amtrup, F. & Honore, E. (1989). Primary carcinoma of the fallopian tube. A retrospective study of patients reported to the Danish Cancer Registry in a five-year period.*Acta Oncol.*, Vol. 28, No. 1, pp. (7-11).

Poynter, J.N.; Amatruda, J.F. & Ross, J. A. (2010). Trends in incidence and survival of pediatric and adolescent patients with germ cell tumors in the United States, 1975 to 2006. *Cancer,* Vol. 116, pp. *(* 4882-4891).

Prat, J.; Ribé, A. & Gallardo A. (2005). Hereditary ovarian cancer. *Hum Pathol.*, Vol. 36, No. 8, (August 2005), pp. (861-70).

Riska, A.; Leminen, A. & Pukkala E. (2003). Sociodemographic determinants of incidence of primary fallopian tube carcinoma, Finland 1953-97. *Int J Cancer*, Vol. 104, No. 5, pp. (643-645).

Smith, H.O.; Berwick, M.; Verschraegen, C.F.; Wiggins, C.; Lansing, L.; Muller, C.Y. & Qualls, C.R. (2006). Incidence and survival rates for female malignant germ cell tumors. *Obstet.Gynecol.*, Vol. 107, No. 5 (May 2006), pp. (1075-1085).

Stewart, S.L.; Wike, J.M.; Foster, S.L. & Michaud, F. (2007). The incidence of primary fallopian tube cancer in the United States. *Gynecol Oncol.*, Vol. 107, No. 3, pp (392-397).

Stiller, C.A. (2007). International patterns of cancer incidence in adolescents. *Cancer Treat.Rev.*, Vol. 33, No. 7. (November 2007), pp. (631-645).

Tamakoshi, K.; Kondo, T.; Yatsuya, H.; Hori, Y.; Kikkawa, F. & Toyoshima, H. (2001). Trends in the mortality (1950-1997) and incidence (1975-1993) of malignant ovarian neoplasm among Japanese women: analyses by age, time, and birth cohort. *Gynecol.Oncol.*, Vol. 83, No. 1, (October 2001), pp. (64-71).

Thun, M.J.; DeLancey, J.O.; Center, M.M.; Jemal, A. & Ward, E.M. (2010). The global burden of cancer: priorities for prevention. *Carcinogenesis*, Vol. 33, No. 1, pp. (100-110).

Thun, M.J.; Jemal, A. & Ward, E. (2011). Global cancer incidence and mortality., In: *DeVita, Hellman, and Rosenberg's Cancer: Principles and Practice of Oncology, 9th Edition.*, DeVita, V.T.; Lawrence, T.S. & Rosenberg, S.A.pp. (241-260) Lippincott, Williams, & Wilkins, ISBN 978-1-4511-0545-2, Philadelphia, PA, USA

U.S. Cancer Statistics Working Group. United States Cancer Statistics: 1999–2007 Incidence and Mortality Web-based Report. Atlanta: U.S. Department of Health and Human Services, Centers for Disease Control and Prevention and National Cancer Institute; 2010. Accessed 07/21/2011. Available at: www.cdc.gov/uscs.

Young, J.L. Jr.; Wu, X.C.; Roffers, S.A.; Howe, H.L.; Correa, C.N. & Weinstein R (2003). Ovarian cancer in children and young adults in the United States, 1992-1997. *Cancer*, Vol 97, No. 10 Suppl., (May 2003), pp.(2694-2700).

Zambon, P., & La Rosa, F. (2004). Gynecological cancers: cervix, corpus uteri, ovary. *Epidemiol Prev.*, Vol. 28(2 Suppl), pp.(68-74).

2

Screening for Ovarian Cancer in Women

Duangmani Thanapprapasr and Sarikapan Wilailak
Department of Obstetrics and Gynecology, Faculty of Medicine,
Ramathibodi Hospital, Mahidol University
Thailand

1. Introduction

Of all the gynecologic cancers, ovarian malignancy represents the greatest clinical challenge because it is difficult for early detection, difficult to cure, and it has the highest fatality to case ratio of all the gynecologic malignancies. Many studies have been tried to find a novel strategy on early detection of ovarian cancer. Ultimately, successful screening in asymptomatic women could increase cure rate and prolong survival among patients who have to live with ovarian cancer.

Estimated age-standardised incidence rate of ovarian cancer per 100,000 women-year, all ages*

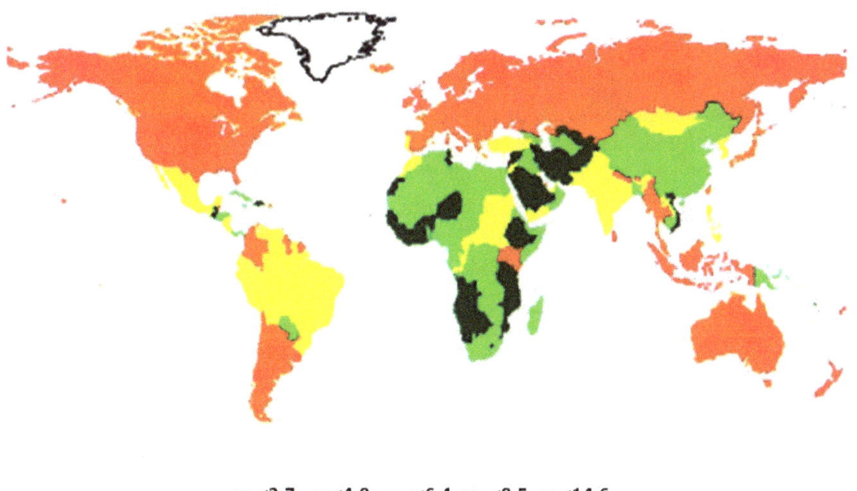

*Ferlay J, Shin HR, Bray F, Forman D, Mathers C and Parkin DM.
GLOBOCAN 2008 v1.2, Cancer Incidence and Mortality Worldwide: IARC CancerBase No. 10 [Internet].
Lyon, France: International Agency for Research on Cancer; 2010. Available from: http://globocan.iarc.fr, accessed on day/month/year.

Fig. 1. Estimated age-standardised incidence rate per 100,000 women-year of ovarian cancer, all ages.

2. Epidemiology and impact

Higher than two hundred thousand women were diagnosed ovarian cancer in 2008 worldwide(Ferlay, Shin et al. 2010). As a result, more than one hundred and forty thousand women accounting for more than fifty percent fatality to case ratio died in this year. Major incidences are in Northern America and Europe. In Asia, higher trend of incidence grows significantly. Unfortunately, ovarian cancer remains mysterious for early detection and cure. Morbidity and mortality from ovarian cancer have been major burdens from the past to the present.

Region	Ovarian cancer		Cervical cancer		Uterine cancer	
	New cases	Death	New cases	Death	New cases	Death
World*	224,747	140,163	530,232	275,008	288,387	73,854
US**	21,990	15,460	12,710	4,290	46,470	8,120
Thailand***	1,384	-	6,954	-	745	-

*Ferlay, Shin et al. 2010
**American Cancer Society. Cancer Facts & Figures 2011. Atlanta: American Cancer Society; 2011.
***Attasara P, Srivatanakul, P, Sriplung, H. cancer incidence in Thailand. In: Khuhaprema T, Srivatanakul P, Attasara P, Sriplung H, Wiangnon S, Sumitsawan Y, editor. Cancer in Thailand 2001-2003 vol.V. 1st ed. Bangkok: Bangkok Medical Publisher. 2010: 3-76.

Table 1. Number of new cases and deaths from ovarian, cervical and uterine cancer in a year.

2.1 The incidence and prevalence of ovarian cancer including the stage distribution

World age-specific incidence rate of ovarian cancer was 6.3 per 100,000 women with a cumulative risk 0-74 year-old of 0.7 in 2008 (Ferlay, Shin et al. 2010). It does not seem to significant lower from the year 2002. The distant and regional stage distributions are higher than localized ovarian cancer in both developed and developing countries as shown in table 2. Overall five year survival rate in the SEER database is 45.9%(SEER).

Ovarian cancer distribution	US*		Thailand**	
	Percent of cases	5 year survival (%)	Percent of cases	5 year survival (%)
Localized	15	94	26	90
Regional	23	73	39	80
Distant	62	28	35	15-25

* American Cancer Society. Cancer Facts & Figures 2011. Atlanta: American Cancer Society; 2011.
**modified from Wilailak S. Epidemiologic report of gynecologic cancer in Thailand. J Gynecol Oncol. 2009;20: 81–83.

Table 2. The ovarian cancer distribution and percent of five-year survival.

2.2 The sequelae and impact of ovarian cancer

Eventually, ovarian cancer impacts on patients' survival and their quality of life. Suffering from gut obstruction and malnutrition, renal failure, liver failure, respiratory failure, severe chronic pain, infection and sepsis are expected during lifetime and at the end of life in women diagnosed with ovarian cancer. Impacts of ovarian cancer are direct from cancer and metastases and indirect from treatments and complications.

Direct sequelae from cancer and metastases

- Primary tumor: intractable pain
- Secondary tumor: Brain, Bone, Lung, Liver, KUB system, GI system, lymph nodes

Indirect sequelae from treatments and complications.

- Surgery: hemorrhage, internal organ injury, gut obstruction.
- Chemotherapy: Leukopenia, thrombocytopenia, sepsis, renal failure, cardiotoxicity, hypersensitivity reaction
- Molecular therapy: hypertension, bowel perforation.

3. Challenges of ovarian cancer

Challenges toward early ovarian cancer diagnosis could increase cure rate, prolong survival and delay suffering from cancer and decreased interventive complications.

3.1 Pre-Cancer lesion has not yet been identified

Ovarian cancer pathogenesis has been hypothesized, but it and also pre-cancerous lesion have not yet been identified.

3.2 Most cases are diagnosed in advanced stage

Asymptomatic women with intra-abdominal concealing of ovarian cancer are most likely having late ovarian cancer diagnosis. Eighty-five percent of patients with ovarian cancer are diagnosed when the cancer cells already metastases out of the ovary to the whole abdomen. Survival and prognosis directly relate to extent of disease. Asymptomatic or nonspecific symptoms always found in women with early ovarian cancer.

3.3 Symptoms are non-specific

Ninety percent of patients with ovarian cancer had non-specific symptoms which mostly were misdiagnosed and delayed proper treatments for some periods.

3.4 Difficulty in palpation by either patients or physicians

Women could not feel abdominal mass or even any abnormalities before the mass enlarged to beyond her pubic symphysis. Physicians could palpate any mass of ovarian cancer during pelvic examination.

3.5 Result of the treatment is poor in advanced stage

Contemporary standard primary treatment is surgery and adjuvant combined chemotherapy for early stages cancer. In advanced cancer, initially exploratory laparotomy with biopsy followed by palliative chemotherapy and/or secondary cytoreductive surgery or neo-adjuvant chemotherapy followed by primary cytoreductive surgery is decided depending on individualized patient. The most reliable prognosis depends on the residual tumor after every attempted surgery.

3.6 The present tumor markers are non-specific

Tumor markers are non-specific. Currently, CA125 is widely used as the most promising tool along with contemporary standard primary treatment. CA125 is a tumor-associated antigen which is detected in 80-85 percent of epithelial ovarian cancer. Only fifty percent of patients with FIGO stage I and 60% of patients with FIGO stage II has shown an increased CA125 level. Moreover, CA125 test has low specificity among women with reproductive age, pregnancy and benign diseases including myoma uteri, endometriosis, and pelvic infection. Data suggest that combined CA125 and transvaginal ultrasonography improved specificity for ovarian cancer screening.

4. Screening target population

Currently, there are no effective screening methods that could decrease mortality from ovarian cancer. They are evidences for ovarian cancer screening in both general and high risk population.

4.1 General population

Mass screening in asymptomatic and general risk population seems to be ineffective and associated with increased rates of surgery and patient anxiety(Fung, Bryson et al. 2004). Two large studies in Europe and Northern America (Menon, Gentry-Maharaj et al. 2009; Buys, Partridge et al. 2011) have shown currently data. The prostate, lung, colorectal and ovarian (PLCO) cancer screening randomized controlled trial was conducted in the United States. Asymptomatic women aged 55-74 years who had no previous diagnosis of lung, colorectal or ovarian cancer were recruited between 1993-2001. Thirty-nine thousand one hundred and five participants received annual screening with transvaginal ultrasounds for four years and CA125 blood tests for six years. On comparison, Thirty-nine thousand one hundred and eleven participants received usual medical care. The positive predictive value was only 23.5%. Sixty percent of invasive cancers would not have been detected by the screening. Only 21 percent of the participants, who were detected cancer by the screening, were stage I/II. It was shown that women who were screened for ovarian cancer with annual transvaginal ultrasound and CA125 blood test had not reduced ovarian cancer mortality. In addition, the screening increased invasive medical procedures and associated harms (Buys, Partridge et al. 2011).

The United Kingdom Collaborative Trial of Ovarian Cancer Screening (UKCTOCS) was studied between 2001-2005 (Menon, Gentry-Maharaj et al. 2009). Post-menopausal women aged 50—74 years were randomly assigned to no treatment (control; n=101 359); annual CA125 screening with transvaginal ultrasound scan as a second-line test (multimodal screening [MMS]; n=50 640); or annual screening with transvaginal ultrasound (USS; n=50 639) alone in a 2:1:1 ratio (Menon, Gentry-Maharaj et al. 2009).

Forty-two women with the annual CA125 screening and transvaginal ultrasound scan and 45 women with annual transvaginal ultrasound were detected primary ovarian and tubal cancers including 28 borderline tumors (eight MMS, 20 USS). 28 (16 MMS, 12 USS) of 58 (48·3%) of the invasive cancers were stage I/II, with no difference in stage distribution between the groups. For primary invasive epithelial ovarian and tubal cancers, the sensitivity, specificity, and positive-predictive values were 89·5%, 99·8%, and 35·1% for MMS, and 75·0%, 98·2%, and 2·8% for USS, respectively. Specificity was higher in the annual CA125 screening with transvaginal ultrasound scan than in the annual screening with transvaginal ultrasound alone group, resulting in lower rates of repeat testing and surgery. The screening strategies might be feasible. However, the results of ongoing screening are awaited to determine the effect of the screening on mortality from ovarian cancer (Menon, Gentry-Maharaj et al. 2009).

4.2 Increased-risk population

Prevalence of ovarian cancer is higher in high risk population. Positive family history of specific cancers, menopause and having adnexal mass are higher probabilities for ovarian cancer. Screening benefits should be more pronounced and encourage. In addition, screening by gynecologic oncologists is feasible and cost effective.

4.2.1 Menopause

Senescence is significantly caused genetic aberration inducing cancer. Postmenopause are high risk for ovarian cancer (Hensley, Robson et al. 2003).

4.2.2 Positive family history

Women with certain family histories have higher risks of ovarian cancer than general population. Ten percent of women with epithelial ovarian cancer have mutations in the BRCA1 and BRCA2 genes with located on chromosome 17 and 13 respectively. Lynch II syndrome is a less common genetic cause of ovarian cancer and endometrial cancer, which is known as the hereditary nonpolyposis colorectal cancer syndrome (HNPCC syndrome). There is a very limited benefit, of screening even in high-risk women with BRCA1 and BRCA2 mutation carriers (Hermsen, Olivier et al. 2007; Woodward, Sleightholme et al. 2007). In addition, annual gynecological screening is unlikely to reduce mortality in women with BRCA1 and BRCA2 mutation carriers (Hogg and Friedlander 2004; Hermsen, Olivier et al. 2007).

4.2.3 Having adnexal mass

Malignant ovarian masses are pathological diagnosed. Occasionally, it is possible to differentiate benign from malignant tumors on the basis of history and physical examination findings.

5. General characteristics of a good cancer screening

Screening for ovarian cancer is a method for secondary prevention by early detection followed with definite treatment. Efficacy screening depends on 5 factors including incidence of disease, effective early treatment, available cost effectiveness method and adequate population target. Impact of ovarian cancer burden and surgically and adjuvant chemotherapeutic effective early treatments are significantly propagated the development of a good ovarian cancer screening. There are general characteristics to consider.

a. High sensitivity, specificity and predictive value

Accuracy for screening is necessary. Ideally, a good cancer screening for ovarian cancer could decrease mortality rate significantly. As this result, it could detect ovarian cancer among women who have the cancer. It could discrete non-ovarian cancer women among truly non-ovarian cancer women. Moreover, the test should be accurate on the results of the tests, it means that truly non-ovarian cancer women would be among negative tests' women and truly asymptomatic women with ovarian cancer would be among positive tests' women. More than 75 percent sensitivity and more than 99 percent specificity of the most effective test is required to achieve a positive predictive value of 10 percent(Moore, MacLaughlan et al. 2010). These mean ten operations of each case of ovarian cancer detected.

b. Safe

Safety set as a priority for mass screening in asymptomatic women.

c. Simple

Simple method screening which is easy and noninvasive is suitable to coverage the target population.

d. Inexpensive

Cost of the screening should be paid on attention other than its effectiveness. Cost could be one of the obstacles to be refused and ignore from the target population.

6. The aim of ovarian cancer screening is an attempt to detect early-stage asymptomatic individuals

6.1 Tools for ovarian cancer screening

Beyond pelvic examination, various tools are proposed including tumor markers, ultrasonography and abdominal imaging.

6.2 Tumor markers

The most extensively evaluated and available tumor marker currently is Cancer Antigen 125 (CA125). It has been firstly introduced as OC125 since 1981(Bast, Feeney et al. 1981). Up to eighty percent of patients with advanced epithelial ovarian cancer had high CA125 levels during diagnosis. However, only 50 percent of patients at early staged ovarian cancer were found higher levels than serum thresholds. Low specificity and variable levels of CA125 resulted in low accurate for screening. Many benign gynecologic and medical conditions compromised the specificity. However, CA125 remains valuable for follow up in women with epithelial ovarian cancer who have ever had high CA125 level.

6.3 Imaging

6.3.1 Ultrasonography

Utrasonographic results could discriminate patients with ovarian malignancy including bilaterality, large cystic structure, any solid lesions (as shown in picture 1), and papillary vegetation on the cyst wall or ascites. Accuracy of ultrasonography is still low for detecting ovarian cancer.

6.3.2 Computerized tomography (CT), Magnetic resonance imaging (MRI)

High false positive rate for detecting ovarian cancer using imaging technology have been reports. Individualized patients who should have benefits from the imaging should be judged by their physicians.

7. Single modality of screening or multiple modalities

7.1 Single/multiple tumor markers

Various types of tumor markers have been study both early staged and late staged of ovarian cancer (Table 3)(Rein, Gupta et al. 2011). High serum levels of HE4, Osteopontin, Mesothelin, B7-H4, Prostatin and VEGF were found in both early staged and late staged ovarian cancer. A number of tumor markers were detected only in late staged of cancer as shown in table 3.

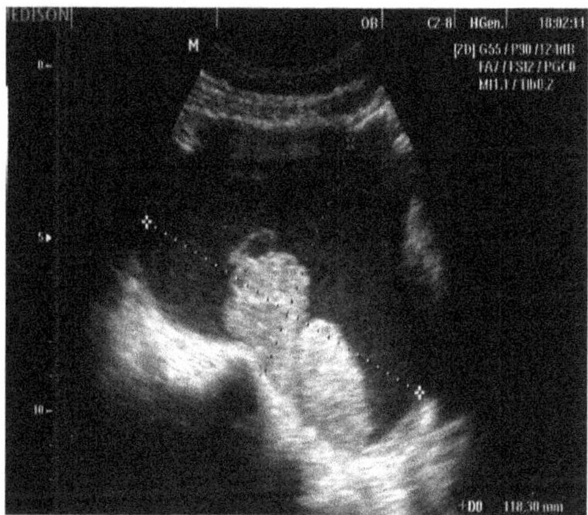

Picture 1. Transabdominal ultrasonography of 44 year-old, single woman with palpable pelvic mass has shown mixed solid cystic mass sized 11.8 cm. Postoperative pathologic diagnosed clear cell adenocarcinoma of ovary, FIGO stage IC.

Tumor markers*	
Early staged	Advanced and late-staged
HE4	HE4
Osteopontin	Osteopontin
Mesothelin	Mesothelin
B7-H4	B7-H4
Prostasin	Prostasin
VEGF	VEGF
IGFBP-3	IGFBP-3
RASSF1A	RASSF1A
BRCA1	BRCA1
LPA	LPA
IL-6, IL-8	Haptoglobin
Eosinophil-derived neurotoxin and COOH-osteopontin fragments	M-CSF
OVX1	Sat2-Chr1, Satα
APOA1 and transthyretin	MCJ
	P53

*modified from Rein BJ, Gupta S, Dada R, Safi J, Michener C, Agarwal A. Potential markers for detection and monitoring of ovarian cancer. J Oncol 2011;2011: 475983. (Rein, Gupta et al. 2011)

Table 3. The tumor markers detect during early staged and late staged of ovarian cancer.

Human epididymis protein 4 (HE4) is elevated in ovarian cancer, especially endometrioid adenocarcinoma and serous cystadenocarcinoma (Scholler, Crawford et al. 2006).
Osteopontin is a glycoprotein and secreted from vascular endothelial cells and osteoblasts. It has an ability to inhibit apoptosis and correlates with metastasis(Denhardt and Noda 1998).
Mesothelin expresses on the surface of mesothelial cells. It is overexpressed in ovarian cancer, mesotheliomas and pancreatic cancer (Hassan, Remaley et al. 2006).
B7-H4 over expressed in T-cells and ovarian cancer including serous cystadenocarcinoma, endometrioid adenocarcinoma and clear cell carcinoma. Its levels were elevated 45% of patients with early stage ovarian cancer (Simon, Zhuo et al. 2006).
Hepatoglobin originated from the liver. It has been shown expression in ascetic fluid and serum of patients with ovarian cancer. Higher levels of hepatoglobin have been associated with poor prognosis(Zhao, Annamalai et al. 2007). The levels also decreased during chemotherapy.
CA125 is only promising tumor marker currently, but it is low specificity. In combination with CA125, other serum tumor markers have been evaluated to improve the accuracy with some limitations (Visintin, Feng et al. 2008; Amonkar, Bertenshaw et al. 2009; Nosov, Su et al. 2009). The study in 2008 evaluated various combinations of 9 markers including CA125, HE4, SMRP, CA72-4, Osteopontin, ERBB2, Inhibin, Activin, and EGFR. Dual marker combination of CA125 and HE4 had a greater sensitivity than either marker alone (Moore, Brown et al. 2008). However, the dual markers are limited in detecting epithelial ovarian cancer of mucinous cell type. Human epididymis protein4 (HE4) has equivalent sensitivities to CA125 for detecting malignancy in women with pelvic masses (Shah, Lowe et al. 2009). In addition, HE4 has greater specificity in premenopausal women due to it does not influence by benign gynecologic conditions. Contrary, another study has shown that in combination of HE4 and CA125 test was no benefit in clinical practice(Jacob, Meier et al. 2011). HE4 is going on studies for ovarian cancer screening.

7.2 The risk of malignancy index (RMI)

The risk of malignancy index (RMI) was introduced for discriminating ovarian cancer from other ovarian mass (Jacobs, Oram et al. 1990). The RMI score is calculated from menstruation status, ultrasonographic result and CA125 level. RMI cut-off level of 200 has 85% sensitivity and 97% specificity to identify ovarian cancer.
RMI indices followed by Histoscanning study, a novel computer aided diagnostic tool, were assessed in 199 women with adnexa masses. A cutoff RMI value of 250 resulted in 74% sensitivity and 86% specificity. The RMI indices with cutoff values between 105-2100 followed by Histoscanning study improved diagnostic accuracy in women with adnexal masses with 88% sensitivity and 95% specificity (Vaes, Manchanda et al. 2011).

7.3 Risk of malignancy algorithm (ROMA)

The risk of malignancy algorithm (ROMA) is a scoring system in combination of CA125 and HE4 which shows excellent diagnostic performance for the detection of epithelial ovarian cancer in post-menopausal women presenting with pelvic mass (Montagnana, Danese et al. 2011).
Using ROMA, 389 women with pelvic mass were measured serum levels of HE4 and CA125 preoperatively. A cutoff of 12.5% for pre-menopausal patients had 67.5% sensitivity and 87.9% specificity. A cutoff of 14.4% for postmenopausal patients had 90.8% sensitivity and 66.3% specificity. However, HE4 and ROMA did not increase the detection of ovarian cancer comparing to CA125 alone (Van Gorp, Cadron et al. 2011).

On comparison, the dual markers using HE4 and CA125, calculated a ROMA value were evaluated preoperatively (Moore, Jabre-Raughley et al. 2010). This study used the following predictive probability algorithm (ROMA):

Premenopausal Predictive index (PI) = -12+2.38*LN (HE4) +0.0626*LN (CA125)
Postmenopausal Predictive index (PI) = -8.09+1.04*LN (HE4) +0.732*LN (CA125)
Predicted probability = exp (PI)/ [1+exp (PI)]

The following equation was used to calculate RMI:

RMI = U X M X serum CA125
Where U = 0 for imaging score of 0
U = 1 for imaging score of 1
U = 3 for imaging score of 2-5
M = 1 if premenopausal
M = 3 if postmenopausal

It shows significant higher sensitivity for detecting epithelial ovarian cancer than RMI as shown in figure 5 (Moore, Jabre-Raughley et al. 2010).

Group	**Sensitivity (%)**			**Positive predictive value (%)**		**Negative predictive value (%)**	
	ROMA	RMI	Pretest *P* value	ROMA	RMI	ROMA	RMI
Benign vs. EOC and LMP	89.0	80.7	0.0113	62.3	59.7	93.6	89.3
Benign vs. EOC stage I-IV	94.3	84.6	0.0029	59.8	56.8	97.1	92.5
Benign vs. EOC stage I-II	85.3	64.7	0.0000	27.1	21.8	97.9	95.1
Benign vs. EOC stage III-IV	98.8	93.0	0.0350	52.1	50.3	99.6	97.5

*modified from Moore. Comparison of a novel multiple marker assay versus the RMI. Am J Obstet Gynecol 2010.

Table 4. The sensitivity, positive predictive value and negative predictive value between Risk of Ovarian Malignancy Algorithm (ROMA) and Risk of Malignancy Index (RMI) of benign tumor and epithelial ovarian cancer (EOC) stage I-IV at a set specificity of 75%. LMP= low malignant potential.

Receiver operating characteristic (ROC) analysis of individual tumor markers and their combinations were evaluated and summarized(Jacob, Meier et al. 2011). HE4 performed best 83.3% sensitivity and 84.6% specificity. Whereas ROMA were 85.4% sensitivity and 85.6% specificity (Table 4).

Tumor markers and their combinations	Borderline tumors and cancer group versus non-malignant group		
	AUC	Sensitivity (%)	Specificity (%)
HE4	0.89	83.3	84.6
CA125	0.87	60.4	91.3
CA125*HE4	0.90	70.8	94.2
ROMA	0.90	85.4	85.6
RMIHE4	0.93	79.1	86.5
RMICA125	0.95	66.7	97.1
RMICA125*HE4	0.95	75.0	98.1

*modified from Jacob F, Meier M, Caduff R, et al. No benefit from combining HE4 and CA125 as ovarian tumor markers in a clinical setting. Gynecol Oncol 2011;121(3): 487-91. (Jacob, Meier et al. 2011)

Table 5. The AUC, sensitivity and specificity of individual tumor markers and their combinations between borderline tumors and cancer group versus non-malignant group.

8. Economic evaluation: Cost effectiveness analysis

During economic crisis around the world, the cost effectiveness should be evaluated. It is estimated the cost-effectiveness of different screening strategies using a stochastic simulation model (Skates and Singer 1991). On prediction, a multimodel strategy would cost 51,000 US dollars per year of life saved. Therefore, it would be potentially cost-effective for ovarian cancer screening (Sfakianos and Havrilesky 2011).

9. Conclusion and recommendations

In conclusion, screening for ovarian cancer would be emerged as a promising strategy to increase cure rate, prolong survival and decrease morbidities in the future. Further evaluations for ovarian cancer screening and early detection should be encouraged. Understanding preclinical ovarian cancer and development of novel effective strategy could lead for early detection, ultimately it will decrease incidence and mortality from ovarian cancer.

10. References

Amonkar, S. D., G. P. Bertenshaw, et al. (2009). "Development and preliminary evaluation of a multivariate index assay for ovarian cancer." *PLoS One* 4(2): e4599.

Bast, R. C., Jr., M. Feeney, et al. (1981). "Reactivity of a monoclonal antibody with human ovarian carcinoma." *J Clin Invest* 68(5): 1331-1337.

Buys, S. S., E. Partridge, et al. (2011). "Effect of screening on ovarian cancer mortality: the Prostate, Lung, Colorectal and Ovarian (PLCO) Cancer Screening Randomized Controlled Trial." *JAMA* 305(22): 2295-2303.

Denhardt, D. T. and M. Noda (1998). "Osteopontin expression and function: role in bone remodeling." *J Cell Biochem Suppl* 30-31: 92-102.

Ferlay, J., H. R. Shin, et al. (2010). "Estimates of worldwide burden of cancer in 2008: GLOBOCAN 2008." *Int J Cancer* 127(12): 2893-2917.

Fung, M. F., P. Bryson, et al. (2004). "Screening postmenopausal women for ovarian cancer: a systematic review." *J Obstet Gynaecol Can* 26(8): 717-728.

Hassan, R., A. T. Remaley, et al. (2006). "Detection and quantitation of serum mesothelin, a tumor marker for patients with mesothelioma and ovarian cancer." *Clin Cancer Res* 12(2): 447-453.

Hensley, M. L., M. E. Robson, et al. (2003). "Pre- and postmenopausal high-risk women undergoing screening for ovarian cancer: anxiety, risk perceptions, and quality of life." *Gynecol Oncol* 89(3): 440-446.

Hermsen, B. B., R. I. Olivier, et al. (2007). "No efficacy of annual gynaecological screening in BRCA1/2 mutation carriers; an observational follow-up study." *Br J Cancer* 96(9): 1335-1342.

Hogg, R. and M. Friedlander (2004). "Biology of epithelial ovarian cancer: implications for screening women at high genetic risk." *J Clin Oncol* 22(7): 1315-1327.

Jacob, F., M. Meier, et al. (2011). "No benefit from combining HE4 and CA125 as ovarian tumor markers in a clinical setting." *Gynecol Oncol* 121(3): 487-491.

Jacobs, I., D. Oram, et al. (1990). "A risk of malignancy index incorporating CA 125, ultrasound and menopausal status for the accurate preoperative diagnosis of ovarian cancer." *Br J Obstet Gynaecol* 97(10): 922-929.

Menon, U., A. Gentry-Maharaj, et al. (2009). "Sensitivity and specificity of multimodal and ultrasound screening for ovarian cancer, and stage distribution of detected cancers: results of the prevalence screen of the UK Collaborative Trial of Ovarian Cancer Screening (UKCTOCS)." *Lancet Oncol* 10(4): 327-340.

Montagnana, M., E. Danese, et al. (2011). "The ROMA (Risk of Ovarian Malignancy Algorithm) for estimating the risk of epithelial ovarian cancer in women presenting with pelvic mass: is it really useful?" *Clin Chem Lab Med* 49(3): 521-525.

Moore, R. G., A. K. Brown, et al. (2008). "The use of multiple novel tumor biomarkers for the detection of ovarian carcinoma in patients with a pelvic mass." *Gynecol Oncol* 108(2): 402-408.

Moore, R. G., M. Jabre-Raughley, et al. (2010). "Comparison of a novel multiple marker assay vs the Risk of Malignancy Index for the prediction of epithelial ovarian cancer in patients with a pelvic mass." *Am J Obstet Gynecol* 203(3): 228 e221-226.

Moore, R. G., S. MacLaughlan, et al. (2010). "Current state of biomarker development for clinical application in epithelial ovarian cancer." *Gynecol Oncol* 116(2): 240-245.

Nosov, V., F. Su, et al. (2009). "Validation of serum biomarkers for detection of early-stage ovarian cancer." *Am J Obstet Gynecol* 200(6): 639 e631-635.

Rein, B. J., S. Gupta, et al. (2011). "Potential markers for detection and monitoring of ovarian cancer." *J Oncol* 2011: 475983.

Scholler, N., M. Crawford, et al. (2006). "Bead-based ELISA for validation of ovarian cancer early detection markers." *Clin Cancer Res* 12(7 Pt 1): 2117-2124.

SEER " Surveillance, Epidemiology, and End Results (SEER) Program(www.seer.cancer.gov) SEER*Stat Database: Populations - Total U.S. (1969-2009) <Single Ages to 85+, Katrina/Rita Adjustment> - Linked To County Attributes - Total U.S., 1969-2009

Counties, National Cancer Institute, DCCPS, Surveillance Research Program, Cancer Statistics Branch, released April 2011.".

Sfakianos, G. P. and L. J. Havrilesky (2011). "A review of cost-effectiveness studies in ovarian cancer." *Cancer Control* 18(1): 59-64.

Shah, C. A., K. A. Lowe, et al. (2009). "Influence of ovarian cancer risk status on the diagnostic performance of the serum biomarkers mesothelin, HE4, and CA125." *Cancer Epidemiol Biomarkers Prev* 18(5): 1365-1372.

Simon, I., S. Zhuo, et al. (2006). "B7-h4 is a novel membrane-bound protein and a candidate serum and tissue biomarker for ovarian cancer." *Cancer Res* 66(3): 1570-1575.

Skates, S. J. and D. E. Singer (1991). "Quantifying the potential benefit of CA 125 screening for ovarian cancer." *J Clin Epidemiol* 44(4-5): 365-380.

Vaes, E., R. Manchanda, et al. (2011). "Differential diagnosis of adnexal masses: A sequential use of the Risk of Malignancy Index and a novel computer aided diagnostic tool." *Ultrasound Obstet Gynecol.*

Van Gorp, T., I. Cadron, et al. (2011). "HE4 and CA125 as a diagnostic test in ovarian cancer: prospective validation of the Risk of Ovarian Malignancy Algorithm." *Br J Cancer* 104(5): 863-870.

Visintin, I., Z. Feng, et al. (2008). "Diagnostic markers for early detection of ovarian cancer." *Clin Cancer Res* 14(4): 1065-1072.

Woodward, E. R., H. V. Sleightholme, et al. (2007). "Annual surveillance by CA125 and transvaginal ultrasound for ovarian cancer in both high-risk and population risk women is ineffective." *BJOG* 114(12): 1500-1509.

Zhao, C., L. Annamalai, et al. (2007). "Circulating haptoglobin is an independent prognostic factor in the sera of patients with epithelial ovarian cancer." *Neoplasia* 9(1): 1-7.

3

Preventive Strategies in Epithelial Ovarian Cancer

Gina M. Mantia-Smaldone and Nathalie Scholler
Penn Ovarian Cancer Research Center
University of Pennsylvania, Philadelphia,
USA

1. Introduction

Despite advances in surgery and chemotherapy, epithelial ovarian cancer (EOC) remains the most lethal gynecologic malignancy [1]. Due to lack of a specific prodromal symptomatology as well as effective screening strategies, the vast majority of EOC patients present with advanced stage disease will ultimately die from their disease [1]. Furthermore, while up to 80% of patients will respond to conventional primary platinum/taxane chemotherapy, greater than 60% will experience disease recurrence, and current reports indicate discouraging response rates of 20% in women with resistance to platinum-based chemotherapy [2]. Preventive strategies, including improvements in early detection of disease as well as in preventing disease recurrence, are, therefore, crucial to improving prognosis.

Ovarian cancer prevention can be defined by two main strategies: 1) early detection of cancer in at-risk patients and 2) prevention of recurrent disease in patients with an established diagnosis of cancer. Through the use of screening tools, such as serum biomarkers and medical imaging, early disease detection offers the promise of identifying cancer while still localized and potentially curable [3]. Secondary preventive approaches aim to maintain patients without evidence of active disease and thereby extend their disease-free survival. Surveillance methods including serial biomarker measurements as well as therapeutic vaccinations have been examined for their impact on survival outcomes. Finally, risk stratification is critical to the success of any cancer prevention strategy; capitalizing on risk-reducing behaviors and intensive screening is most likely to improve individuals at greatest risk for disease-related morbidity and mortality.

Current research in the early detection of ovarian cancer largely focuses on biomarker discovery, using transcriptome analysis, proteomics, epigenomics, metabolomics and glycomics of differentially expressed molecules between women with disease and healthy controls. Biomarkers already approved by the FDA (i.e., CA125 and HE4) or those under investigation, including osteopontin, MUC1 and mesothelin, offer hope for women at risk for disease development, especially those with predisposing genetic mutations [4]. As part of this effort, we have generated site-specific biotinylated recombinant antibodies secreted by yeast (Biobodies [5]) to cost- and time-effectively generate antibodies for developing screening tools for large populations of women [6]. In addition, biomarkers, especially tumor associated antigens, may also serve as targets for vaccination [7].

Immune-driven therapies are currently under investigation for the prevention of ovarian cancer recurrence[8-12]. Therapeutic vaccinations, targeting molecules specific to an individuals' disease through the use of whole tumor lysates and tumor-pulsed dendritic cells, are currently under investigation for women with recurrent disease; such immunotherapeutic strategies are an additional research interest in our group (NCT00683241, NCT01132014, NCT00603460) [13, 14]. Preventive approaches targeting individuals at risk for ovarian cancer as well as those with advanced stage disease may significantly impact disease incidence and prognostic outcomes. In this chapter, we will discuss these current approaches in detail.

2. Challenges in ovarian cancer prevention

In 1968, the World Health Organization (WHO) established guidelines for disease screening, including that the screened condition should be an important health problem with available treatment [15]. Ovarian cancer arguably satisfies these principles as it ranks as one of the top ten most common cancers amongst women in the US with more than 21,000 diagnosed annually [1]. Further, ovarian cancer is the fifth most common cause of cancer mortality and remains the most lethal gynecologic cancer [1]. Platinum/taxane chemotherapy is available for women with this disease, and approximately 70-80% will respond to this regimen [1]. However, more than 75% of women are diagnosed when disease has already spread from the ovary, and advanced stage disease at presentation carries an overall poor prognosis [1]. Improved ovarian cancer screening methods are therefore needed to detect disease in its earliest stages when treatment is more effective, translating into improved overall five year survival rates ranging from 60% to 90% [3, 16, 17].

The prevention strategy applied in cervical cancer demonstrates that successful disease screening significantly diminishes disease-related morbidity and mortality. The understanding of the natural history of cervical cancer led to the introduction of screening cervical cytology via Papnicolaou smears and guidelines for the early detection of preneoplastic cervical lesions. Since the introduction of these strategies, the incidence of cervical cancer has declined by more than 75% [18]. Furthermore, vaccination against the oncogenic Human papillomavirus (HPV) will also aid in eliminating this disease.

However, preventive strategies in ovarian cancer, unlike those in cervical cancer, have been met with several challenges. First, compared to cervical cancer which ranks as the second most common gynecologic cancer worldwide, ovarian cancer has a low prevalence with 40 cases per year per 100,000 women over the age of 50 years; this mandates that an effective screening test for ovarian cancer has both a high sensitivity and specificity in order to significantly impact disease incidence [19]. Second, current screening methods for early detection of ovarian cancer, including routine physical examination, CA125 serum assessment, and transvaginal ultrasound, have high false-positive rates and low positive predictive values (**Table 1**) [20]. In fact, for a positive predictive value (PPV) of 10%, an ovarian cancer screening test would require a sensitivity of at least 75% and a specificity of greater than 99% [22]. Further, current methods of screening have not resulted in a significant impact on disease morbidity or mortality [21].

While it is known that persistent HPV infection is responsible for virtually all cervical cancer and its immediate precursors worldwide [23], the exact etiology for ovarian cancer remains largely debated. Precursors for ovarian cancer should be "morphologically recognizable lesions that are reproducible thereby permitting early clinical intervention" [24]. It has been generally accepted that ovarian cancer originates from the ovarian surface epithelium (OSE) or from postovulatory inclusion cysts, and one hypothesis is that incessant ovulation is the main pathogenic mechanism [25, 26]. Yet, recent evaluation of pathologic specimens has also suggested that a greater proportion of "ovarian" cancers may actually originate in the fimbriated end of the fallopian tube with metastasis to the ovary [26, 27]. Further, a dualistic classification system has been proposed in which ovarian cancers are divided into two groups: type I tumors which consist of low-grade neoplasms and type II tumor which are aggressive and progress rapidly [28]. Precursor lesions, including borderline malignant tumors and endometriosis, have been identified for type I tumors and may serve to improve early detection of these ovarian tumors especially given their indolent nature; a slower transition time between early and later stage of disease may afford opportunities to detect disease when it is still localized to the ovary. However, type II tumors do not have well-characterized precursor lesions, which is perhaps due to their high level of genetic instability [24]. Because the transition time between stage I and stage III is unknown, it is uncertain whether these tumors rapidly progress from an early stage to an advanced stage or whether these tumors develop as a result of a diffuse peritoneal process [19]. At this point in time and despite a large body of work, no consensus has been reached regarding ovarian cancer precursors, which contributes to the challenge of creating an effective preventive strategy for ovarian cancer.

Finally, screening can carry some significant disadvantages, including an increased cost to society for over-utilized medical resources as well as psychological stress/anxiety especially in cases of false positive screening resulting in unnecessary operative intervention for benign pathology. However, thanks to stratifying approaches based on reproducible risk factors enabling maximized efficiency and balanced cost-effectiveness, this last hurdle may be easier to overcome.

Method	Sensitivity	Specificity	PPV
Symptomatology	57-83%[31, 75]	86.7-90% [31, 75]	1% [34]
Bimanual Exam	28%[145]	93%[145]	64%[145]
Ultrasound	75-95%[54, 56, 58]	73-98.7% [54, 56, 58]	1-46% [54, 58]
CA125	57%[68]	85-93%[68]	96-100%[68]

Table 1. Current Ovarian Cancer Screening Methods.

3. Available modalities in prevention of late stage ovarian cancers and of disease recurrence

The goal of preventive strategies is to reduce ovarian cancer-related morbidity and mortality. Disease screening aims to detect ovarian cancer while it is still confined to the ovary and the five-year survival rates are 80-90% [1], thus to prevent incurable, late stage disease. Disease surveillance following conventional adjuvant chemotherapy allows for early detection of recurrent ovarian cancer and therefore permits prevention of clinically apparent recurrence. Current screening modalities include symptom recognition, bimanual exam, serial CA125 levels and pelvic ultrasound, while disease surveillance typically relies on physical exam, CA125 levels and imaging.

3.1 Do symptoms correspond with the onset of disease or with recurrence?

Ovarian cancer is referred to as the "silent killer" due to non-specific symptoms which often go unrecognized until the disease has significantly spread. Although there is limited data to support symptomatology as a sole screening modality for ovarian cancer, recognition of ovarian cancer symptoms by both patients and caregivers may help to identify individuals with early stage disease [29] and in 2007 the Gynecologic Cancer Foundation, American Cancer Society and Society of Gynecologic Oncologists issued a consensus statement supporting the recognition of symptoms as a modality in the evaluation of ovarian cancer [30].

Patient symptoms have been correlated with the onset of disease [31-33]. Symptoms commonly attributed to ovarian cancer include abdominal bloating, increased abdominal size and urinary symptoms [32]. In a case-control study of women at risk for developing ovarian cancer symptoms, specifically pelvic/abdominal pain, urinary urgency/frequency, increased abdominal size/bloating and difficulty eating/early satiety, were significantly associated with ovarian cancer when they occurred more than 12 days per month for less than one year duration [31]. Further, a symptom index was more sensitive in women with advanced stage disease (79.5% vs. 56.7% early stage disease) and more specific in women greater than 50 years of age (90% vs. 86.7% for women less than 50 years old). The authors also applied this symptom index to a sample of 1709 women at average risk and reported a positive screening rate of 2.6%.

In a large population-based study [34], Rossing and colleagues reported a positive symptom index in 62.3% of women with early stage disease compared to 70.7% with late-stage disease and 5.1% of controls. While symptoms were more likely to occur in women with ovarian cancer, there only was a short interval (less than 5 months) from symptom onset to diagnosis. This suggests that the symptom index may not provide a critical help to diagnose early stage ovarian cancer. In addition, the PPV of the symptom index was approximately 1%; thus the use of a positive symptom index alone would only result in the diagnosis of ovarian cancer in 1 out of 100 women in the general population presenting with the same symptoms.

Further complicating this screening technique is the fact that symptom presentation and duration may be influenced by the histological subtype of ovarian cancer [35]. In a recent population-base study, women with serous histology (the major histologic subtype) were less likely to report symptoms, were more often diagnosed at advanced stage (compared to mucinous tumors) and had a shorter duration of symptoms compared to women with early stage disease. This study also further highlights the difficulty in diagnosing ovarian cancer at an early stage due to rapid progression of disease.

Finally, monitoring symptoms in women with established ovarian cancer has also been considered for early intervention for disease recurrence. However, in a recent systematic review [36], approximately 67% of a patients identified with recurrent disease had no concurrent clinical symptoms. Other surveillance modalities, including clinical examination, biomarker determination and imaging, should therefore be used in conjunction with symptoms in order to diagnose recurrent ovarian cancer.

3.2 Can bimanual examination diagnose early stage ovarian cancer and/or recurrent disease?

Routine pelvic examination is a key component of annual gynecologic health assessment. Palpation of the uterus and ovaries by bimanual examination may allow for the earlier detection of ovarian cancer; exam findings may initiate further evaluation with ultrasound and ultimately surgery, potentially detecting cancers before they become clinically evident. Further, a pelvic exam has little adverse consequences [37].

However, pelvic examination is generally recommended only for the evaluation of symptomatic patients and only in conjunction with ultrasonography [38]. Routine pelvic exam is considered as being neither a sensitive nor a specific means for detecting ovarian cancer in asymptomatic women [39, 40] and may thus result in unnecessary surgical intervention for benign ovarian lesions. Further supporting this view, bimanual examination, which was originally included in the screening protocol of asymptomatic, postmenopausal women in the Prostate, Lung, Colorectal and Ovarian Screening Trial of the National Cancer Institute (NCI), was eliminated as a screening modality from the trial as it became evident that it failed to detect the first onset of ovarian cancer [41].

In contrast, pelvic examination is recommended for disease surveillance of ovarian cancer per the NCCN guidelines, as 26-50% of recurrences occur within the pelvis [42]. Physical examination is an inexpensive, safe and practical tool that can trigger further evaluation with other modalities, but it must be kept in mind that the detection rates of recurrent ovarian cancer vary widely [43, 44] and physical examination may fail to detect common sites of recurrence, including the upper abdomen, the retroperitoneum and the thorax [45].

3.3 How effective is ultrasound in detecting early stage ovarian cancer?

Pelvic ultrasound has been utilized for predicting the likelihood of malignancy, especially in women with a known pelvic mass. Transvaginal ultrasound (TVUS) can detect changes in ovarian size and morphology and is superior to physical examination in evaluating ovarian size, especially in women who are postmenopausal, obese or who have an enlarged uterus[46]. Primary screening studies with TVUS in both asymptomatic and symptomatic at-risk women have been successful in identifying early stage ovarian cancers [47-50].

Ovarian volume is inversely related to age; thus an enlarged ovary in post-menopausal women can be a sign of an evolving ovarian cancer. Mean ovarian volume is significantly greater in premenopausal women compared to postmenopausal women [51]; the upper limit of normal ovarian volume is 20 cm^3 and 10cm^3 in premenopausal and postmenopausal women, respectively. Other ovarian characteristics, including complex or solid morphology, cyst papillations, septae and increased blood flow, have also been suggested as findings suspicious for malignancy [52, 53].

To decrease the number of false-positive results, morphology scoring indices have been introduced for ovarian cancer screening. Investigators at the University of Kentucky have developed a morphology scoring index based on ovarian volume, wall structure and septal structure as a means to improve the PPV of TVUS for ovarian cancer screening [54]. In a multi-institutional sample of patients undergoing surgical intervention for ovarian tumors, this morphology index implemented during preoperative ultrasound evaluation, yielded a sensitivity of 89%, a specificity of 73%, and a positive predictive value of 46% [55].

The International Ovarian Tumor Analysis (IOTA) study has also provided a reproducible standardized methodology for the ultrasound evaluation of adnexal masses and has further identified features with increased risk of malignancy: the presence of an irregular solid tumor, the presence of papillary or solid components, the presence of ascites, an irregular multilocular solid tumor and the presence of pronounced blood flow [53]. Prospective validation of these simple ultrasound rules in a sample of women with adnexal masses yielded a sensitivity of 95%, a specificity of 91%, positive likelihood ratio of 10.37 and negative likelihood ratio of 0.06

[56]. This study has also demonstrated that although pattern recognition of ultrasound findings by an experienced examiner can not only reproducibly discriminate between benign and malignant adnexal masses, it is superior to serum CA125 [57] .

The United Kingdom Collaborative Trial of Ovarian Cancer Screening (UKCTOCS) is a randomized control trial evaluating the effect of screening on mortality [58]. Patients are randomized to screening with CA125 and transvaginal ultrasound or with transvaginal ultrasound alone. At the prevalence screen, the results were promising for transvaginal ultrasound, which yielded a sensitivity, specificity and PPV of 75.0%, 98.2%, and 2.8%, respectively, for primary invasive epithelial ovarian and tubal cancers [58]. The impact of ultrasound screening on mortality is still pending at this time.

Ultrasound has also been examined for its role in the detection of ovarian cancer recurrence [45]. While sensitivity ranges 45-85% and specificity ranges 60-100% [45], ultrasound has user variability and limited visibility [59]. For this reason, CT scans are often employed in surveillance protocols [42] and are typically only performed when indicated by clinical findings. In summary, although it is not the imaging modality of choice for ovarian cancer surveillance, TVUS is a useful tool to prevent the discovery of late stage ovarian cancer in women who are at increased risk for developing ovarian cancer.

3.4 What role do biomarkers play in the screening of ovarian cancer and the detection of disease recurrence?

Biomarkers are substances which help to indicate the presence of a disease. Soluble biomarkers differentially expressed between individuals with disease and normal controls are convenient tools of disease detection. The perceived advantages of biomarkers compared to other disease screening modalities such as physical exam or ultrasound, include availability, reproducibility, objectivity (operator-independent) and cost-effectiveness. Biomarkers for early detection aim to identify ovarian cancer in individuals who are symptomatic (Phase II specimens) or who are asymptomatic before a clinical diagnosis is made (Phase III specimens). However, the identification of such biomarkers is challenging. Discovery methods often use patient samples with clinically diagnosed and advanced stage disease, thus making it necessary to extrapolate findings of advanced disease to early-stage disease, and biomarkers discovered in diagnostic samples may not be validated in prediagnostic samples [60].

CA125 (or MUC16) glycoprotein is the most studied tumor marker, alone and/or in combination with other biomarkers, for ovarian cancer screening. Approximately 80% of ovarian cancer tumors are CA125 positive [61]. Elevated serum CA125 levels (>35 units/mL) can be detected in asymptomatic women with ovarian cancer using a monoclonal antibody (OC 125) [62] and carry a specificity of 98.5% for postmenopausal women [63]. An elevation in CA125 levels, especially twice the upper limits of normal, can often occur 2 to 5 months prior the clinical detection of an ovarian cancer recurrence [45], with sensitivity and specificity for recurrence detection ranging from 62-94% and 91-100% [45, 64-66]. Recent work has further shown that CA125 levels may begin to rise as early as 3 years prior to clinical diagnosis, but will likely only reach detectable levels in the final year before diagnosis [67].

While CA125 is the most predictive marker of ovarian cancer [67] and remains the single-best marker [68], studies have generally indicated that CA125 serum testing performs poorly in the detection of early stage disease [69]. CA125 levels are only elevated in approximately 50% of stage I ovarian cancers [62]. Further, false positive CA125 levels can occur in women with benign conditions, including menstruation, appendicitis, benign ovarian cysts, endometriosis and pelvic inflammatory disease, as well as with other malignancies, including breast, lung, endometrial and pancreatic cancers [61]. Thus, multimodal strategies, particularly the combination of CA125 with pelvic ultrasound, have been examined in order to improve sensitivity and PPV of ovarian cancer screening.

The combination of CA125 and ultrasound has been examined in several studies [70]. In a prospective pilot study, 144 women with an elevated risk of ovarian cancer, as defined by a Receiver Operating Characteristic (ROC) curve based on age and CA125, underwent TVUS [71]. Sixteen women were recommended for surgery and 3 women were found to have primary invasive ovarian cancer, thus yielding a specificity of 99.8% and a PPV of 19%. This algorithm was subsequently incorporated into the United Kingdom Collaborative Trial of Ovarian Cancer Screening, which is a randomized controlled trial designed to assess the effect of screening on mortality [58]. Women are randomized to three arms: no treatment, CA125 with TVUS screening or TVUS alone screening. At the prevalence screen, CA125 combined with TVUS achieved sensitivity, specificity, and positive-predictive values of 89.5%, 99.8% and 35.1%, respectively [58]. The specificity was higher in this combined screening group compared to the TVUS alone group (89.4% vs. 75.0%), suggesting that this screening would result in lower rates of repeat testing and surgery. In an additional study, an elevated serum CA125 (≥35 units/mL) and preoperative ultrasound findings of solid or complex tumors yielded a PPV of 84.7%, a NPV of 92.4% and correctly identified 77.3% of patients with early stage disease [70].

Additional potential serum biomarkers have been identified [72-74] and extensively examined for the detection of ovarian cancer [75-77]. Human epididymis protein 4 (HE4) is a biomarker overexpressed by both serous and endometrioid ovarian cancers [78] and is expressed by 32% of ovarian cancers lacking CA125 expression [76]. HE4 has been FDA approved to monitor for disease recurrence (June 2008) and was recently incorporated into the clinical evaluation of ovarian cancer patients. Studies have also indicated that HE4 may also improve prediction of malignancy in ovarian masses when combined with CA125 measurements [75-76]. Furthermore, Anderson and colleagues have demonstrated an increase in CA125, HE4 and mesothelin in ovarian cancer patients compared to matched controls, with a differential expression noted as early as 3 years preceding diagnosis; these results suggest that a multimarker profile may improve detection of early stage disease [67].

Several panels of biomarkers have been published during the past ten years. One of them, a multiplex, bead-based, immunoassay system, examined serum concentrations of leptin, prolactin, osteopontin, insulin-like growth factor II, macrophage inhibitory factor and CA125. This blood test, called OvaSure™, was reported to achieve a sensitivity of 95.3% and specificity of 99.4%, providing a significant improvement over CA125 alone for ovarian cancer detection in a cohort of women newly diagnosed with ovarian cancer compared to healthy controls [79]. OvaSure™ was proposed as a screening tool for women at risk for ovarian cancer, but, due to some concerns [80], further investigation is warranted prior to the commercial use of this biomarker panel as a screening tool for the early detection of ovarian cancer.

The use of CA125 for detection of relapsed disease is not supported by the recent results of a randomized control trial [81]. This multi-institutional European randomized control trial failed to demonstrate a survival advantage for women with recurrent disease who received early intervention based on rising CA125 levels compared to those who received treatment when symptoms developed [81]. The authors thus questioned the value of routine CA125 measurements for surveillance of women with ovarian cancer who attain a complete response after first line therapy. Yet, the conclusions of this study have been underplayed by several concerns, including failure to address the role of secondary cytoreduction, lack of stratification by residual disease following primary cytoreduction, lack of radiographic confirmation of recurrence and non-standardized second-line therapies. Thus, the prevention of clinically detectable relapses using serial CA125 measurements will likely continue at the discretion of the patient and her physician [82].

4. Biomarker discovery for ovarian cancer prevention

Various techniques are currently under investigation in order to identify new biomarkers which may improve the detection of early stage ovarian cancer as well as improve the detection of recurrent disease [83-87]. Proteomic analysis of serum and ascites samples by mass spectrometry is a strategy under investigation for the detection of differentially expressed proteins or protein fragments in women with ovarian cancer compared to healthy controls [83, 88, 89]. Biomarkers and respective panels identified with proteomics have the potential to influence ovarian cancer prevention; further development and validation, however, are necessary before they may introduced into clinical practice [89].

Evolving technologies, including transcriptomics [84], epigenomics [85, 86], metabolomics [90] and glycomics [87], are also under investigation in ovarian cancer. Transcriptomics, or expression profiling, studies the impact of RNA molecules, including mRNA, rRNA, tRNA and non-coding RNAs, in diseases. Using techniques based on DNA microarrays, these molecules can be identified to help pinpoint genes which may be differentially expressed in ovarian cancer compared to normal tissue [84]. Gene expression profiling can be performed using both serum and formalin-fixed paraffin-embedded tissue biopsies and may help to identify genes associated with early-stage disease thereby improving screening [84].

Epigenomics focuses on the role of DNA methylation, histone modifications, RNA interference and nucleosome remodeling in the development and progression of ovarian cancer [86]. Epigenetic alterations can be used as candidate targets for early detection and for monitoring of ovarian cancer recurrence [85]. Aberrant DNA hypermethylation of CpG islands in the promoter of tumor suppressor genes and other cancer genes as well as microRNAs (miRNAs) are currently being identified in both body fluids and tissue biopsies and may help to demonstrate the importance of specific genes involved in ovarian tumorigenesis [85].

Metabolomics examines the role of small molecules ("metabolites") which are unique to a specific cellular process. Metabolic fingerprints of ovarian cancer can be measured in serum and/or other bodily fluids using mass spectrometry and has the potential to improve detection of early stage and recurrent disease [90]. Lysophosphatidic acid [91] and lipid associated sialic acid [92] are metabolites which are currently under investigation for ovarian cancer detection.

Glycosylation is the most common post-translational modification of proteins. Aberrant glycosylation patterns of proteins, such as MUC1 [93], have been identified in ovarian cancer and may play a key role in promoting tumor cell invasion and metastasis as well as stimulating anti-tumor immune responses [94]. Therefore, glycoproteins are currently being examined for their potential as biomarker as well as for treatment [87].

In addition to these efforts, we have generated a cost- and time-effective method for generating site-specific *in vivo* biotinylated recombinant antibodies secreted by yeast

(Biobodies [5, 95]). Biobodies have been generated against HE4 [95] and mesothelin [96]. We have also demonstrated that this technology can be used reliably in a highly-sensitive bead-based ELISA assay for screening large populations of women for ovarian cancer [5, 67] and for serum biomarker discovery [6].
These novel approaches to biomarker discovery offers promise for improved ovarian cancer screening and for detection of recurrences. The impact of these biomarkers on clinical outcomes warrants further investigation in prospective clinical trials.

5. Current recommendations for ovarian cancer prevention

Given its low prevalence in the general population, universal screening for ovarian cancer is neither feasible nor cost-effective. Risk assessment is inherent to the success of any screening approach, and women at highest risk for disease are likely to benefit the most from preventive strategies. Several risk factors have been identified for epithelial ovarian cancer (**Table 2**) [25], and current screening recommendations are often stratified by an individual's risk of developing disease. While the exact pathogenesis of this disease is still unclear, it is generally postulated that an increase in ovulation and/or an increase in estrogen exposure is associated with an increased lifetime risk of disease. Thus, factors, such as nulliparity, menarche at an early age, menopause at a late age, fertility drug use and hormone replacement therapy use, are believed to put individuals at risk for disease [25, 97-101]. Age, Caucasian race, ethnicity (especially Ashkenazi Jewish heritage), living in an industrialized country, and a history of endometriosis are other factors predisposing to ovarian cancer [25]. In addition, several factors, particularly multiparity, oral contraceptive use, breastfeeding and tubal ligation, have been linked with a decreased incidence of ovarian cancer and are therefore believed to be protective against developing ovarian cancer [102, 103].

Protective Factors	Risk Factors
Hysterectomy	Age
Tubal Ligation	Caucasian race
Multiparity	Early menarche
Lactation	Ethnicity (Ashkenazi Jewish, Icelandic, Hungarian)
Oral Contraceptive use	Family history
	Fertility drug use
	Hormone replacement therapy
	Late menopause
	Nulliparity
	Personal history of breast cancer
	Residence in North America and Northern Europe
	Talc
	Endometriosis

Table 2. Protective and Risk factors for Ovarian Cancer [25].

Perhaps, the single most important risk factor for ovarian cancer is family history. Hereditary ovarian cancers account for approximately 10% of all EOC cases. Compared to controls, women with one first or second-degree relative with ovarian cancer have a threefold increase in risk [104]. Hereditary ovarian cancers are commonly attributed to genetic mutations which are transmitted in families in an autosomal dominant fashion. Germline mutations in *BRCA1* and *BRCA2*, tumor suppressors which participate in homologous recombination repair of double-stranded DNA breaks, account for approximately 95% of all hereditary EOC cases [105] and carry a 25 to 50% lifetime risk of ovarian cancer [106]. Further, *BRCA1/2* mutations are highly prevalent amongst women of Ashkenazi Jewish descent; 35-40% of Ashkenazi women with ovarian cancers have a *BRCA1 or BRCA2* mutation [107]. These mutations may also be suspected in individuals with a personal history of breast cancer before age 50, dual breast cancer or ovarian cancer [108]. Women with *BRCA*- associated ovarian cancer typically present with high grade serous cancers at an earlier age compared to non-hereditary controls; however, these individuals more often have higher response rates to platinum-based chemotherapy and improved overall survival [109].

The remaining hereditary EOC cases are attributed to Lynch Syndrome II, also referred to as hereditary nonpolyposis colorectal cancer (HNPCC) syndrome; these individuals with mutations in DNA mismatch repair genes *MLH1, MSH2, MSH6 and PMS2* are at increased risk for colon cancer as well as numerous other cancers, including endometrial and ovarian cancer [110]. Women with this autosomal dominant genetic background have a 3 to 14% lifetime risk of ovarian cancer [110].

5.1 Recommendations for ovarian cancer prevention in women at average risk

In the absence of significant risk factors, a typical woman carries a 1 in 72 lifetime risk of ovarian cancer [111] and is considered at average risk of developing ovarian cancer.

5.1.1 Prevention by risk reducing behaviors

Epidemiologic studies of women with ovarian cancer risk have identified several protective factors, including oral contraceptive pill use (OCP), parity, lactation, and tubal ligation (**Table 2**). These protective factors should be considered for women with any risk of ovarian cancer as an additional preventive strategy. Patients should be counseled regarding the impact of these factors on their risk of ovarian cancer. Specifically, (1) the use of OCPs for 5 or more years results in a 50% reduction in the incidence of ovarian cancer [102], and this benefit may last for up to 30 years following use [112]. This benefit has also been reported in women with *BRCA1* or *BRCA2* mutations [113] and for most histological subtypes [114]. It is estimated that OCPs have prevented 200,000 ovarian cancers and 100,000 deaths [25]. (2) Parity is a protective factor for ovarian cancer [25]. The risk for ovarian cancer decreases with each live birth, but there is no additional benefit once a women achieves grand multiparity [115]. Parous women with *BRCA1* mutations can also experience a reduced risk of ovarian cancer with each additional full-term pregnancy [116]. (3) Lactation also results in a decreased incidence of ovarian cancer[117]. However, there is no additional benefit for individual episodes of lactation beyond 12 months. The relative risk of ovarian cancer decreases by 2% for each month of breastfeeding [118]. (4) Tubal ligation may also substantially reduce the risk of ovarian cancer [119]. Given a greater than 60% risk reduction, women with *BRCA1* mutations should be counseled regarding this option especially when they have completed childbearing [120].

5.1.2 Prevention by routine screening

Given a low incidence and prevalence of ovarian cancer in the general population, large study cohorts are necessary to evaluate the utility of an ovarian cancer screening test [121]. The results of initial clinical trials, while failing to evaluate the impact of screening on cancer-related mortality, emphasize limitations on the specificity and PPV of available screening strategies for women at average risk.

A pilot randomized control trial evaluated a multimodal screening approach with serial CA125 and pelvic ultrasound in a sample of almost 22,000 postmenopausal women [121]. Combined CA125 and ultrasound (US) screening was not only feasible but also preliminarily resulted in a survival advantage (median survival 72.9 months in the screened group vs. 41.8 months in the control group, $p = 0.0112$). Data from this trial have paved the way for larger randomized-control trials [21, 58, 122] which aim to examine the impact of screening on mortality.

The Shizuoka Cohort Study of Ovarian Cancer Screening (SCSOCS) trial was a prospective, randomized trial examining ovarian screening, via CA125 and US, in asymptomatic postmenopausal Japanese women between 1985 and 1999 [122]. Of more than 41,000 women who underwent screening, only 27 had detected ovarian cancer; at the prevalent screen, screening produced a detection rate of 0.31 per 1000. Ovarian cancer screening also identified a higher proportion of stage I cancers (63% vs. 38%, p=0.23) when compared to the control group.

The Prostate, Lung, Colorectal and Ovarian Cancer (PLCO) screening trial is a randomized controlled cancer screening trial evaluating screening tests for the 4 PLCO cancers [41]. More than 78,000 healthy women between 55 and 74 years of age from across the United States were randomized to a screening or usual care arm at 10 screening sites between 1993 and 2001. The primary objective of this trial was to determine whether routine screening via transvaginal ultrasound (TVUS) and/or CA125 can reduce ovarian cancer-specific mortality. Twenty-nine neoplasms were identified in almost 29,000 women who received any screening test, producing a PPV for TVUS of 1.0%, 3.7% for CA125, and 23.5% for combined TVUS and CA125. Overall, these screening tests were associated with a high number of false-positive tests, especially for women who were younger, heavier, and had a history of prior hysterectomy [123]. Further, TVUS and CA125 failed to produce a significant impact on ovarian cancer mortality, and 15% of women with false-positive screening experienced serious resulting complications [21]. The results of this trial suggest that routine screening with CA125 and TVS should not be performed in asymptomatic women at low-risk for ovarian cancer.

The United Kingdom Collaborative Trial of Ovarian Cancer Screening (UKCTOCS) is a large randomized control trial evaluating TVUS and/or CA125 versus no screening in sample of more than 200,000 postmenopausal women between 2001 and 2005 [58]. The primary objective of this study is to determine whether screening affected ovarian cancer-related mortality. In the prevalence screen, 42 primary ovarian and 45 fallopian tube cancers were identified with 48.3% of these cancers reported as stage I or II disease. The sensitivity, specificity and PPV for primary invasive epithelial ovarian and tubal cancers were 89.5%, 99.8% and 35.1% for combined TVUS and CA125 versus 75.0%, 98.2%, and 2.8% for TVUS alone, respectively. Thus, combination screening methods yielded the lowest number of false-positive screens, translating into lower rates of repeat testing and surgery. While this initial screen indicates that these screening strategies are feasible, the impact of these tests on mortality is still pending at this time.

In summary, the latest studies suggest that risk reducing behaviors can provide significant prevention of ovarian cancer, while routine screening for ovarian cancer in women at average risk does not improve the prevention of late-stage disease and is currently not recommended by any professional society [25].

5.2 Recommendations for ovarian cancer prevention in women at increased risk

Women with a strong family history of either ovarian or breast cancer alone are considered to be at higher-than-average risk, while women with confirmed mutations in *BRCA1 or BRCA2* and those with Lynch syndrome are at the highest risk of developing ovarian cancer. Genetic risk assessment should be performed in individuals to provide "individualized and quantified assessment of risk as well as options for tailored screening and prevention strategies" [108]. The Society of Gynecologic Oncologists recommends genetic screening in women with a 20-25% risk of having an inherited predisposition to breast and ovarian cancer: (1) women with a personal history of both breast and ovarian cancer (including those with primary peritoneal or fallopian tube cancers; (2) women with ovarian cancer and a close relative with breast cancer at ≤ 50 years or ovarian cancer at any age; (3) women with ovarian cancer at any age who are of Ashkenazi Jewish ancestry; (4) women with breast cancer at ≤50 years and a close relative with ovarian or male breast cancer at any age; (5) women of Ashkenazi Jewish ancestry and breast cancer at ≤ 40 years; or (6) women with a first or second degree relative with a known *BRCA1* or *BRCA2* mutation [108]. Further, risk assessment is recommended if women have a 20-25% of having an inherited predisposition to endometrial, colorectal and related cancers, including: those patients meeting the revised Amsterdam criteria [124] and those with personal or family history concerning for Lynch Syndrome [108].

5.2.1 Prevention by risk reducing behaviors and surgery

In addition to the risk reducing behaviors described earlier for women at average risk,, prophylactic surgery should be strongly considered in women at high risk for ovarian cancer. Risk-reducing salpingo-oophorectomy (RRSO) is associated with an 80% risk reduction in *BRCA1/2*-associated ovarian, fallopian tube or primary peritoneal cancer [125, 126]. Women with *BRCA* germline mutations have a significant survival advantage following risk-reducing surgery compared to disease surveillance [125, 126]. This approach has also been reported as a cost-effective strategy [127, 128]. Women with *BRCA1/2* germline mutations should be counseled on risk-reducing strategies, and RRSO should be recommended upon completion of childbearing or by age 40 [25].

Risk-reducing hysterectomy and bilateral salpingo-oophorectomy is also a feasible preventive approach in women with Lynch Syndrome, with risk reduction approaching 100% [129] . Recent cost-effective analyses demonstrated that risk-reducing surgery is the most cost-effective gynecologic cancer prevention strategy in this patient population [128, 130].

5.2.2 Prevention by routine screening

Current opinion suggests that screening may be appropriate for women in these increased risk categories. However, while intensive screening is recommended for women with *BRCA1* and *2* mutations, studies have indicated that screening with CA125 and TVUS are ineffective [131, 132] because the majority of cancers are still detected at advanced stages. In a retrospective study of 241 women with confirmed *BRCA1* or *BRCA2* mutations, surveillance with annual pelvic exam, transvaginal ultrasound and serum CA125 level failed to effectively identify women with early stage disease [131].

Currently, women with HNPCC/Lynch Syndrome are offered active disease surveillance including annual TVUS, endometrial biopsy and CA125 [108]. Auranen and colleagues performed a systematic review of the literature to determine the role of screening in women with HNPCC or with a family history of HNPCC [133]. Of five studies meeting inclusion criteria, only three examined the utility of CA125 surveillance for ovarian cancer in this patient population. In total, five ovarian cancer cases, none of which were reported as early stage disease, were detected by CA125 surveillance. Based on the current available published evidence, the authors concluded that there is no benefit for ovarian cancer screening in this patient population.

In summary, while studies have failed to demonstrate a benefit for screening in high risk patients, risk-reducing surgery is the most cost-effective gynecologic cancer prevention strategy and screening with serial CA125 levels and TVUS is generally recommended until risk-reducing surgery can be performed.

5.3 Recommendations for ovarian cancer prevention in women with pelvic masses

Several investigators have introduced risk models which would allow for the preoperative risk assessment of women with pelvic masses [134-137]. The Risk of Malignancy Index (RMI) is a diagnostic model combining CA125 levels, imaging and menopausal status; at a cutoff level of 200, the RMI produced a sensitivity of 85% and a specificity of 97% and was an effective model for discriminating between cancer and benign lesions [137]. The Risk of Ovarian Malignancy Algorithm (ROMA) is another model which predicts the likelihood of ovarian cancer in women with pelvic masses by the combination of HE4 and CA125 serum levels with menopausal status [136]. This algorithm has shown promising diagnostic performance for the detection of ovarian cancer in postmenopausal women, with a sensitivity of 82.5% [136], and has also been shown to perform better than the RMI model for risk prediction of ovarian cancer [134, 135]. This model may therefore be an effective strategy for triaging patients with pelvic masses.

5.4 Current recommendations for preventing disease recurrence

5.4.1 Role of disease surveillance

Active disease surveillance aims to detect recurrent ovarian cancer in asymptomatic women in order to provide opportunities for early intervention and ultimately improved outcomes. However, current surveillance recommendations are often based on expert opinions and practice patterns. The National Comprehensive Cancer Network (NCCN) recommends routine visits every 2 to 4 months for 2 years, then every 3 to 6 months for 3 years, followed by annual visits after 5 years [42]. A physical examination, serum CA125 and laboratory and imaging (as clinically indicated) are to be performed at each visit.

In response to the MRC OV05/EORTC 55955 trial [81], the Society of Gynecologic Oncologists issued a statement on the use of CA125 for monitoring ovarian cancer in June 2009: "Although there may not presently be a major survival advantage to the use of CA125 monitoring for earlier diagnosis of recurrence, patients and their physicians should still have the opportunity to choose this approach as integral to a philosophy of active management" and that "patients and their physicians should be encouraged to actively discuss the pros and cons of CA125 monitoring and the implications for subsequent treatment and quality of life" [82].

A systematic review of the literature demonstrated that routine surveillance was able to detect 67% of asymptomatic recurrences with a lead time of 3 months but that published studies failed to demonstrate a survival advantage of early detection of ovarian cancer by routine surveillance [36]. The authors suggest that routine surveillance should be reconsidered in current practice.

5.5 Immunoprevention of disease recurrence

While 70-80% of patients with advanced EOC will initially respond to conventional platinum/taxane therapy, more than 60% will experience a recurrence of disease and 70-90% will ultimately die of their disease [2]. Immune-driven vaccines are currently under investigation for the prevention of ovarian cancer recurrence [8-12].

Host anti-tumor immune responses have the potential to significantly influence prognosis in ovarian cancer patients. The presence of tumor-infiltrating lymphocytes (TILs) has been correlated with significantly improved progression-free and overall survival rates in women with advanced stage ovarian cancer compared to women without TILs [138, 139]. Thus, given that ovarian cancer is intrinsically immunogenic, it may be possible to enhance host anti-tumor immune responses by using vaccines which strengthen TIL responses and thereby improve patient outcomes by preventing recurrent disease.

Therapeutic vaccinations derived from autologous whole tumor cell lysates may help to enhance host antigen-specific anti-tumoral immune responses [14]. The main advantages of these vaccines are "the opportunity to induce immunity to a personalized and broad range of antigens" and the incorporation of yet unidentified tumor antigens [140]. A recent meta-analysis of 173 immunotherapy trials, including ovarian and other primary cancers, demonstrated a higher objective clinical response in individuals receiving whole tumor antigen-based vaccines compared to those receiving synthetic antigens (8.1% vs. 3.6%, respectively; p <0.001) [141]. The Penn Ovarian Cancer Research Center is currently conducting a phase I/II randomized study to determine the feasibility, safety and immunogenicity of a vaccine derived from autologous oxidized tumor cell lysate (OC-L) in combination with Ampligen, a Toll-like receptor 3 agonist (NCT01312389).

Vaccination with antigen-specific dendritic cells (DCs) can enhance anti-tumor immunity via specific tumor-antigen presentation and activation of effector T cells [142]. There are several approaches to DC-based vaccines, including exposure of DCs to whole tumor cell lysates, defined ovarian tumor peptides, and ovarian tumor cells, to induce a cytotoxic T lymphocyte (CTL) response [143]. In a phase I trial, three of six patients with progressive or recurrent ovarian cancer experienced stabilization of disease following administration of autologous tumor antigen-pulsed DCs with reported progression-free intervals of 8-45 months [144]. Given these promising data, DC-based vaccines are currently the focus of several new trials (NCT00703105, NCT00683241, and NCT01132014) which will hopefully demonstrate an impact on long-term prognosis. The Penn Ovarian Cancer Research Center is currently examining the feasibility and immunogenicity of a DC vaccine loaded with autologous tumor lysate administered intranodally, alone or in combination with intravenous Bevacizumab (NCT01132014). A phase I/II trial is also underway at our institution in which patients with recurrent EOC or primary peritoneal cancer will undergo adoptive transfer of ex vivo CD3/CD28-costimulated autologous peripheral blood T cells along with tumor lysate-pulsed DC vaccination (DCVax®-L) (NCT00603460) in order to determine the feasibility and safety of this combination and progression-free survival at 6 months.

6. Conclusion

Ovarian cancer is the most lethal gynecologic cancer in the United States. Given the low prevalence of this disease in the general population, risk assessment is crucial to the success of available preventive strategies. However, current primary preventive strategies, even in women at high risk, have not proven reliable in the detection of early stage disease nor have they significantly impacted disease related mortality. Thus, risk-reducing behaviors and surgery should be considered in women at high risk for ovarian cancer.

In the near future, novel technologies may help to better characterize critical pathways in ovarian carcinogenesis and therefore result in biomarkers and/or multimarker panels more effective than CA125 alone, in both detecting early stage disease as well as recurrences. Validations of proposed strategies are under investigation in ongoing studies (**Table 3**).

Trial Name	Trial Identifier	Primary Investigator	Study Status	Study Population	Method(s) under investigation	Objective
Prospective Study of Risk-Reducing Salpingo-Oophorectomy and Longitudinal CA-125 Screening Among Women at Increased Genetic Risk of Ovarian Cancer[146]	NCT00049049	Green, M.H.	Closed	Increased genetic risk	Screening (TVUS, CA125, ROCA) vs. RR surgery (RRSO + screening)	Compare the prospective incidence of ovarian cancer, breast cancer, fallopian tube cancer, primary peritoneal cancer, and all cancer in participants at increased genetic risk of ovarian cancer who undergo risk-reducing salpingo-oophorectomy (RRSO) or screening
The UK Familial Ovarian Cancer Screening Study	NCT00033488	Mackay, J.	Closed to Accrual (as of 3/31/2010)	Increased risk due to strong family history	TVUS, CA125	Determine an optimal screening procedure for ovarian cancer, in terms of the most appropriate screening test, criteria for interpretation of results and screening intervals, in women at high genetic risk for developing ovarian cancer
Quality of Life Associated With a Low-Risk Screening Program for Ovarian Cancer	NCT00511641	Bodurka, D.C.	Currently Recruiting	Average risk, postmenopausal women	CA125	The goal of this research study is to learn more about how women feel about an ovarian cancer screening program that involves getting a blood test to measure CA 125 levels. This includes finding out about women's quality of life and whether they are concerned or worried about their risk of developing cancer. This study also seeks to find out whether elevated CA 125 levels affect participants in terms of cancer worries or concerns.

Trial Name	Trial Identifier	Primary Investigator	Study Status	Study Population	Method(s) under investigation	Objective
United Kingdom Collaborative Trial Of Ovarian Cancer Screening[58, 147]	NCT00058032	Menon, U.	Closed	Average risk, postmenopausal women	CA125, US	Randomized clinical trial to study the effectiveness of ultrasound with or without measuring CA 125 levels in detecting ovarian cancer in postmenopausal women.
Ovarian Cancer Screening Pilot Trial in High Risk Women	NCT00039559	Skates, S.J.	Active	At increased genetic risk	CA125, ROCA	Screening trial to determine the significance of CA 125 levels in detecting ovarian cancer in participants who have a high genetic risk of developing ovarian cancer
Northwestern Ovarian Cancer Early Detection & Prevention Program	NCT00005095	Shulman, L.P.	Active	At high risk due to family or personal medical history	Symptoms, biomarkers, CA125, physical exam, TVUS	This clinical trial is studying screening methods for identifying women who are at increased risk for developing ovarian cancer
Specialized Program Of Research Excellence (SPORE) In Ovarian Cancer/Cancer Genetics Network Collaborative Ovarian Cancer Screening Pilot Trial In High Risk Women	NCT00080639	Patridge, E.E.	Closed	At high risk due to family history, genetic mutation or ethnic background	CA125	This phase II trial is studying CA-125 levels in screening for cancer in women who are at high risk of developing ovarian cancer
A Randomized Controlled Trial Using Novel Markers to Predict Malignancy in Elevated-Risk Women[67, 75, 148]	NCT01121640	Urban, N. and Karlan, B.	Recruiting	At increased risk due to BRCA mutation, personal or family history or elevated biomarker screen	CA125, HE4, TVUS	The Novel Markers Trial will compare the safety, feasibility and effectiveness of two different epithelial ovarian cancer screening strategies that use CA125 and add HE4 as either a first or second line screen. This study is the next step in a larger research effort to develop a blood test that can be used as a screening method for the early detection of epithelial ovarian cancer.
Cancer Screening and Prevention Program for High Risk Women	NCT00849199	Muggia, F.	Recruiting	At increased risk due to personal or family history or who are perceived at increased risk	Questionnaire, pelvic exam, Pap smear, mammogram, TVUS, CA125	The purpose of this study is to evaluate screening and prevention in women with high risk of ovarian or breast cancer.

Trial Name	Trial Identifier	Primary Investigator	Study Status	Study Population	Method(s) under investigation	Objective
Efficacy of a Combined Program for Early Detection of Breast and Gynecological Cancers in Low Resource Countries[31, 32, 49, 58]	NCT01178736	Yang W, Singh D, and Filho A.	Not Yet Recruiting	Symptomatic postmenopausal women age 50-64	TVUS, PE	The purpose of this study is to implement a community-based combined program for early detection of breast, cervical, ovarian and endometrial cancer in low-resource countries delivered through a free standing or a mobile Well Woman Clinic
Screening and Identification of Novel Diagnostic and Prognostic Biomarkers on Ovarian Cancers	NCT00854399	Cheng, W.F.	Recruiting	Women with documented ovarian cancer	mesothelin	To further evaluate the role of mesothelin in ovarian cancer and elucidate the potential of mesothelin as a target antigen for immunotherapy.
Ovarian Cancer Early Detection Screening Program	NCT01292733	Paley, P.	Recruiting	At increased risk due to family history, Ashkenazi Jewish ethnicity, male relative with breast cancer or high likelihood of BRCA mutation	CA125, TVUS, Health Status Questionnaire	The main purpose of this program is to see whether periodically measuring CA-125 (tumor marker) levels in the blood and undergoing transvaginal ultrasounds over time will be effective in the early detection of ovarian cancer
Development of an Assay for the Early Detection of Ovarian Cancer	NCT00986206	Brard, L.	Recruiting	Pelvic Mass, diagnosed EOC or known BRCA carrier	Lyso phosphatidic acid (LPA)	This clinical trial is studying using the lysophosphatidic acid assay to see how well it works in early detection of ovarian cancer in patients with ovarian cancer or who are at risk for ovarian cancer.
The University of Louisville Ovarian Screening Study	NCT00267072	Helm, C.W.	Completed	Asymptomatic Postmenopausal women or premenopausal women at risk due to personal or family history, BRCA mutation, or prior fertility drug use	Tumor membrane fragments	The objectives of this study are: To identify women at increased risk for developing ovarian cancer To detect ovarian cancers at an early stage To investigate the role of tumor membrane fragments as tumor markers for early ovarian carcinoma

Trial Name	Trial Identifier	Primary Investigator	Study Status	Study Population	Method(s) under investigation	Objective
Assessment of Screening Modalities for Gynecologic Cancers	NCT00879840	Sherman, M.E.	Recruiting	Postmenopausal women with confirmed or suspected ovarian cancer who will be having surgery	Assess alternative tissue sampling techniques; DNA methylation pattern	DNA will be extracted from samples collected using a vaginal Tampon and an endometrial brushing using an FDA approved device (Tao brush) prior to surgery. A panel of methylation markers will be analyzed from samples yielding sufficient DNA. The results of the methylation analysis will be compared to the final histology for all patients in the study.
NYU Ovarian Cancer Early Detection Program Blood and Genetics	NCT00531778	Pothuri, B.	Terminated	At increased risk due to personal or family history of breast and/or ovarian cancer or due to genetic mutations in BRCA or mismatch repair genes (i.e., Lynch syndrome), or fertility drug use	molecular, biochemical, functional, and genetic markers	To identify and develop highly sensitive and specific tumor markers that can be applied to population-based screening for the early detection of ovarian cancer.
PROTOCOL FOR THE NCI PROSTATE, LUNG, COLORECTAL, AND OVARIAN (PLCO) CANCER SCREENING TRIAL[41, 123, 149, 150]	NCT00002540	Berg, C.	Ongoing, Closed to recruitment	Average risk, postmenopausal women	CA125, TVUS	Determine whether screening with CA 125 and transvaginal ultrasound can reduce mortality from ovarian cancer in women aged 55-74
Use of the CA 125 Algorithm for the Early Detection of Ovarian Cancer in Low Risk Women	NCT00539162	Lu, K.	Recruiting	Average risk, postmenopausal women	CA125	To evaluate the longitudinal CA-125 algorithm for the early detection of ovarian cancer in a low risk cohort of women

Trial Name	Trial Identifier	Primary Investigator	Study Status	Study Population	Method(s) under investigation	Objective
A Pilot Study of Short Non-coding RNA Biomarkers of Predisposition to Ovarian Cancer	NCT01187602	Jazaeri, A.	Recruiting	Women at average risk, increased risk and with ovarian cancer	sncRNA	The purpose of this study is to create new tests to identify biomarkers for ovarian cancer so that a screening test can be developed. For patients who have a diagnosis of ovarian Cancer, researchers will use blood samples before and after treatment to see if disease status can be determined by measuring the amount of biomarker.
Study to Assess the Effectiveness of the CAAb Test With Ovarian Cancer Patients	NCT00327925	Hayka, A.	Unknown	Women with ovarian cancer	Ovarian Cancer Associated Antibodies (CAAb)	The expectation of the CAAb in the cancer population differs from that of the control population
Mesothelin as a New Tumor Marker for Ovarian Cancer	NCT00155740	Chen, C.	Unknown	Women with ovarian cancer vs. benign adnexal pathology	mesothelin	We will evaluate that if mesothelin can be a new potential tumor marker for ovarian cancer in this proposal. We will evaluate the amount of mesothelin in pre- and post-treatment serum samples of patients with epithelial ovarian cancer. We will also correlate the clinicopathologic items and the prognosis of ovarian cancer patients and evaluate whether mesothelin can be a new rumor marker for ovarian cancer patients.

Table 3. Ongoing Clinical Trials (as of June 2011).

7. References

[1] Jemal A, Siegel R, Xu J, Ward E. Cancer statistics, 2010. CA Cancer J Clin;60:277-300.

[2] Cannistra SA. Cancer of the ovary. N Engl J Med 2004;351:2519-29.

[3] Etzioni R, Urban N, Ramsey S, et al. The case for early detection. Nat Rev Cancer 2003;3:243-52.

[4] Husseinzadeh N. Status of tumor markers in epithelial ovarian cancer has there been any progress? A review. Gynecol Oncol 2011;120:152-7.

[5] Scholler N, Lowe KA, Bergan LA, et al. Use of yeast-secreted in vivo biotinylated recombinant antibodies (Biobodies) in bead-based ELISA. Clin Cancer Res 2008;14:2647-55.

[6] Scholler N, Gross JA, Garvik B, et al. Use of cancer-specific yeast-secreted in vivo biotinylated recombinant antibodies for serum biomarker discovery. J Transl Med 2008;6:41.

[7] Liu B, Nash J, Runowicz C, Swede H, Stevens R, Li Z. Ovarian cancer immunotherapy: opportunities, progresses and challenges. J Hematol Oncol 2010;3:7.
[8] Benencia F, Courreges MC, Coukos G. Whole tumor antigen vaccination using dendritic cells: comparison of RNA electroporation and pulsing with UV-irradiated tumor cells. J Transl Med 2008;6:21.
[9] Chianese-Bullock KA, Irvin WP, Jr., Petroni GR, et al. A multipeptide vaccine is safe and elicits T-cell responses in participants with advanced stage ovarian cancer. J Immunother 2008;31:420-30.
[10] Tsuda N, Mochizuki K, Harada M, et al. Vaccination with predesignated or evidence-based peptides for patients with recurrent gynecologic cancers. J Immunother 2004;27:60-72.
[11] Aoki Y, Takakuwa K, Kodama S, et al. Use of adoptive transfer of tumor-infiltrating lymphocytes alone or in combination with cisplatin-containing chemotherapy in patients with epithelial ovarian cancer. Cancer Res 1991;51:1934-9.
[12] Fujita K, Ikarashi H, Takakuwa K, et al. Prolonged disease-free period in patients with advanced epithelial ovarian cancer after adoptive transfer of tumor-infiltrating lymphocytes. Clin Cancer Res 1995;1:501-7.
[13] Courreges MC, Benencia F, Conejo-Garcia JR, Zhang L, Coukos G. Preparation of apoptotic tumor cells with replication-incompetent HSV augments the efficacy of dendritic cell vaccines. Cancer Gene Ther 2006;13:182-93.
[14] Kandalaft LE PJD, Lori Smith, et al. Autologous whole-tumor antigen combinatorial immunotherapy for recurrent ovarian cancer. In: Society of Gynecologic Oncologists Annual Meeting on Women's Cancer March 14-17, 2010; San Francisco, CA.
[15] Wilson JM, Jungner YG. [Principles and practice of mass screening for disease]. Bol Oficina Sanit Panam 1968;65:281-393.
[16] Schwartz PE. Current diagnosis and treatment modalities for ovarian cancer. Cancer Treat Res 2002;107:99-118.
[17] Lu KH, Patterson AP, Wang L, et al. Selection of potential markers for epithelial ovarian cancer with gene expression arrays and recursive descent partition analysis. Clin Cancer Res 2004;10:3291-300.
[18] Scarinci IC, Garcia FA, Kobetz E, et al. Cervical cancer prevention: new tools and old barriers. Cancer 2010;116:2531-42.
[19] Clarke-Pearson DL. Clinical practice. Screening for ovarian cancer. N Engl J Med 2009;361:170-7.
[20] Badgwell D, Bast RC, Jr. Early detection of ovarian cancer. Dis Markers 2007;23:397-410.
[21] Buys SS, Partridge E, Black A, et al. Effect of screening on ovarian cancer mortality: the Prostate, Lung, Colorectal and Ovarian (PLCO) Cancer Screening Randomized Controlled Trial. JAMA 2011;305:2295-303.
[22] Nossov V, Amneus M, Su F, et al. The early detection of ovarian cancer: from traditional methods to proteomics. Can we really do better than serum CA-125? Am J Obstet Gynecol 2008;199:215-23.
[23] Schiffman M, Castle PE, Jeronimo J, Rodriguez AC, Wacholder S. Human papillomavirus and cervical cancer. Lancet 2007;370:890-907.
[24] Kurman RJ, McConnell TG. Precursors of endometrial and ovarian carcinoma. Virchows Arch 2010;456:1-12.

[25] Schorge JO, Modesitt SC, Coleman RL, et al. SGO White Paper on ovarian cancer: etiology, screening and surveillance. Gynecol Oncol 2010;119:7-17.
[26] Crum CP, Drapkin R, Kindelberger D, Medeiros F, Miron A, Lee Y. Lessons from BRCA: the tubal fimbria emerges as an origin for pelvic serous cancer. Clin Med Res 2007;5:35-44.
[27] Kindelberger DW, Lee Y, Miron A, et al. Intraepithelial carcinoma of the fimbria and pelvic serous carcinoma: Evidence for a causal relationship. Am J Surg Pathol 2007;31:161-9.
[28] Shih Ie M, Kurman RJ. Ovarian tumorigenesis: a proposed model based on morphological and molecular genetic analysis. Am J Pathol 2004;164:1511-8.
[29] Vine MF, Calingaert B, Berchuck A, Schildkraut JM. Characterization of prediagnostic symptoms among primary epithelial ovarian cancer cases and controls. Gynecol Oncol 2003;90:75-82.
[30] . (Accessed June 25, 2011, at http://www.wcn.org/articles/types_of_cancer/ovarian/symptoms/index.html.)
[31] Goff BA, Mandel LS, Drescher CW, et al. Development of an ovarian cancer symptom index: possibilities for earlier detection. Cancer 2007;109:221-7.
[32] Goff BA, Mandel LS, Melancon CH, Muntz HG. Frequency of symptoms of ovarian cancer in women presenting to primary care clinics. JAMA 2004;291:2705-12.
[33] Olson SH, Mignone L, Nakraseive C, Caputo TA, Barakat RR, Harlap S. Symptoms of ovarian cancer. Obstet Gynecol 2001;98:212-7.
[34] Rossing MA, Wicklund KG, Cushing-Haugen KL, Weiss NS. Predictive value of symptoms for early detection of ovarian cancer. J Natl Cancer Inst 2010;102:222-9.
[35] Lurie G, Wilkens LR, Thompson PJ, Matsuno RK, Carney ME, Goodman MT. Symptom presentation in invasive ovarian carcinoma by tumor histological type and grade in a multiethnic population: a case analysis. Gynecol Oncol 2010;119:278-84.
[36] Geurts SM, de Vegt F, van Altena AM, et al. Considering early detection of relapsed ovarian cancer: a review of the literature. Int J Gynecol Cancer 2011;21:837-45.
[37] Westhoff CL, Jones HE, Guiahi M. Do new guidelines and technology make the routine pelvic examination obsolete? J Womens Health (Larchmt) 2011;20:5-10.
[38] Committee Opinion No. 477: the role of the obstetrician-gynecologist in the early detection of epithelial ovarian cancer. Obstet Gynecol 2011;117:742-6.
[39] Westhoff C, Clark CJ. Benign ovarian cysts in England and Wales and in the United States. Br J Obstet Gynaecol 1992;99:329-32.
[40] Grover SR, Quinn MA. Is there any value in bimanual pelvic examination as a screening test. Med J Aust 1995;162:408-10.
[41] Buys SS, Partridge E, Greene MH, et al. Ovarian cancer screening in the Prostate, Lung, Colorectal and Ovarian (PLCO) cancer screening trial: findings from the initial screen of a randomized trial. Am J Obstet Gynecol 2005;193:1630-9.
[42] Morgan RJ, Jr., Alvarez RD, Armstrong DK, et al. Ovarian cancer. Clinical practice guidelines in oncology. J Natl Compr Canc Netw 2008;6:766-94.
[43] von Georgi R, Schubert K, Grant P, Munstedt K. Post-therapy surveillance and after-care in ovarian cancer. Eur J Obstet Gynecol Reprod Biol 2004;114:228-33.
[44] Fehm T, Heller F, Kramer S, Jager W, Gebauer G. Evaluation of CA125, physical and radiological findings in follow-up of ovarian cancer patients. Anticancer Res 2005;25:1551-4.

[45] Gadducci A, Cosio S. Surveillance of patients after initial treatment of ovarian cancer. Crit Rev Oncol Hematol 2009;71:43-52.

[46] Ueland FR, Depriest PD, Desimone CP, et al. The accuracy of examination under anesthesia and transvaginal sonography in evaluating ovarian size. Gynecol Oncol 2005;99:400-3.

[47] Sato S, Yokoyama Y, Sakamoto T, Futagami M, Saito Y. Usefulness of mass screening for ovarian carcinoma using transvaginal ultrasonography. Cancer 2000;89:582-8.

[48] Bourne TH, Campbell S, Reynolds KM, et al. Screening for early familial ovarian cancer with transvaginal ultrasonography and colour blood flow imaging. BMJ 1993;306:1025-9.

[49] van Nagell JR, Jr., DePriest PD, Ueland FR, et al. Ovarian cancer screening with annual transvaginal sonography: findings of 25,000 women screened. Cancer 2007;109:1887-96.

[50] van Nagell JR, Jr., DePriest PD, Reedy MB, et al. The efficacy of transvaginal sonographic screening in asymptomatic women at risk for ovarian cancer. Gynecol Oncol 2000;77:350-6.

[51] Pavlik EJ, DePriest PD, Gallion HH, et al. Ovarian volume related to age. Gynecol Oncol 2000;77:410-2.

[52] Granberg S, Wikland M, Jansson I. Macroscopic characterization of ovarian tumors and the relation to the histological diagnosis: criteria to be used for ultrasound evaluation. Gynecol Oncol 1989;35:139-44.

[53] Timmerman D, Valentin L, Bourne TH, Collins WP, Verrelst H, Vergote I. Terms, definitions and measurements to describe the sonographic features of adnexal tumors: a consensus opinion from the International Ovarian Tumor Analysis (IOTA) Group. Ultrasound Obstet Gynecol 2000;16:500-5.

[54] DePriest PD, Shenson D, Fried A, et al. A morphology index based on sonographic findings in ovarian cancer. Gynecol Oncol 1993;51:7-11.

[55] DePriest PD, Varner E, Powell J, et al. The efficacy of a sonographic morphology index in identifying ovarian cancer: a multi-institutional investigation. Gynecol Oncol 1994;55:174-8.

[56] Timmerman D, Testa AC, Bourne T, et al. Simple ultrasound-based rules for the diagnosis of ovarian cancer. Ultrasound Obstet Gynecol 2008;31:681-90.

[57] Van Calster B, Timmerman D, Bourne T, et al. Discrimination between benign and malignant adnexal masses by specialist ultrasound examination versus serum CA-125. J Natl Cancer Inst 2007;99:1706-14.

[58] Menon U, Gentry-Maharaj A, Hallett R, et al. Sensitivity and specificity of multimodal and ultrasound screening for ovarian cancer, and stage distribution of detected cancers: results of the prevalence screen of the UK Collaborative Trial of Ovarian Cancer Screening (UKCTOCS). Lancet Oncol 2009;10:327-40.

[59] Salani R BF, Fung M, Holschneider CH, Parker LP, Bristow RE and Goff BA. Posttreatment surveillance and diagnosis of recurrence in women with gynecologic malignancies: Society of Gynecologic Oncologists recommendations. Am J Obstet Gynecol 2011;204:466-78.

[60] Zhu CS, Pinsky PF, Cramer DW, et al. A framework for evaluating biomarkers for early detection: validation of biomarker panels for ovarian cancer. Cancer Prev Res (Phila) 2011;4:375-83.

[61] Bast RC, Jr., Klug TL, St John E, et al. A radioimmunoassay using a monoclonal antibody to monitor the course of epithelial ovarian cancer. N Engl J Med 1983;309:883-7.
[62] Jacobs I, Bast RC, Jr. The CA 125 tumour-associated antigen: a review of the literature. Hum Reprod 1989;4:1-12.
[63] Einhorn N, Sjovall K, Knapp RC, et al. Prospective evaluation of serum CA 125 levels for early detection of ovarian cancer. Obstet Gynecol 1992;80:14-8.
[64] Vaidya AP, Curtin JP. The follow-up of ovarian cancer. Semin Oncol 2003;30:401-12.
[65] Prat A, Parera M, Adamo B, et al. Risk of recurrence during follow-up for optimally treated advanced epithelial ovarian cancer (EOC) with a low-level increase of serum CA-125 levels. Ann Oncol 2009;20:294-7.
[66] Rustin GJ, Nelstrop AE, Tuxen MK, Lambert HE. Defining progression of ovarian carcinoma during follow-up according to CA 125: a North Thames Ovary Group Study. Ann Oncol 1996;7:361-4.
[67] Anderson GL, McIntosh M, Wu L, et al. Assessing lead time of selected ovarian cancer biomarkers: a nested case-control study. J Natl Cancer Inst 2010;102:26-38.
[68] Cramer DW, Bast RC, Jr., Berg CD, et al. Ovarian cancer biomarker performance in prostate, lung, colorectal, and ovarian cancer screening trial specimens. Cancer Prev Res (Phila) 2011;4:365-74.
[69] Helzlsouer KJ, Bush TL, Alberg AJ, Bass KM, Zacur H, Comstock GW. Prospective study of serum CA-125 levels as markers of ovarian cancer. JAMA 1993;269:1123-6.
[70] McDonald JM, Doran S, DeSimone CP, et al. Predicting risk of malignancy in adnexal masses. Obstet Gynecol 2010;115:687-94.
[71] Menon U, Skates SJ, Lewis S, et al. Prospective study using the risk of ovarian cancer algorithm to screen for ovarian cancer. J Clin Oncol 2005;23:7919-26.
[72] McIntosh MW, Drescher C, Karlan B, et al. Combining CA 125 and SMR serum markers for diagnosis and early detection of ovarian carcinoma. Gynecol Oncol 2004;95:9-15.
[73] Schorge JO, Drake RD, Lee H, et al. Osteopontin as an adjunct to CA125 in detecting recurrent ovarian cancer. Clin Cancer Res 2004;10:3474-8.
[74] Woolas RP, Xu FJ, Jacobs IJ, et al. Elevation of multiple serum markers in patients with stage I ovarian cancer. J Natl Cancer Inst 1993;85:1748-51.
[75] Andersen MR, Goff BA, Lowe KA, et al. Use of a Symptom Index, CA125, and HE4 to predict ovarian cancer. Gynecol Oncol 2010;116:378-83.
[76] Rosen DG, Wang L, Atkinson JN, et al. Potential markers that complement expression of CA125 in epithelial ovarian cancer. Gynecol Oncol 2005;99:267-77.
[77] Sturgeon CM, Hoffman BR, Chan DW, et al. National Academy of Clinical Biochemistry Laboratory Medicine Practice Guidelines for use of tumor markers in clinical practice: quality requirements. Clin Chem 2008;54:e1-e10.
[78] Drapkin R, von Horsten HH, Lin Y, et al. Human epididymis protein 4 (HE4) is a secreted glycoprotein that is overexpressed by serous and endometrioid ovarian carcinomas. Cancer Res 2005;65:2162-9.
[79] Visintin I, Feng Z, Longton G, et al. Diagnostic markers for early detection of ovarian cancer. Clin Cancer Res 2008;14:1065-72.

[80] McIntosh M, Anderson G, Drescher C, et al. Ovarian cancer early detection claims are biased. Clin Cancer Res 2008;14:7574; author reply 7-9.
[81] Rustin GJ, van der Burg ME, Griffin CL, et al. Early versus delayed treatment of relapsed ovarian cancer (MRC OV05/EORTC 55955): a randomised trial. Lancet 2010;376:1155-63.
[82] Society of Gynecologic Oncologists Statement on Use of CA125 for Monitoring Ovarian Cancer. (Accessed June 28, 2011, at *www.sgo.org/WorkArea/linkit.aspx?LinkIdentifier=id&ItemID=3664.*)
[83] Petricoin EF, Ardekani AM, Hitt BA, et al. Use of proteomic patterns in serum to identify ovarian cancer. Lancet 2002;359:572-7.
[84] Chon HS, Lancaster JM. Microarray-based gene expression studies in ovarian cancer. Cancer Control 2011;18:8-15.
[85] Maradeo ME, Cairns P. Translational application of epigenetic alterations: Ovarian cancer as a model. FEBS Lett 2011;585:2112-20.
[86] Maldonado L, Hoque MO. Epigenomics and ovarian carcinoma. Biomark Med 2010;4:543-70.
[87] Wang H, Wong CH, Chin A, et al. Integrated mass spectrometry-based analysis of plasma glycoproteins and their glycan modifications. Nat Protoc 2011;6:253-69.
[88] Kozak KR, Amneus MW, Pusey SM, et al. Identification of biomarkers for ovarian cancer using strong anion-exchange ProteinChips: potential use in diagnosis and prognosis. Proc Natl Acad Sci U S A 2003;100:12343-8.
[89] Zhang B, Barekati Z, Kohler C, et al. Proteomics and biomarkers for ovarian cancer diagnosis. Ann Clin Lab Sci 2010;40:218-25.
[90] Guan W, Zhou M, Hampton CY, et al. Ovarian cancer detection from metabolomic liquid chromatography/mass spectrometry data by support vector machines. BMC Bioinformatics 2009;10:259.
[91] Baker DL, Morrison P, Miller B, et al. Plasma lysophosphatidic acid concentration and ovarian cancer. JAMA 2002;287:3081-2.
[92] Schutter EM, Visser JJ, van Kamp GJ, et al. The utility of lipid-associated sialic acid (LASA or LSA) as a serum marker for malignancy. A review of the literature. Tumour Biol 1992;13:121-32.
[93] Vlad AM, Kettel JC, Alajez NM, Carlos CA, Finn OJ. MUC1 immunobiology: from discovery to clinical applications. Adv Immunol 2004;82:249-93.
[94] Taylor AD, Hancock WS, Hincapie M, Taniguchi N, Hanash SM. Towards an integrated proteomic and glycomic approach to finding cancer biomarkers. Genome Med 2009;1:57.
[95] Scholler N, Garvik B, Quarles T, Jiang S, Urban N. Method for generation of in vivo biotinylated recombinant antibodies by yeast mating. J Immunol Methods 2006;317:132-43.
[96] Bergan L, Gross JA, Nevin B, Urban N, Scholler N. Development and in vitro validation of anti-mesothelin biobodies that prevent CA125/Mesothelin-dependent cell attachment. Cancer Lett 2007;255:263-74.
[97] Brinton LA, Westhoff CL, Scoccia B, et al. Causes of infertility as predictors of subsequent cancer risk. Epidemiology 2005;16:500-7.

[98] Kallen B, Finnstrom O, Lindam A, Nilsson E, Nygren KG, Olausson PO. Malignancies among women who gave birth after in vitro fertilization. Hum Reprod 2011;26:253-8.
[99] Ness RB, Cramer DW, Goodman MT, et al. Infertility, fertility drugs, and ovarian cancer: a pooled analysis of case-control studies. Am J Epidemiol 2002;155:217-24.
[100] Rossing MA, Tang MT, Flagg EW, Weiss LK, Wicklund KG. A case-control study of ovarian cancer in relation to infertility and the use of ovulation-inducing drugs. Am J Epidemiol 2004;160:1070-8.
[101] Tortolero-Luna G, Mitchell MF. The epidemiology of ovarian cancer. J Cell Biochem Suppl 1995;23:200-7.
[102] Franceschi S, Parazzini F, Negri E, et al. Pooled analysis of 3 European case-control studies of epithelial ovarian cancer: III. Oral contraceptive use. Int J Cancer 1991;49:61-5.
[103] Negri E, Franceschi S, Tzonou A, et al. Pooled analysis of 3 European case-control studies: I. Reproductive factors and risk of epithelial ovarian cancer. Int J Cancer 1991;49:50-6.
[104] Kerlikowske K, Brown JS, Grady DG. Should women with familial ovarian cancer undergo prophylactic oophorectomy? Obstet Gynecol 1992;80:700-7.
[105] Boyd J. Molecular genetics of hereditary ovarian cancer. Oncology (Williston Park) 1998;12:399-406; discussion 9-10, 13.
[106] Antoniou A, Pharoah PD, Narod S, et al. Average risks of breast and ovarian cancer associated with BRCA1 or BRCA2 mutations detected in case Series unselected for family history: a combined analysis of 22 studies. Am J Hum Genet 2003;72:1117-30.
[107] Khoury-Collado F, Bombard AT. Hereditary breast and ovarian cancer: what the primary care physician should know. Obstet Gynecol Surv 2004;59:537-42.
[108] Lancaster JM, Powell CB, Kauff ND, et al. Society of Gynecologic Oncologists Education Committee statement on risk assessment for inherited gynecologic cancer predispositions. Gynecol Oncol 2007;107:159-62.
[109] Tan DS, Rothermundt C, Thomas K, et al. "BRCAness" syndrome in ovarian cancer: a case-control study describing the clinical features and outcome of patients with epithelial ovarian cancer associated with BRCA1 and BRCA2 mutations. J Clin Oncol 2008;26:5530-6.
[110] Barrow E, Robinson L, Alduaij W, et al. Cumulative lifetime incidence of extracolonic cancers in Lynch syndrome: a report of 121 families with proven mutations. Clin Genet 2009;75:141-9.
[111] *SEER Cancer Statistics Review, 1975-2008.*, 2011. (Accessed at http://seer.cancer.gov/csr/1975_2008/.)
[112] Beral V, Doll R, Hermon C, Peto R, Reeves G. Ovarian cancer and oral contraceptives: collaborative reanalysis of data from 45 epidemiological studies including 23,257 women with ovarian cancer and 87,303 controls. Lancet 2008;371:303-14.
[113] Narod SA, Risch H, Moslehi R, et al. Oral contraceptives and the risk of hereditary ovarian cancer. Hereditary Ovarian Cancer Clinical Study Group. N Engl J Med 1998;339:424-8.
[114] La Vecchia C. Oral contraceptives and ovarian cancer: an update, 1998-2004. Eur J Cancer Prev 2006;15:117-24.

[115] Hinkula M, Pukkala E, Kyyronen P, Kauppila A. Incidence of ovarian cancer of grand multiparous women--a population-based study in Finland. Gynecol Oncol 2006;103:207-11.

[116] Antoniou AC, Rookus M, Andrieu N, et al. Reproductive and hormonal factors, and ovarian cancer risk for BRCA1 and BRCA2 mutation carriers: results from the International BRCA1/2 Carrier Cohort Study. Cancer Epidemiol Biomarkers Prev 2009;18:601-10.

[117] Jordan SJ, Siskind V, A CG, Whiteman DC, Webb PM. Breastfeeding and risk of epithelial ovarian cancer. Cancer Causes Control 2010;21:109-16.

[118] Danforth KN, Tworoger SS, Hecht JL, Rosner BA, Colditz GA, Hankinson SE. Breastfeeding and risk of ovarian cancer in two prospective cohorts. Cancer Causes Control 2007;18:517-23.

[119] Hankinson SE, Hunter DJ, Colditz GA, et al. Tubal ligation, hysterectomy, and risk of ovarian cancer. A prospective study. JAMA 1993;270:2813-8.

[120] Narod SA, Sun P, Ghadirian P, et al. Tubal ligation and risk of ovarian cancer in carriers of BRCA1 or BRCA2 mutations: a case-control study. Lancet 2001;357:1467-70.

[121] Jacobs IJ, Skates SJ, MacDonald N, et al. Screening for ovarian cancer: a pilot randomised controlled trial. Lancet 1999;353:1207-10.

[122] Kobayashi H, Yamada Y, Sado T, et al. A randomized study of screening for ovarian cancer: a multicenter study in Japan. Int J Gynecol Cancer 2008;18:414-20.

[123] Nyante SJ, Black A, Kreimer AR, et al. Pathologic findings following false-positive screening tests for ovarian cancer in the Prostate, Lung, Colorectal and Ovarian (PLCO) cancer screening trial. Gynecol Oncol 2011;120:474-9.

[124] Vasen HF, Watson P, Mecklin JP, Lynch HT. New clinical criteria for hereditary nonpolyposis colorectal cancer (HNPCC, Lynch syndrome) proposed by the International Collaborative group on HNPCC. Gastroenterology 1999;116:1453-6.

[125] Finch A, Beiner M, Lubinski J, et al. Salpingo-oophorectomy and the risk of ovarian, fallopian tube, and peritoneal cancers in women with a BRCA1 or BRCA2 Mutation. JAMA 2006;296:185-92.

[126] Rebbeck TR, Kauff ND, Domchek SM. Meta-analysis of risk reduction estimates associated with risk-reducing salpingo-oophorectomy in BRCA1 or BRCA2 mutation carriers. J Natl Cancer Inst 2009;101:80-7.

[127] Anderson K, Jacobson JS, Heitjan DF, et al. Cost-effectiveness of preventive strategies for women with a BRCA1 or a BRCA2 mutation. Ann Intern Med 2006;144:397-406.

[128] Yang KY, Caughey AB, Little SE, Cheung MK, Chen LM. A cost-effectiveness analysis of prophylactic surgery versus gynecologic surveillance for women from hereditary non-polyposis colorectal cancer (HNPCC) Families. Fam Cancer 2011.

[129] Schmeler KM, Lynch HT, Chen LM, et al. Prophylactic surgery to reduce the risk of gynecologic cancers in the Lynch syndrome. N Engl J Med 2006;354:261-9.

[130] Kwon JS, Sun CC, Peterson SK, et al. Cost-effectiveness analysis of prevention strategies for gynecologic cancers in Lynch syndrome. Cancer 2008;113:326-35.

[131] van der Velde NM, Mourits MJ, Arts HJ, et al. Time to stop ovarian cancer screening in BRCA1/2 mutation carriers? Int J Cancer 2009;124:919-23.

[132] Olivier RI, Lubsen-Brandsma MA, Verhoef S, van Beurden M. CA125 and transvaginal ultrasound monitoring in high-risk women cannot prevent the diagnosis of advanced ovarian cancer. Gynecol Oncol 2006;100:20-6.
[133] Auranen A, Joutsiniemi T. A systematic review of gynecological cancer surveillance in women belonging to hereditary nonpolyposis colorectal cancer (Lynch syndrome) families. Acta Obstet Gynecol Scand 2011;90:437-44.
[134] Moore RG, Jabre-Raughley M, Brown AK, et al. Comparison of a novel multiple marker assay vs the Risk of Malignancy Index for the prediction of epithelial ovarian cancer in patients with a pelvic mass. Am J Obstet Gynecol 2010;203:228 e1-6.
[135] Moore RG, McMeekin DS, Brown AK, et al. A novel multiple marker bioassay utilizing HE4 and CA125 for the prediction of ovarian cancer in patients with a pelvic mass. Gynecol Oncol 2009;112:40-6.
[136] Montagnana M, Danese E, Ruzzenente O, et al. The ROMA (Risk of Ovarian Malignancy Algorithm) for estimating the risk of epithelial ovarian cancer in women presenting with pelvic mass: is it really useful? Clin Chem Lab Med 2011;49:521-5.
[137] Jacobs I, Oram D, Fairbanks J, Turner J, Frost C, Grudzinskas JG. A risk of malignancy index incorporating CA 125, ultrasound and menopausal status for the accurate preoperative diagnosis of ovarian cancer. Br J Obstet Gynaecol 1990;97:922-9.
[138] Zhang L, Conejo-Garcia JR, Katsaros D, et al. Intratumoral T cells, recurrence, and survival in epithelial ovarian cancer. N Engl J Med 2003;348:203-13.
[139] Adams SF, Levine DA, Cadungog MG, et al. Intraepithelial T cells and tumor proliferation: impact on the benefit from surgical cytoreduction in advanced serous ovarian cancer. Cancer 2009;115:2891-902.
[140] Kandalaft LE, Powell DJ, Jr., Singh N, Coukos G. Immunotherapy for ovarian cancer: what's next? J Clin Oncol 2011;29:925-33.
[141] Buckanovich RJ, Facciabene A, Kim S, et al. Endothelin B receptor mediates the endothelial barrier to T cell homing to tumors and disables immune therapy. Nat Med 2008;14:28-36.
[142] Steinman RM. Dendritic cells: understanding immunogenicity. Eur J Immunol 2007;37 Suppl 1:S53-60.
[143] Cannon MJ, O'Brien TJ. Cellular immunotherapy for ovarian cancer. Expert Opin Biol Ther 2009;9:677-88.
[144] Hernando JJ, Park TW, Kubler K, Offergeld R, Schlebusch H, Bauknecht T. Vaccination with autologous tumour antigen-pulsed dendritic cells in advanced gynaecological malignancies: clinical and immunological evaluation of a phase I trial. Cancer Immunol Immunother 2002;51:45-52.
[145] Padilla LA, Radosevich DM, Milad MP. Limitations of the pelvic examination for evaluation of the female pelvic organs. Int J Gynaecol Obstet 2005;88:84-8.
[146] Greene MH, Piedmonte M, Alberts D, et al. A prospective study of risk-reducing salpingo-oophorectomy and longitudinal CA-125 screening among women at increased genetic risk of ovarian cancer: design and baseline characteristics: a Gynecologic Oncology Group study. Cancer Epidemiol Biomarkers Prev 2008;17:594-604.

[147] Jacobs I, Gentry-Maharaj A, Burnell M, et al. Sensitivity of transvaginal ultrasound screening for endometrial cancer in postmenopausal women: a case-control study within the UKCTOCS cohort. Lancet Oncol 2011;12:38-48.
[148] Lowe KA, Andersen MR, Urban N, Paley P, Dresher CW, Goff BA. The temporal stability of the Symptom Index among women at high-risk for ovarian cancer. Gynecol Oncol 2009;114:225-30.
[149] Lacey JV, Jr., Greene MH, Buys SS, et al. Ovarian cancer screening in women with a family history of breast or ovarian cancer. Obstet Gynecol 2006;108:1176-84.
[150] Partridge E, Kreimer AR, Greenlee RT, et al. Results from four rounds of ovarian cancer screening in a randomized trial. Obstet Gynecol 2009;113:775-82.

4

Borderline and Malignant Surface Epithelial – Stromal Tumors of the Ovary

Susanna Syriac[1], Faith Ough[2] and Paulette Mhawech-Fauceglia[3]
[1]*Roswell Park Cancer Institute, Department of Pathology, Division of Surgical Oncologic Pathology Buffalo,*
[2]*University of Southern California, Department of Pathology, Division of Cytopathology, Los Angeles,*
[3]*University of Southern California, Department of Pathology, Division of Gynecologic Oncologic Pathology, Los Angeles*
USA

1. Introduction

Epithelial ovarian carcinoma (EOC) is the fourth leading cause of cancer mortality among women in western countries. The incidence of newly diagnosed EOC in the US is estimated to be 22,430 cases per year with 15,280 deaths **(Jamel A et al., 2006)**. Surface epithelial-stromal tumors are the most common neoplasms of the ovary. Their origin is likely the epithelium lining the ovarian surface and/or invaginations of this lining into the superficial cortex of the ovary. They occur in women of reproductive age and older. They are usually subclassified as benign, borderline and malignant. Due to the numerous histologic types of ovarian neoplasms, we will limit our discussion to the most common epithelial stromal tumors. We will be discussing the gross appearances, microscopic patterns and differential diagnosis.
Based on the 2002 World Health Organization (WHO) classification of ovarian tumors **(Tavassoli FA and Devilee P, 2003)**, Borderline and Malignant Surface-epithelial stromal tumors are classified as:

1.1 WHO classification

Serous tumors

- Malignant
  - Adenocarcinoma
  - Surface papillary adenocarcinoma
  - Adenocarcinofibroma
- Borderline tumor
  - Papillary cystic tumor
  - Adenofibroma and cystadenofibroma

Mucinous tumors

- Malignant
  - Adenocarcinoma

Adenocarcinofibroma
Borderline tumor
Intestinal type
Endocervical type
Mucinous cystic tumor with mural nodules
Mucinous cystic tumor with pseuodomyxoma peritonei

Endometrioid tumors including variants with squamous differentiation

Malignant
Adenocarcinoma, NOS
Adenocarcinofibroma
Malignant mullerian mixed tumor (carcinosarcoma)
Adenosarcoma
Endometrial stromal sarcoma, low grade
Undifferentiated sarcoma
Borderline tumor
Cystic tumor
Adenofibroma and cystadenofibroma

Clear cell tumors

Malignant
Adenocarcinoma
Adenocarcinofibroma
Borderline tumor
Cystic tumor
Adenofibroma and cystadenofibroma

Transitional cell tumors

Malignant
Transitional cell carcinoma (non-Brenner type)
Malignant Brenner tumor
Borderline
Borderline Brenner tumor

Squamous cell tumors

Squamous cell carcinoma

Mixed epithelial tumors

Undifferentiated and unclassified tumors.

2. Serous tumors

2.1 Borderline tumors

Serous borderline tumors (SBT) represent 25% to 30% of non benign serous tumors and occur in women 30-50 years of age. In the majority of cases they are unilateral and usually present at an early stage (stage I) **(Prat J and de Nictolis M., 2002).** The WHO defines SBT as an "ovarian tumor of low malignant potential exhibiting an atypical epithelial proliferation of serous type cells greater than that seen in its benign counterpart but without destructive stromal invasion".

Grossly, the mass is usually partially cystic and partially solid. Polypoid excrescences are present on the outer surface of the ovary or within the cyst lumen **Fig.2.1.a,b**.

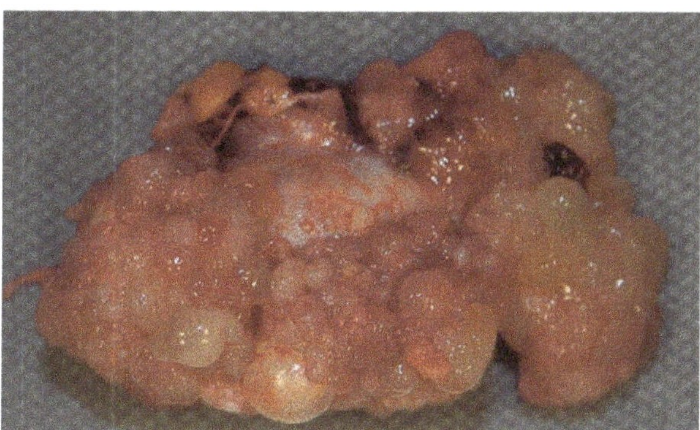

Fig. 2.1.a. Borderline serous tumor (BST). The ovary shows polypoid excrescences on its outer surface.

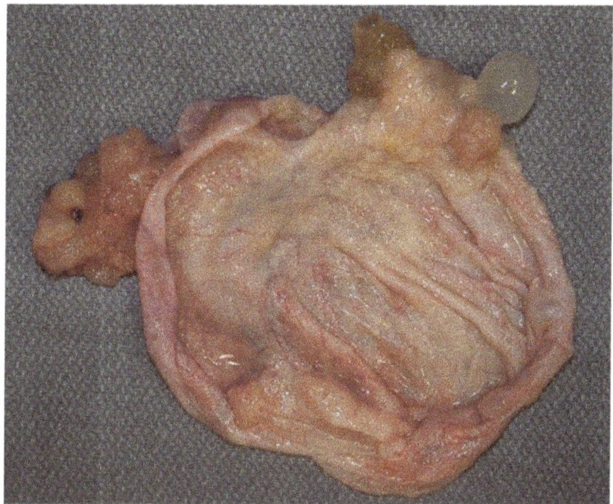

Fig. 2.1.b. BST. In another case, instead of polypoid excrescences on the outer surface of the ovary, papillary projections are seen within the cyst lumen of the ovary.

The papillary structures are yellowish, soft and friable. Grossly, SBT should be differentiated from the hard, stocky, white excrescences that are usually a characteristic of serous cystadenofibroma.
SBTs are divided into typical and micropapillary patterns.

2.1.1 Typical SBT

Typical SBT makes up the majority of SBT (90%). Microscopically, the papillae are lined by stratified cuboidal to columnar epithelial cells. These papillae show branching and complex structure. The epithelial cells have high nuclear cytoplasmic ratio (N/C), and the nuclei are hyperchromatic with prominent nucleoli. Mitotic figures are frequently present **Fig 2.1.1 a,b.**

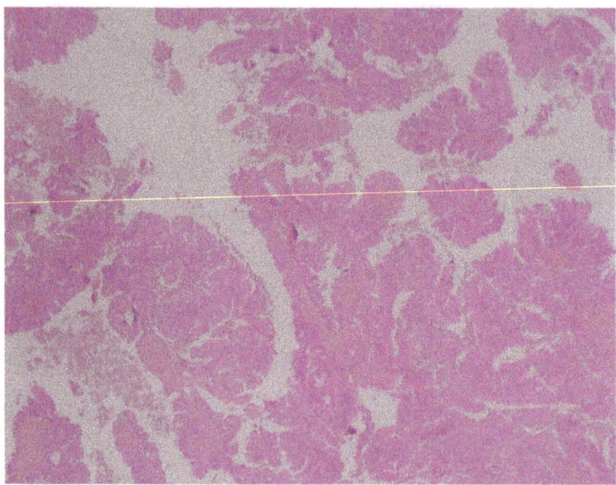

Fig. 2.1.1.a. BST: At the low magnification, the tumor is composed of papillary projections.

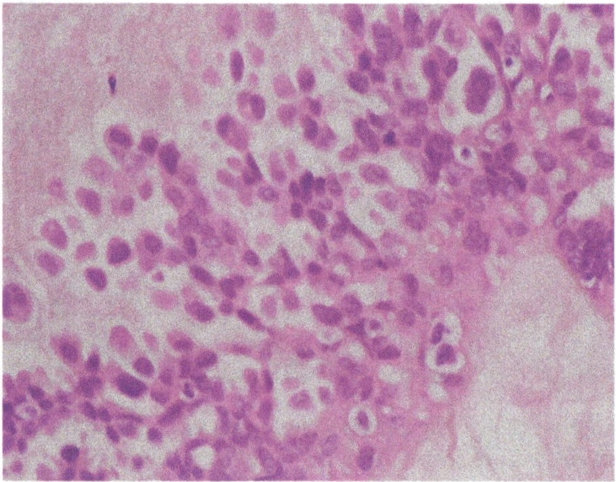

Fig. 2.1.1.b. BST: At higher magnification, the papillae are lined by epithelial cells exhibiting severe pleomorphism with moderate to severe atypia and with high nuclear/cytoplasmic ratio. They have big round nuclei and prominent nucleoli.

Caution should be practiced when one sees what appears to be epithelial proliferation without cytologic atypia, because tangential sectioning of the lining of a benign serous cystadenoma can give the impression of proliferation of the epithelial lining.

By definition, SBT lack stromal invasion. This is a major criterion to differentiate SBT from serous adenocarcinoma. Careful gross examination, as well several sections (1 section/1 cm of the tumor diameter) is needed. Finally, invasion of the stalk of the papillae should not be considered as ovarian stromal invasion.

2.1.2 SBT with micropapillary pattern or micropapillary SBT (MSBT)

SBT with micropapillary pattern or micropapillary SBT (MSBT) accounts 5-10% of all SBTs. The significance of this subtype has generated a lot of debate in pathology. Some authors have found a close association between MSBT and invasive implants and urged to call this entity as "micropapillary serous carcinoma". Yet others prefer the terminology of MSBT, avoiding the use of the term of "carcinoma", to minimize the possibility of over treating patients (**Chang SJ et al., 2008; Sehdev S et al., 2003**). The general agreement on the significance of micropapillary architecture in SBTs is that there is a significant increase in incidence of invasive peritoneal implants (**Burks R et al., 1996**). Molecular studies show that MSBT has a similar gene expression profile as low-grade serous carcinoma (LG-serous carcinoma) and distinct from typical SBT [**May T et al., 2010**]. The underlying genes involved in the pathogenesis of LG-serous carcinoma, and in MBST include mutations in a number of different genes including *KRAS* and *BRAF*. Actually, MSBT is the only surface-epithelial stromal tumor with a well defined adenoma-carcinoma sequence, where LG serous is thought to arise in a stepwise fashion from a benign cystadenoma through BST to an invasive LG-serous carcinoma (**Kurman RJ et al., 2008**). Microscopically, MSBTs shows highly complex micropapillary growth in a filigree pattern, growing in a nonhierarchical fashion from stalk. It has been described as "Medusa head" like appearance. Micropapillae are at least five times as long as they are wide. **Fig 2.1.2 a,b.**

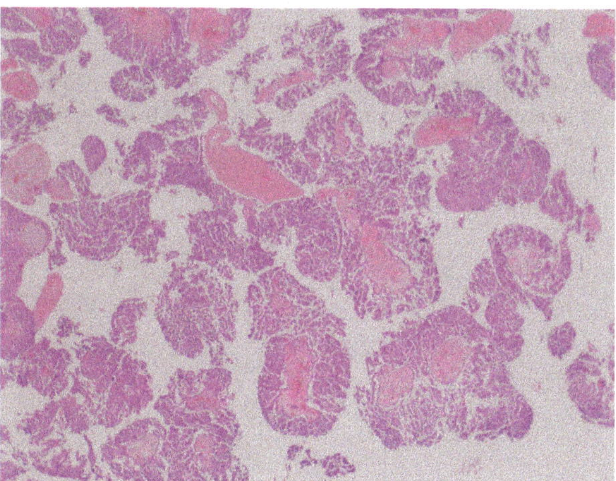

Fig. 2.1.2.a. Micropapillary SBT: Microscopic examination shows highly complex micropapillary growth in a filigree pattern, which is defined by a growth in a nonhierarchical fashion from fibrous stalk forming what we say "Medusa head' like appearance.

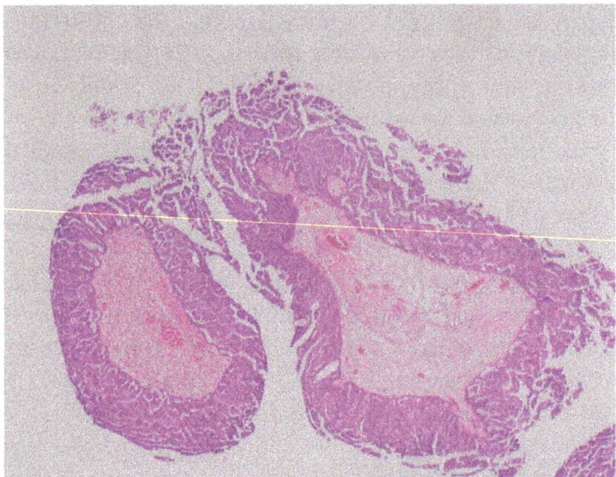

Fig. 2.1.2.b. Micropapillary SBT: The micropapillae are at least five times as long as they are wide.

Micropapillary foci should occupy an area of at least 5 mm, since micropapillary foci of less than 5 mm have no bearing on clinical outcome (**Slomovitz MB et al., 2002**).

2.1.3 Peritoneal implants

Peritoneal implants are classified into epithelial invasive and non-invasive implants, and desmoplastic invasive and non-invasive implants. Implants are a hetergenous group and various types may coexist, therefore, multiple biopsies of numerous foci of suspicious lesions at the time of surgery and extensive tumor sampling by the pathologist, is the main key to exclude an invasive implant.

Epithelial non-invasive implants are characterized by the presence of branching, complex papillae within cystic spaces with no stromal reaction or destruction **Fig 2.1.3.a.**

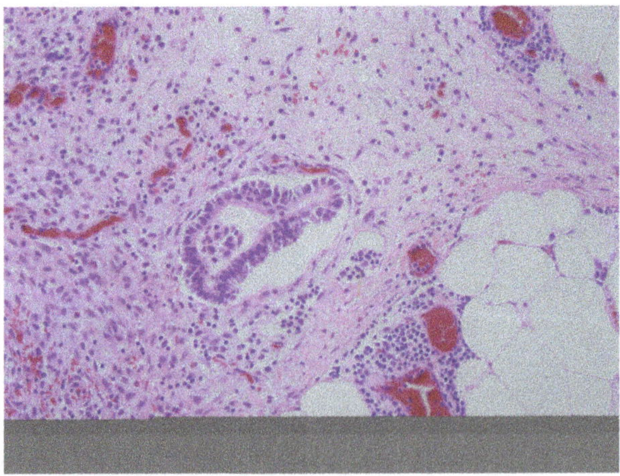

Fig. 2.1.3.a. Non-invasive peritoneal implant: The implant is defined by papillary structure in a space like structure with no evidence of invasion or destruction of the ovarian stroma.

SBT with non-invasive implants have been considered indolent, with 5-year survival rate of 95% and recurrence rate ranging from 8% to 32% **(Silva EG et al., 2006).**

Epithelial invasive implants are characterized by haphazardly distributed glands and clusters of branching papillae infiltrating the adipose tissue and stroma. The epithelial cells should have marked cytologic atypia. The associated stroma is composed of dense fibrous tissue **Fig 2.1.3.b.** Patients with SBT with invasive implants may develop low grade carcinomas many years after initial diagnosis. **(McCluggage WG, 2010)**

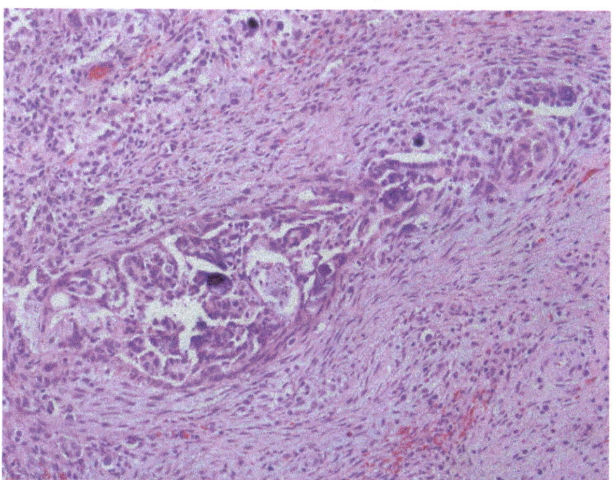

Fig. 2.1.3.b. Invasive implant: it is defined by complex structure of papillae where the neoplastic cells exhibit severe cytologic atypia and they seem to infiltrate a very dense stroma.

Desmoplastic non invasive implants are defined by clusters of tumor cells that are present in a loose fibrous stroma. The stroma may have granulation tissue like features with neutrophilic infiltrates and hemorrhage.

Differential diagnosis: Implants should be distinguished from benign epithelial inclusions or endosalpingiosis. Inclusions are defined by small glands lined by a single cell layer without atypia. Endosalpingiosis is characterized by a lining typical for tubal epithelium such as ciliated and intercalated cells.

2.1.4 SBT with microinvasion

Microinvasion is defined as single cells or few clusters of cells similar to those seen in the overlying SBT that infiltrate the stroma. One or more foci may be present but none should exceed 10 mm^2. SBT with microinvasion appears to have no significance on disease outcome, with 10 year survival rate is of 86% (**Slomovitz BM et al, 2002**).

2.1.5 Implants in a lymph node

Approximately 27% of surgically staged patients with SBT present with lymph node involvement by tumor. The most common lymph nodes involved are the pelvic and paraaortic groups. Recent molecular and morphologic data suggest that although most nodal implants are indeed metastatic from a concurrent ovarian neoplasms, small subsets arises de novo from nodal endosalpingiosis. It has also been suggested that the route of spread from an ovarian

SBT to lymph nodes might be via a peritoneal route and not lymphatic. The morphology of the implant is similar to that occurring in the ovary. Lymph node involvement does not adversely impact the overall survival of patients with SBT of the ovary **[Fadare O, 2009]**. The major differential diagnosis is endosalpingiosis and the criteria are cited previously in the text.

2.2 Serous carcinoma

Serous adenocarcinoma occurs in women a bit older than women with SBT, with an average age of 56 years. Patients with serous adenocarcinoma often present with advanced stage disease (stage III and IV) at first presentation.

Grossly, the tumor varies considerably in size from a few cm to 30 cm. The cut surface may be partially cystic and partially solid or it may be solid with areas of necrosis and hemorrhage **Fig 2.2.a**. When infiltrating the omental adipose tissue, the tumor creates what is called "omental caking" **Fig 2.2.b**.

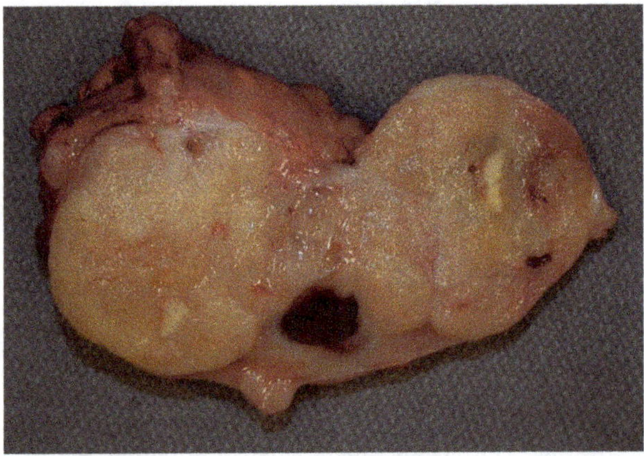

Fig. 2.2.a. Serous adenocarcinoma: the ovarian mass is solid with few cystic areas. The cut surface is firm, white with areas of necrosis and hemorrhage.

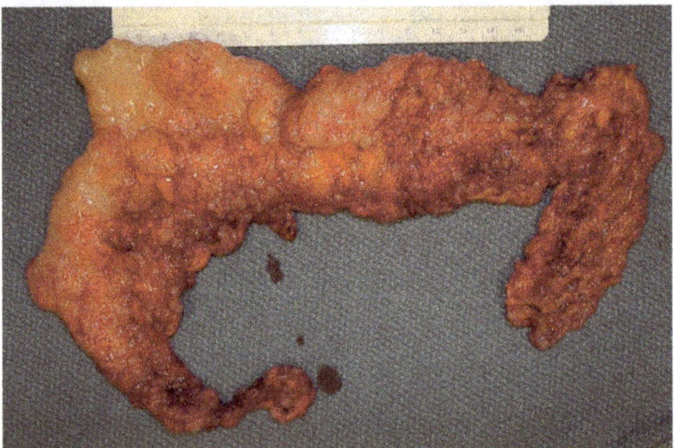

Fig. 2.2.b. Omentum: The tumor involves the omentum and create "omental cake" which is characterized by tumoral seeding of the adipose tissue. The cut surface is white, firm and homogenous.

2.2.1 Grading

Grading of surface epithelial stromal tumors is still performed haphazardly with several systems and non-systems used in different institutes and in different research studies. The lack of uniformity in grading has resulted in little consensus as to whether ovarian tumor grade has any significance in predicting disease outcome. The grading systems used most commonly worldwide are the International Federation of Gynecology and Obstetrics (FIGO) system, and the World Health Organization (WHO) system. The **FIGO** grading system for the ovary is similar to the grading system used in the uterus. It is based on architectural features. The grade depends on the ratio of glandular or papillary structures versus solid tumor growth. Grade 1 is equivalent to <5% solid growth, grade 2 to 5-50% solid growth and grade 3 to =>50% solid growth **(International federation of Gynecology & Obstetrics, 1971**). In the **WHO** system, the grade is assessed by both the architectural and cytologic features, without any quantitative values **(Tavassoli FA and Devilee P., 2003).** The Gynecologic Oncology (GOG) system is the most commonly used system in the United States **(Benda JA et al., 1994).** It employs a method based on the histologic type. For example, ovarian carcinoma of endometrioid type is graded similarly to the endometrial adenocarcinoma of endometrioid type. Ovarian carcinoma of transitional type is graded similar to transitional cell carcinoma (TCC) of the bladder. Clear cell carcinomas are not graded at all. Silverberg's et al proposed a new grading system similar to that used in breast carcinoma and it depends on architectural features (glandular 1, papillary 2 and solid 3), cytologic atypia (mild 1, moderate 2, severe 3), and mitotic rate (1 0-9 mitosis/10HPF, 2 10-24, 3 >25). A score is given by adding the parameters, a score of 3-5, is grade 1, a score of 6-7 is grade 2, and a score of 8 -9 is grade 3 (**Silverberg S, 200**). **Fig 2.2.1a and Fig 2.2.1.b** are examples of grade 1 and grade 3 serous carcinomas.

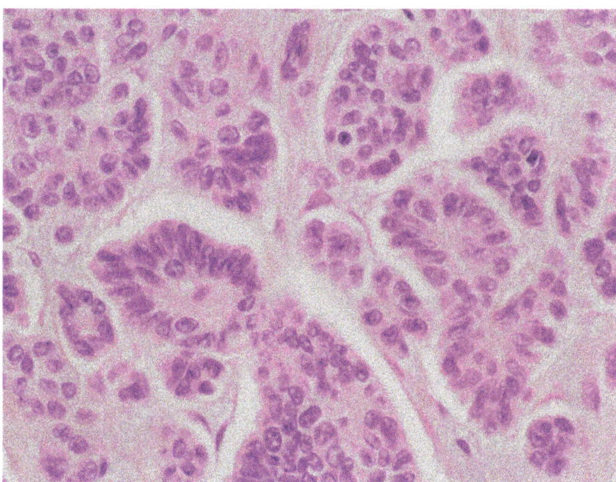

Fig. 2.2.1.a. Low grade serous carcinoma: The tumor has papillary features. The neoplastic cells have mild to moderate atypia and rare mitotic figures.

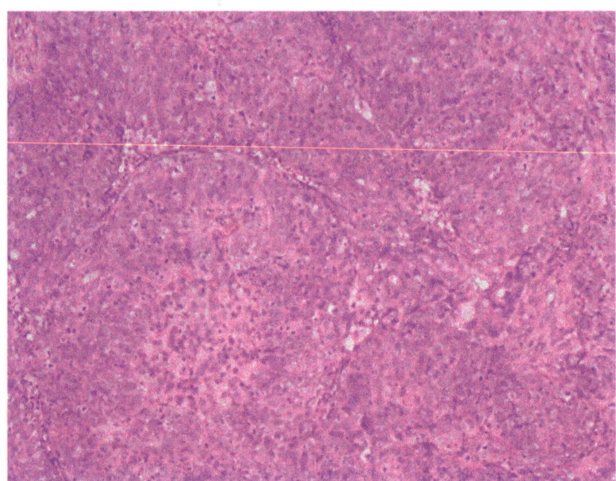

Fig. 2.2.1.b. High grade serous carcinoma: The tumor cells are arranged in solid sheets with very rare foci of papillary architecture. The cells exhibit severe atypia and frequent mitotic figures.

This grading system was confirmed to be reproducible in subsequent studies (**Ishioka SI et al., 2002**). Another study from MD Anderson cancer center group suggested adopting a two-tier system that is based primarily on the assessment of nuclear atypia (uniformity vs. pleomorphism) in the worst area of the tumor (**Malpica A et al., 2004**). The tumor is graded into low grade and high grade. A few years after its introduction, the authors confirmed its reproducibility and urged its use to facilitate the clinical trials and protocols (**Malpica A et al., 2007**).

3. Mucinous tumors

3.1 Mucinous borderline tumors

Mucinous borderline tumors (MBT) (mucinous tumors of low malignant potential) as defined by the WHO, are tumors exhibiting an epithelial proliferation of mucinous type cells greater than that seen in their benign counterparts but without evidence of stromal invasion. MBT can be of intestinal type or endocervical-like type.

3.1.1 Mucinous borderline tumors of intestinal type

The intestinal type tumors are the most common type of MBTs, accounting for 85-90% of cases. They are not associated with peritoneal implants or lymph node involvement. Similar to low- grade serous tumors, intestinal type MBTs are thought to arise from a cystadenoma and to progress to carcinoma, following the adenoma-carcinoma sequence model. Grossly, they are usually a very large unicystic or multicystic mass filled with mucoid-gelatinous material **Fig 3.1.1a**.

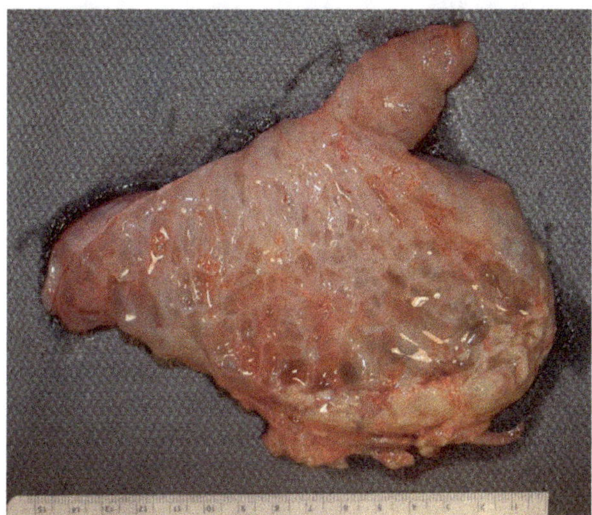

Fig. 3.1.1.a. Mucinous borderline tumor (MBT): The cut surface of the ovarian mass shows multiple cysts filled with gelatinous material. However in some areas the wall of the cyst seemed to be thickened.

Histologically, the lining of the cyst is composed of stratified lining of epithelial cells having high N/C ratio and prominent nucleoli **Fig 3.1.1.b,c**. Goblet cells and Paneth cells are present. No stromal invasion is seen.

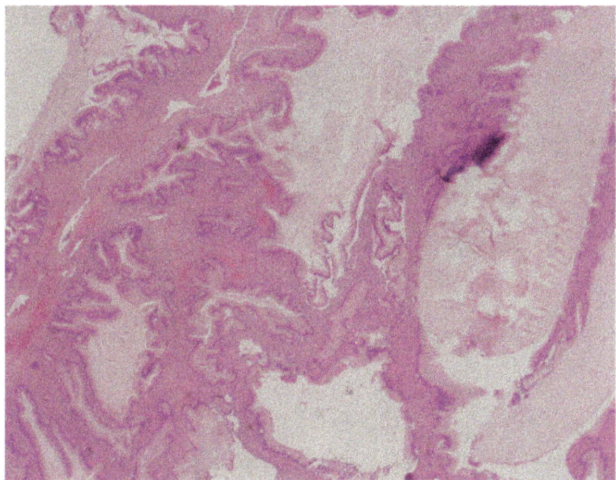

Fig. 3.1.1.b. MBT: At low magnification, the tumor is composed of proliferation of glands which some are cystically dilated separated by abundant intervening stroma.

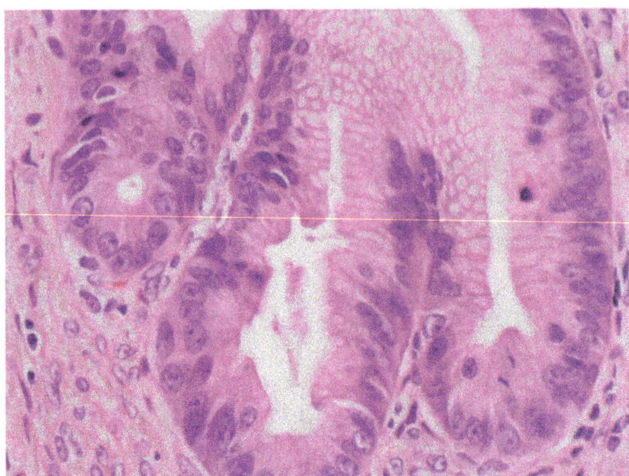

Fig. 3.1.1.c. Higher magnification showed that the glands are lined by mucin secreting cells exhibiting moderate to severe atypia, big nuclei and prominent nucleoli. In some areas, the cytoplasm shows mucin depletion. Mitotic figures are frequently present.

3.1.2 Mucinous borderline tumors of endocervical type

The endocervical type tumors are a less common and make up 10-15% of MBTs. They are usually smaller in size than their intestinal type counterparts and they are commonly bilateral (40%). They are thought to arise from endometriosis. Microscopically, the epithelial cells lining the cyst wall contain intracytoplasmic mucin, resembling endocervical cells.

3.1.3 Mucinous tumors with mural nodules

Mucinous tumors of the ovary, whether benign, borderline or malignant, may contain one or more nodules. These nodules are morphologically different than the overlying mucinous neoplasm. Grossly, nodules are yellow, pink with areas of hemorrhage and necrosis **Fig 3.1.3.a.**

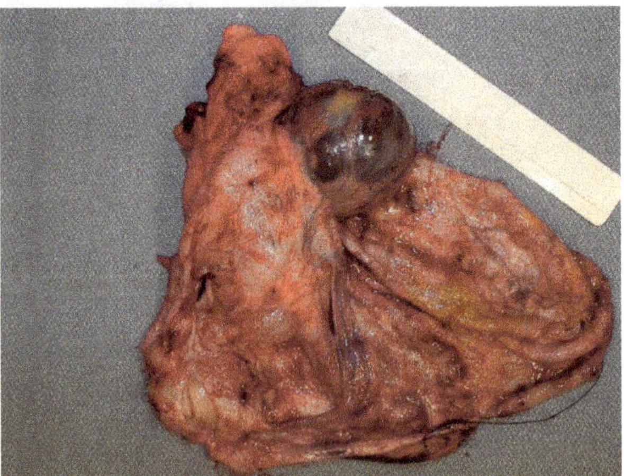

Fig. 3.1.3.a. Mural nodules: Mural nodules are grossly characterized by a well defined mass within the wall of the cyst. The cut surface is often hemorrhagic.

Microscopically, the mural nodules may be malignant (anaplastic, sarcoma or carcinosarcoma) or benign (sarcoma-like). It is important to distinguish between benign and malignant mural nodules, because benign mural nodules are of no prognostic significance. Immunohistochemistry is a very helpful tool for this purpose. Sarcoma-like nodules are composed of a heterogenous cell population of cells including spindle cells, giant cells, mononuclear cells and inflammatory cells. The cells of the sarcoma- like nodules are negative or very weakly positive for cytokeratin **Fig3.1.3.b**.

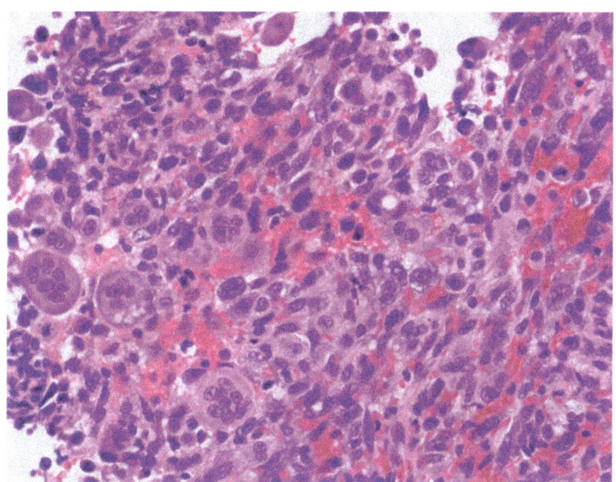

Fig. 3.1.3.b. Sarcoma-like nodules: They are composed of heterogenous cell population including spindle cells, giant cells, mononuclear cells and inflammatory cells.

Anaplastic sarcoma mural nodules are composed of diffuse sheets of spindled or large rhabdoid-looking cells with abundant eosinophilic cytoplasm and prominent nucleoli **fig 3.1.3.c,d**. These cells are usually strongly positive for cytokeratin **fig 3.1.3.e.**

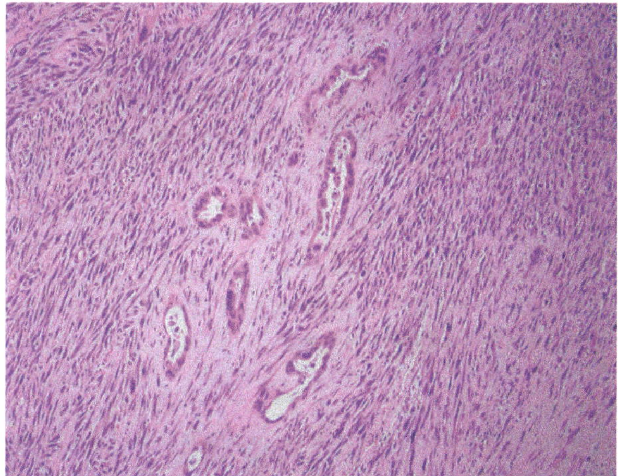

Fig. 3.1.3.c. Anaplastic nodules: They are characterized by proliferation of spindle cells.

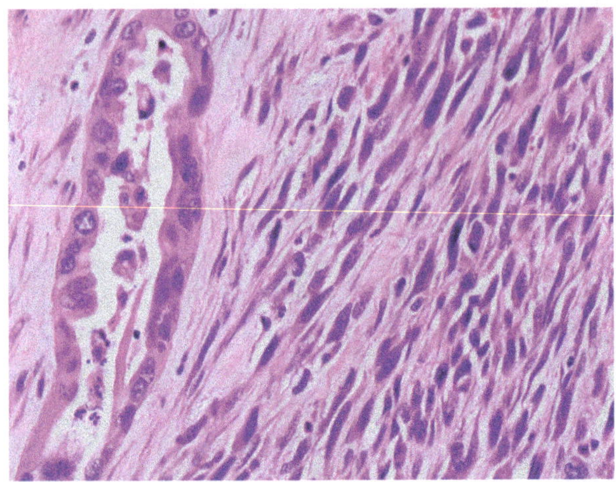

Fig. 3.1.3.d Anaplastic nodules: At higher magnification, the spindle cells exhibit severe atypia, hyperchromasia and numerous mitoses.

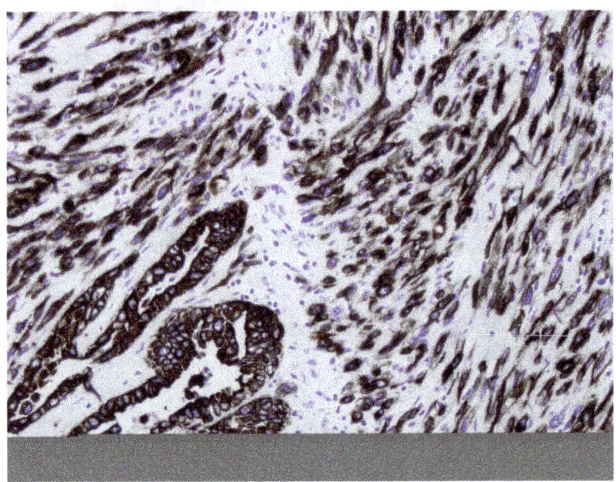

Fig. 3.1.3.e. Anaplastic nodules: The spindle cells in are strongly positive for total cytokeratin immunostain.

Lastly Sarcoma nodules exhibit a variety of patterns such as fibrosarcoma, rhabdomyosarcoma and undifferentiated sarcoma.

3.2 Mucinous adenocarcinoma

Mucinous adenocarcinomas (MAC) are very large tumors; many are 15 to 30 cm in diameter and weigh as much as 4 kgs. The cut surface can be cystic or solid and the content is composed of gelatinous, mucoid material **Fig 3.2a.**

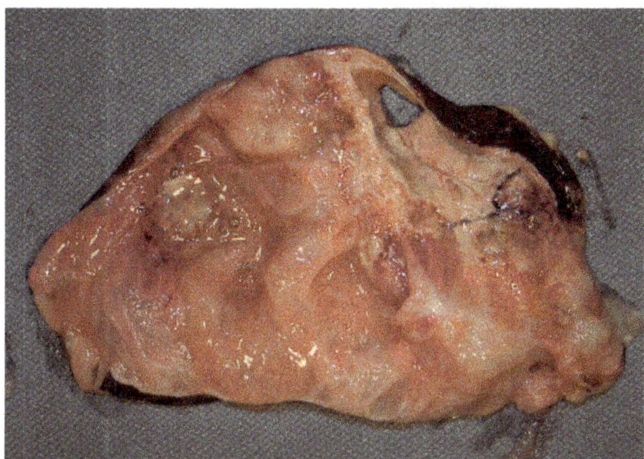

Fig. 3.2.a. Mucinous cystadenocarcinomas: Grossly, they are characterized by partially cystic and partially solid mass. The cysts content is composed of gelatinous material.

These tumors are defined by invasion and adequate sampling is a key factor to document invasion process. Numerous sections (2 to 3 sections /1cm of tumor diameter) are required. Invasion can be defined as infiltration of ovarian stroma by neoplastic cells arranged in nests or as single cells with a stromal desmoplastic reaction **Fig 3.2.b,c**.

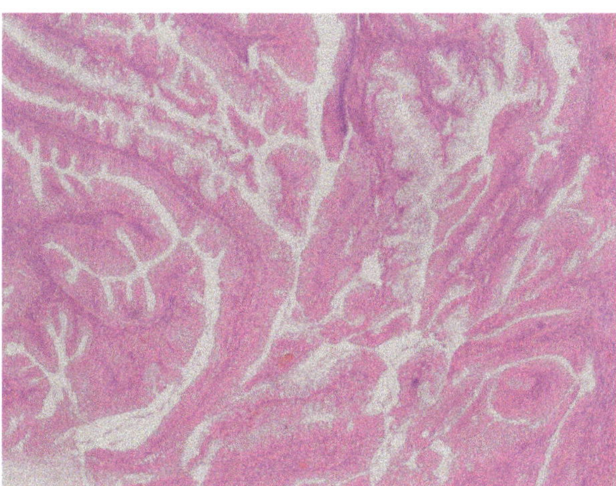

Fig. 3.2.b. Mucinous adenocarcinoma: It is also defined by proliferation of back to back glands with no or little interfering stroma.

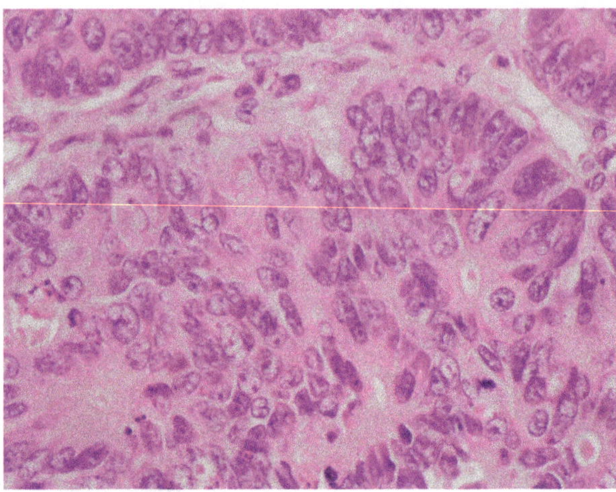

Fig. 3.2.c. Mucinous adenocarcinoma: These glands are cytologically malignant with severe atypia, large nucleoli, loss of cytoplasmic mucin and numerous mitosis.

However, one needs not to see typical stromal invasion with desmoplastic reaction to diagnose MAC, because invasion can also be defined as neoplastic glands which are back to back with no intervening stroma **Fig 3.2d**. Similar to MBTs, the epithelial lining in MAC can be of intestinal or endocervical type. MAC should be distinguished from metastatic adenocarcinoma from colonic origin. Metastatic colonic carcinomas are usually bilateral. Morphologically, they are characterized by glandular proliferation with abundant dirty necrosis and nuclear debris within amorphous necrotic tissue. The glands are lined by stratified cells with prominent atypia and mitosis **Fig 3.2.e**

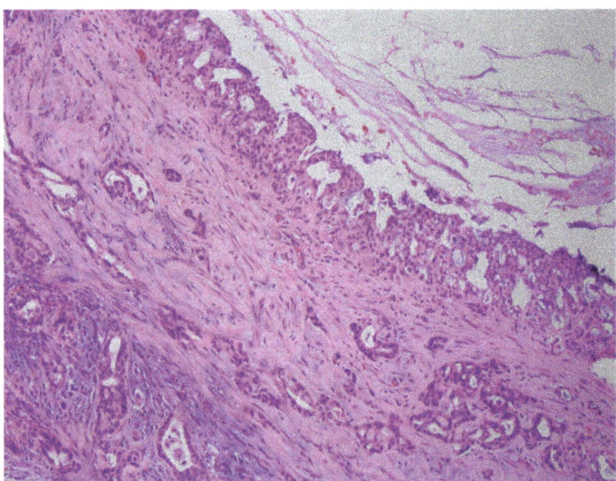

Fig. 3.2.d. Mucinous cystadenocarcinoma: It is defined by invasion of the ovarian stroma by small glands and nests of tumor cells . These glands are cytologically malignant and infiltrate the stroma in disorderly fashion.

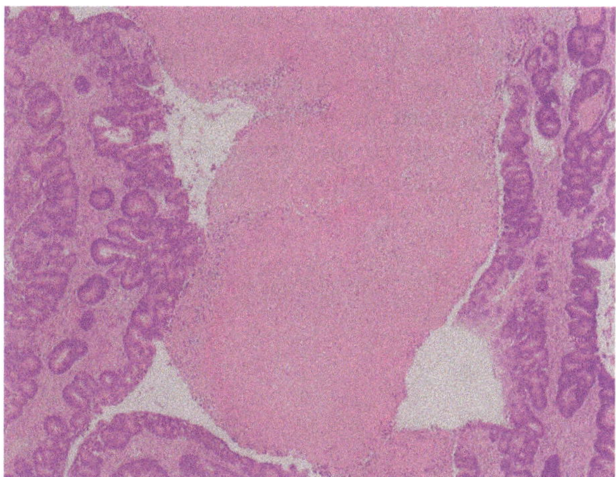

Fig. 3.2.e. Metastatic colon carcinoma: It is characterized by large glands with center "dirty" necrosis and nuclear debris within amorphous necrotic tissue.

3.3 Pseudomyxoma peritonei

Pseudomyxoma peritonei (PP) is a clinical term used to describe the finding of mucoid, gelatinous material in the abdominal cavity, often accompanied by an ovarian or gastrointestinal tumor. In 1995, Ronnett et al classified PP into low-grade variety "diffuse peritoneal adenomucinosis" (DPAM) and to high-grade variety "peritoneal mucinous carcinomatosis" (PMCA) **(Ronnett BM et al, 1995).** DPAM is defined as pools of mucin with few strips of mucinous epithelium exhibiting minimal cytologic atypia and rare mitotic figures **Fig3.3.a.** On the other hand, PMCA is characterized by abundant mucinous epithelium, glands or signet ring cells, showing severe atypia which are clearly malignant **Fig3.3.b**.

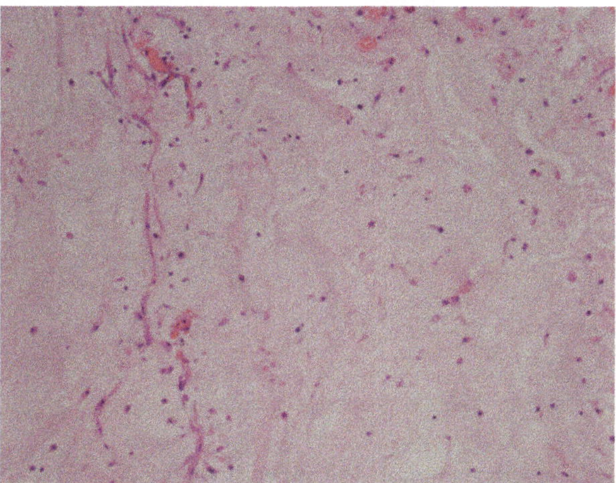

Fig. 3.3.a. Peritoneal mucinosis; It is characterized by pool of acellular mucin.

This classification is prognostically significant with 5-year survival rates of 84% for DPAM and 6.7% for PMCA (**Ronnett BM et al, 2001).** PP may originate from an ovarian primary or from an appendiceal primary. An appendectomy is necessary in those circumstances. Grossly, the appendix shows a dilated lumen filled with mucinous material. Histologically, depending upon the cytologic atypia, the appendiceal tumor may be a mucinous adenocarcinoma or a mucinous tumor of low malignant potential **Fig3.3.c,d. (Misdraji J, 2009).**

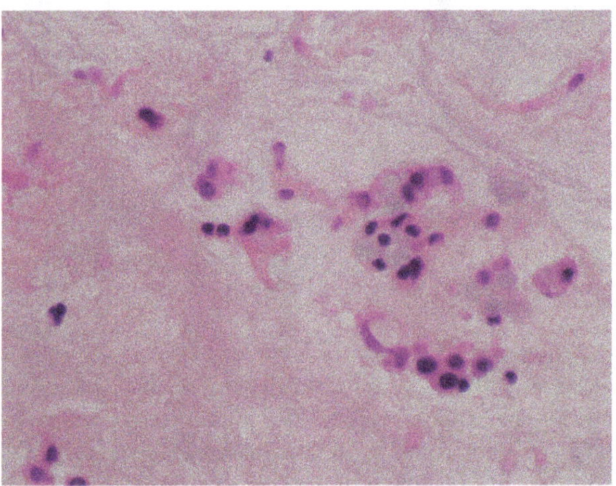

Fig. 3.3.b. Peritoneal adenocarcinomatosis: It is characterized by pool of mucin and clusters of malignant cells with signet-ring features.

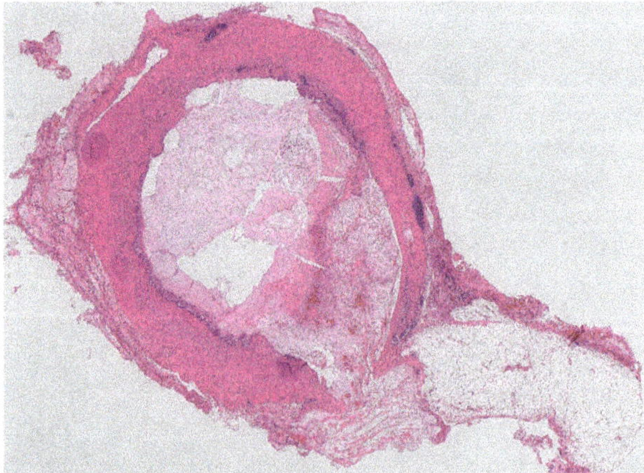

Fig. 3.3.c. Appendiceal mucinous tumor: The appendiceal lumen is dilated and filled with mucin which is dissecting the entire thickness of the wall.

In many cases, the appendix is encased by a very large mucinous mass, and histologically, the appendix is replaced by tumor, rendering the diagnosis of appendiceal primary very difficult.

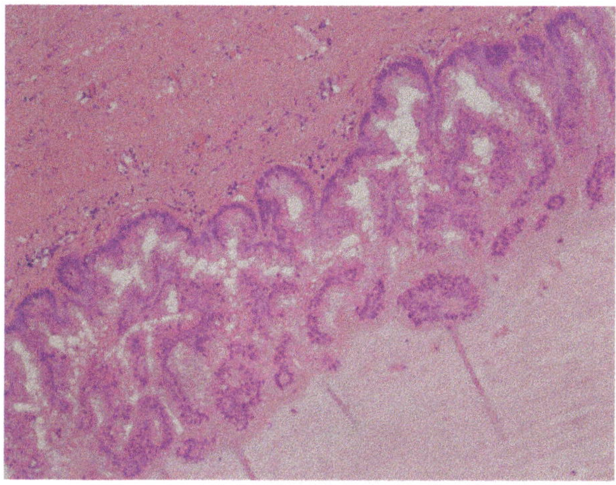

Fig. 3.3.d. Appendiceal mucinous tumor: The appendiceal mucosa shows proliferation of mucin-secreting cells that they are not frankly malignant. Due to the absence of glandular cribriform and submucosal invasion, this lesion is classified as mucinous tumor of low malignant potential.

Not so long ago, there was a considerable controversy about the origin of mucin in PP, in women with concomitant mucinous tumors of the appendix and the ovaries. Recent immunohistochemical, molecular, and genetic evidence supports the appendix as the primary tumor and secondary involvement of the ovary **(Ronnet BM et al, 2004)** In difficult cases, immunohistochemistry study including cytokeratin 7 (CK7), cytokeration 20 (CK20) and CDX2 are useful to discriminate between primary appendix from primary ovarian mucinous tumors. At first CDX2 seemed to be a promising marker and its positivity was found to be very specific for lower gastrointestinal carcinomas but as more studies have been published, more cases of ovarian mucinous tumors have been found to be positive for CDX2 rendering its use of little value. On the other hand CK7/CK20 is more useful, as ovarian mucinous tumor are CK7+/CK20+ and appendiceal/ colon tumors are CK7-/CK20+. Thus, CK7/CK20 is the most useful and reliable combination in distinguishing appendiceal versus ovarian primary **(Chu P et al., 2000; Kaimaktchiev et al., 2004).**

4. Endometrioid tumors

4.1 Endometrioid adenocarcinoma

Endometrioid adenocarcinoma (EAC) account for 10-20% of ovarian carcinomas. They occur in postmenauposal women, with average age of 56 years. The frequent association with endometriosis and endometrioid adenocarcinoma of the endometrium suggested that some EAC of the ovary might have the same risk factors as those occurring in the endometrium. In contrary to serous carcinomas, about half of EAC cases present as early stage disease (stage I and II). They are bilateral in 20% of cases. Microscopically, these tumors are usually well differentiated tumors (grade I). The tumor is microscopically very similar to those occurring in the endometrium, where back to back glands with no intervening stroma and squamous differentiation in the form of squamous morules and keratin pearls are present. **Fig 4.1a., b**

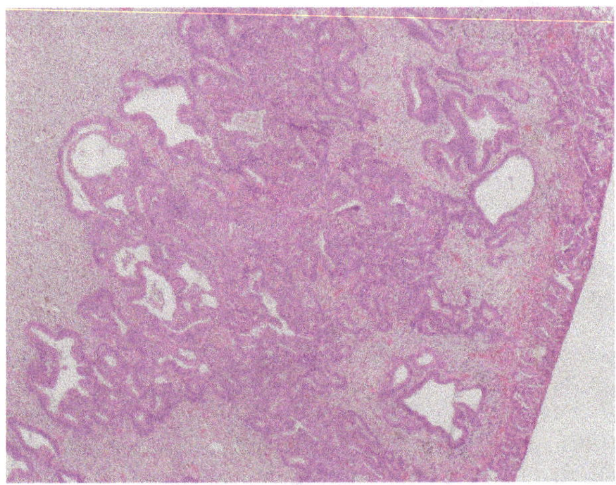

Fig. 4.1.a. Endometrioid adenocarcinoma (EAC): The morphologic features of this tumor are very similar to those occurring in the endometrium where back to back glands with no intervening stroma.

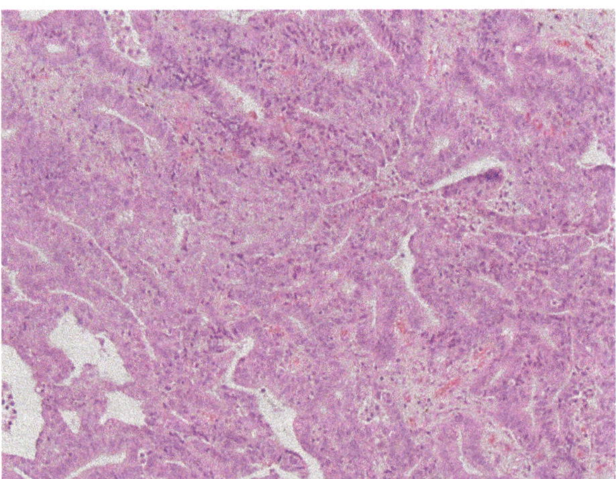

Fig. 4.1.b. EAC: The glands are cribriform and they are cytologcially malignant.

Rare examples of mucin-rich, secretory, ciliated, and oxyphilic types have been described. Occasionally the tumor may resemble granulosa cell tumor, with the cells arranged in ribbons, and small glands, creating the illusion of Call-Exner bodies. Also, rare cases exhibit tubular glands resembling a Sertoli-Leydig cell tumor. In both cases alpha-inhibin is excellent marker to differentiate between EAC and sex-cord tumors, where it is negative in EAC of the ovary and it is positive in sex-cord stromal tumors such as Sertoli-Leydig tumors and granulosa cell tumors **Fig 4.1.c.d (Zhao C et al., 2007; Pelkey TJ et al., 1998).**

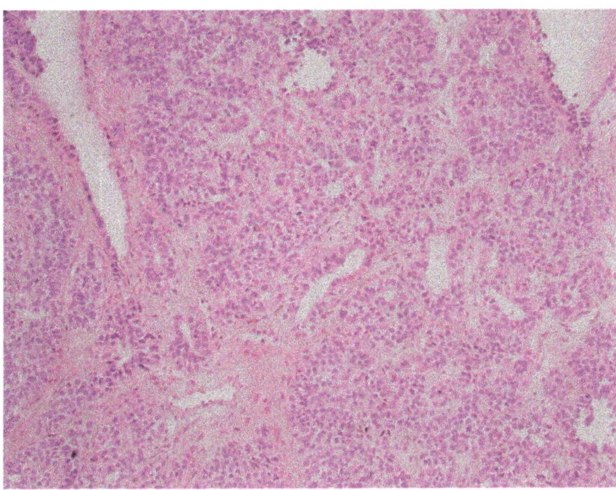

Fig. 4.1.c. Sertoli-Leydig cell tumor: They may be arranged in irregular tubules lined by stratified epithelium resembling endometrial adenocarcinoma.

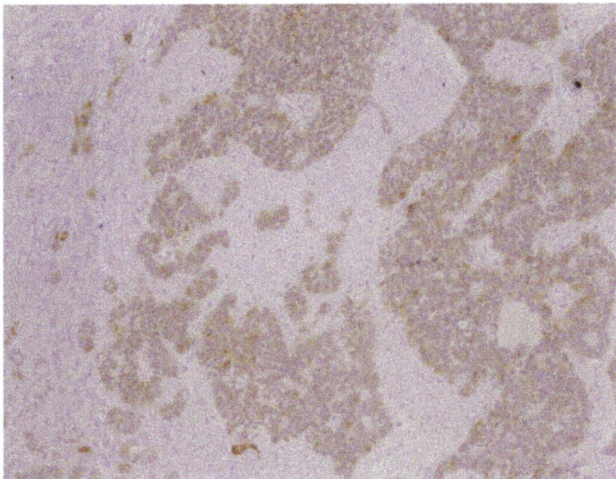

Fig. 4.1.d. Sertoli-Leydig cell tumor: Tumor cells are positive for inhibin immunostain.

4.2 Carcinosarcoma (mixed malignant mullerian tumor/MMMT)

Carcinosarcomas account for <1% of all ovarian cancers and occur in the sixth to eight decades. They are composed of two components; a malignant epithelial component and sarcomatous elements. The sarcomatous component may be homologous (tissue native to the ovary) or heterologous elements (skeletal muscle, cartilage and bone). Molecular studies support a clonal origin of both components, leading some to propose designating carcinosarcoma as a "metaplastic carcinoma" **(Thompson L et al, 1996; Mayall F et al, 1994)**. The epithelial component is usually of endometrioid type adenocarcinoma but other types like serous or mucinous may be found **Fig 4.2.a.** The sarcomatous component may be a homologous type such as fibrosarcoma, high-grade endometrial stromal sarcoma, or a heterologous type including chondrosarcoma or rhabdomyosarcoma **Fig 4.2.b.**

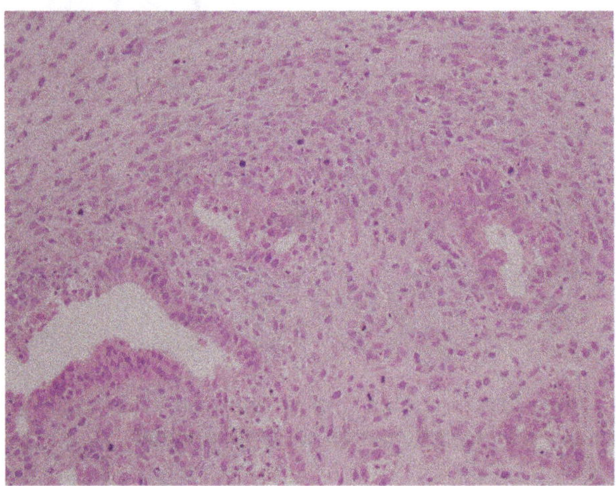

Fig. 4.2.a. MMMT: the tumor is composed of two components which are malignant, the epithelial component (adenocarcinoma) and the mesenchymal component (sarcoma).

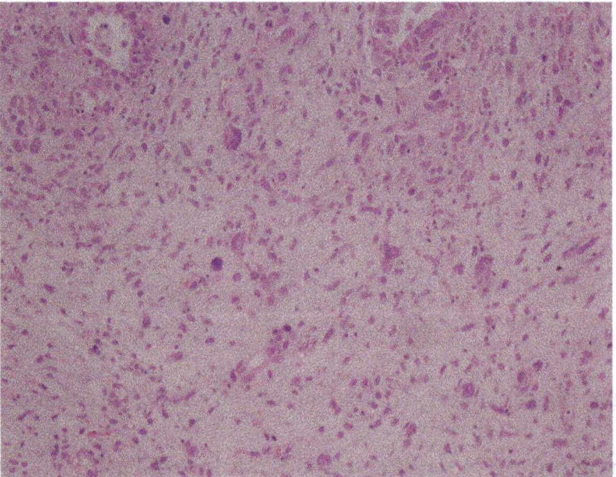

Fig. 4.2.b. MMMT: the mesenchymal component (sarcoma) is composed of very atypical, hyperchromatic cells. These cells have a high mitotic rate.

5. Clear cell tumors

Clear cell carcinoma

Clear cell carcinomas (CCC) represent 6% of surface-epithelial tumors. They occur in postmenopausal women, with a mean age of 57 years. CCC of the ovary has a few notable characteristics 1- they are almost always unilateral, 2- they are admixed with endometrioid type adenocarcinoma in 20-25% of cases, 3- they are often accompanied by endometriosis of the same ovary, 4- they may be associated with paraneoplastic hypercalcemia and 5- they have frequent mutations of ARID1A and PIK3CA genes **(Anglesio MS et al., 2011)**. Histologically, CCC may exhibit various patterns of growth, including tubulo-cystic, papillary and solid patterns **Fig 5.a.** The papillae of CCC are unique in that they are composed of an extensive hyaline core which is different from the small, fibrovascular core papillae as seen in serous adenocarcinoma. In addition, CCC can display numerous cell types such as clear, hobnail, cuboidal, flat, oxyphilic and signet-cell types. The most common type, clear cell type, is defined by round to polygonal cells with a clear cytoplasm, eccentric nuclei and prominent nucleoli **Fig5.b, c.** The cytoplasm contains abundant glycogen which is Periodic acid-Schiff (PAS) positive, diastase digestion resistant. Numerous intracytoplasmic hyaline globules may be seen. Mucin can be found in the lumens of tubules and cysts and it is very abundant in the cytoplasm of the signet ring cell types.

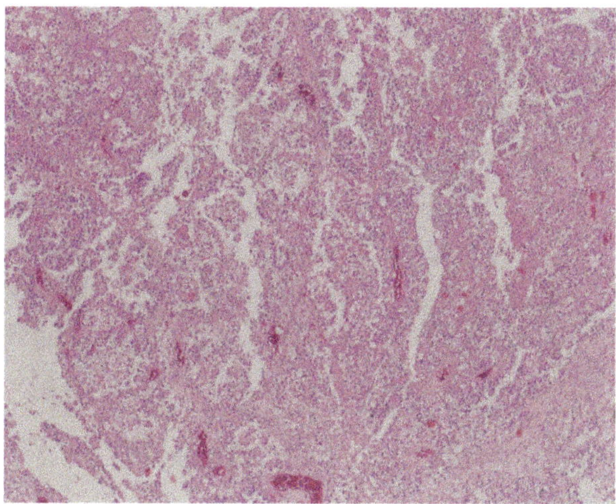

Fig. 5.a. Clear cell carcinoma (CCC): low magnification shows proliferation of neoplastic cells in form of solid sheets and papillary patterns.

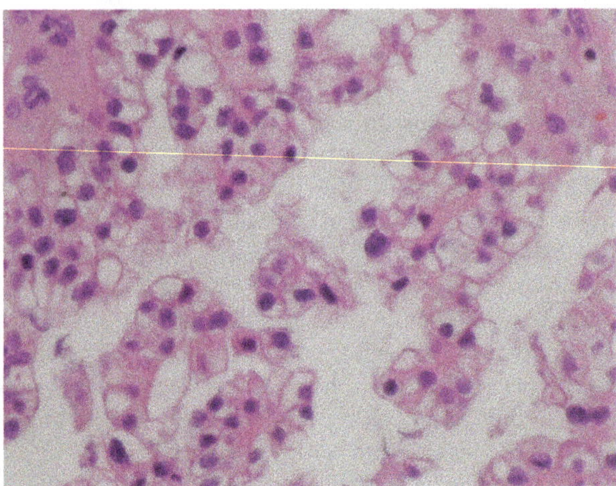

Fig. 5.b. CCC: The cells have a clear cytoplasm, and eccentrically located round nuclei.

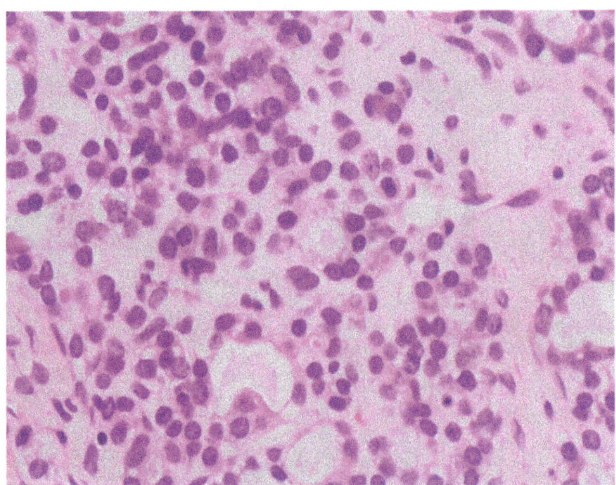

Fig. 5.c. CCC: some cells contain inspissated secretion that is mucicarmine positive creating a targetoid appearance.

Due to these various patterns, CCC can be mistaken for germ cell tumors including dysgerminoma, yolk sac tumors, endometrioid adenocarcinoma with secretory changes, and with metastatic renal cell carcinoma (RCC) **Fig 5.d,e**.

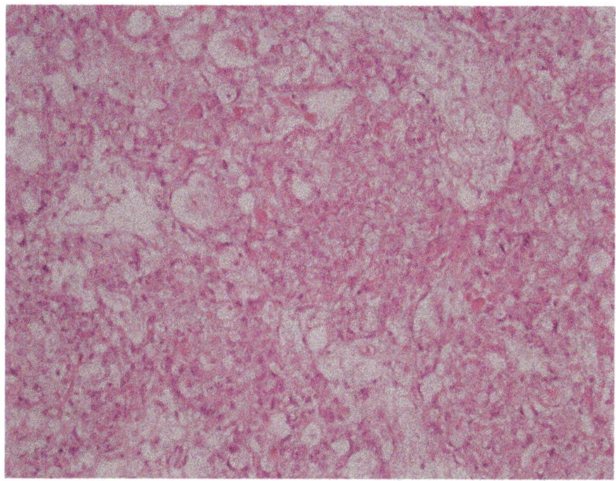

Fig. 5.d. Yolk sac tumor: The tumor is arranged in a loose stroma with small cystic structures.

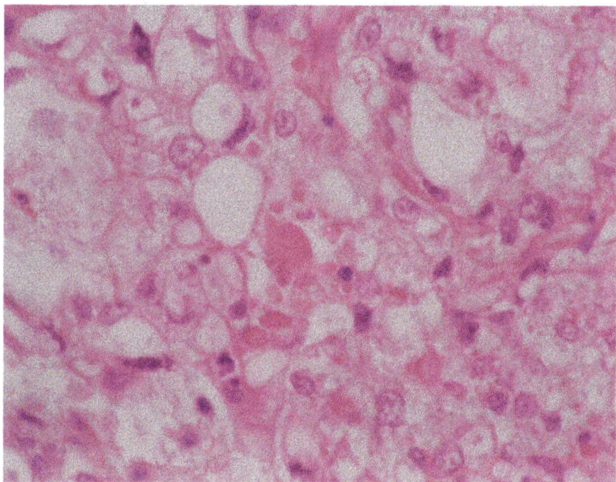

Fig. 5.e. Yolk sac tumor: The tumor cells have abundant eosinophilic cytoplasm and contain hyaline bodies.

Alpha-fetoprotein (AFP), placenta alkaline phosphatse (PLAP), cytokeratins and epithelial membrane antigen (EMA) are helpful immunohistochemistry stains to distinguish CCC from germ cell tumors. In germ cell tumors, AFP and PLAP are positive and cytokeratin and EMA are negative, while CCC cells are negative for AFP and PLAP and positive for cytokeratin and EMA **(Mittal k et al 2008).**

Metastatic RCC to the ovary, though rare, creates a major diagnostic challenge, when CCC of the ovary is of clear cell type. It is almost impossible to differentiate the two based solely on morphology. Therefore, IHC is helpful as RCC is usually negative for CK7 and positive for CD10 and CCC of the ovary is typically positive for CK7 and negative for CD10. In addition, correlation with radiologic findings is necessary to rule out metastatic RCC (**Mittal K et al, 2008**).

6. Transitional cell tumors

Transitional cell carcinoma and malignant Brenner tumors

The group of transitional cell tumors includes benign Brenner tumors, borderline and malignant Brenner tumors, and transitional cell carcinoma. By definition, transitional cell carcinoma of the ovary (TCC-O) and malignant Brenner tumors are composed of epithelial cells morphologically resembling urothelium. TCC-O is the least common surface epithelial tumor of the ovary, accounting 1-2% of all ovarian tumors. It may sometimes be associated with germ cell tumors. They are bilateral in 15% of the cases. Grossly they are cystic with intracystic papillary projections **Fig 6.a.**

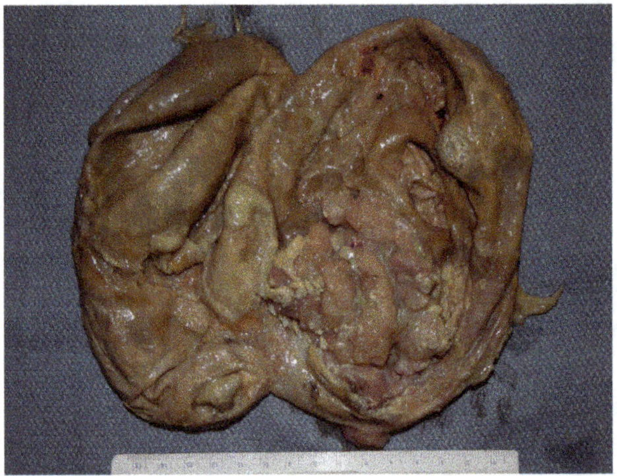

Fig. 6.a. Transitional cell carcinoma of the ovary (TCC-O): The mass is mostly composed of one large cystic where a large vegetating tumoral mass protrudes in the lumen.

TCC-O can be already widespread disease at the time of diagnosis, however, malignant Brenner tumors are usually stage I disease at first presentation. Histologically, TCC-O and malignant Brenner tumors resemble TCC occurring in the urinary tract. They are composed of papillary projections protruding into a cystic lumen, lined by multilayered malignant transitional epithelium **Fig 6.b.c.**

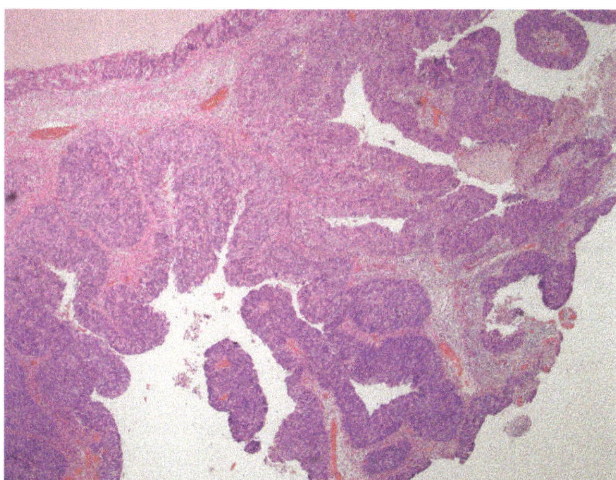

Fig. 6.b. TCC-O: The tumor is composed of broad undulating macropapillae with smooth borders.

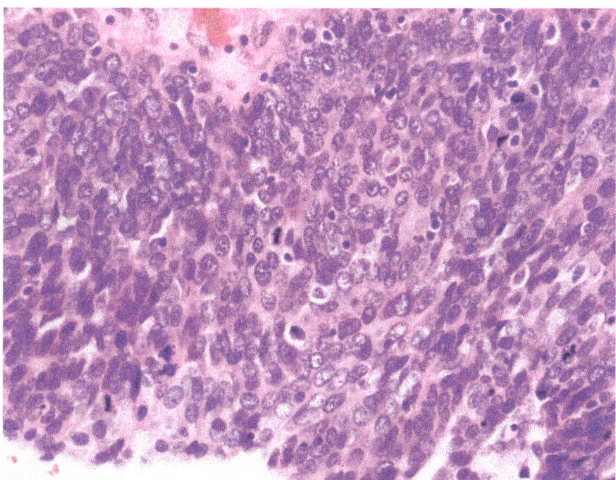

Fig. 6.c. TCC-O: At higher magnification, the macropapillae are composed of multilayered transitional cells resembling that of papillary transitional cell carcinoma of the bladder. These cells have high grade nuclei and numerous mitotic figures.

Foci of glandular differentiation and squamous metaplasia may also be seen. Very often, TCC can be mixed with serous adenocarcinoma. At matched stage, TCC-O has a worse prognosis compared to malignant Brenner tumors. Therefore, TCC-O should be differentiated from malignant Brenner tumors. Morphologically, TCC-O lack an associated benign or borderline Brenner tumor, whereas, malignant Brenner tumors are always accompanied by benign or borderline Brenner tumors **(Eichhorn JH et al., & Young RH, 2004).** Thus, extensive tumor sampling is needed to make an accurate diagnosis. The major differential diagnosis is metastatic TCC from the urinary tract and immunohistochemistry can be very helpful. Numerous studies have dealt with this issue and concluded that the best IHC panel is CK20, uroplakin, and Wilm's tumor (WT). TCC-O are CK20-, uroplakin- and WT1+, whereas, metastatic TCC from the bladder are CK20+, Uroplakin + and WT1- (**Logani S et al., 2003; Delair D et al., 2011 ; Ordonez NG, 2000).**

7. Squamous cell carcinoma

Squamous cell carcinomas (SCCs) of the ovary are very rare. They arise most commonly from the lining of a dermoid cyst, endometrioisis or a Brenner tumor (**Acien P et al, 2010; Bal A et al, 2007**). They have similar morphology to squamous cell carcinoma occurring in the cervix or vagina. **Fig 7.a**

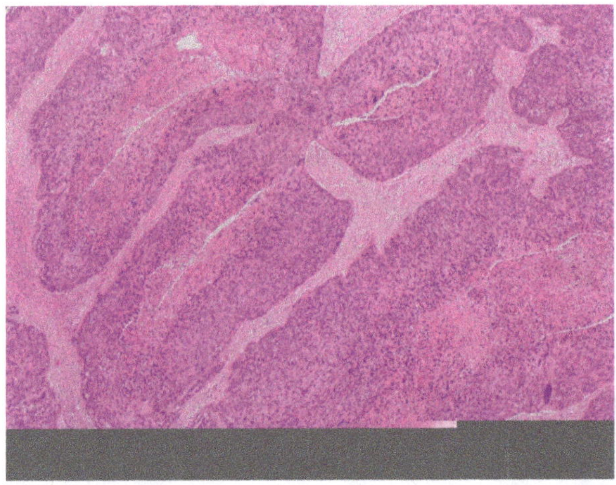

Fig. 7.a. Squamous cell carcinoma. Tumor cells are arranged in large nests. Keratin pearls and necrotic debris is also present. The tumor cells resembling squamous cell carcinoma of the cervix or squamous cell carcinoma of any origin.

Before the diagnosis of primary squamous cell carcinoma of the ovary is made, metastatic SCC from the cervix should be excluded. In addition, primary SCCs of the ovary should be distinguished from endometrioid adenocarcinoma with extensive squamous differentiation. Thus, extensive sampling is recommended. Cases of primary SCCs of the ovary frequently have spread beyond ovary at the time of presentation, leading to poor prognosis.

8. Ovarian carcinoma after neoadjuvant therapy

Traditionally, advanced stage ovarian carcinoma is treated by debulking surgery followed by chemotherapy. In some circumstances, neoadjuvant chemotherapy followed by debulking surgery may be done. Neoadjuvant chemotherapy is increasingly being used in the management of patients with advanced ovarian cancer and pathologists should be aware of the morphologic changes in ovarian cancer after neoadjuvant chemotherapy. For the inexperienced or those with no knowledge of the patients' history, treated tumors may be mistaken for metastatic carcinoma from breast primary or other sites. The morphologic changes seen in response to neoadjuvant chemotherapy include small groups or single tumor cells in a densely fibrotic stroma **Fig 8.a.** The tumor cells are characterized by nuclear and cytoplasmic alteration making the grading and sometimes the tumor typing impossible and inaccurate. Nuclear changes include nuclear enlargement, hyperchromasia, irregular nuclear outlines and chromatin smudging. Cytoplasmic alterations include eosinopholic cytoplasm, vacuolation and foamy cell changes **Fig 8.b.** The stroma may have pronounced fibrosis, inflammation, foamy histiocytic infiltrates, hemosiderin deposits, necrosis, calcification and numerous free psammoma bodies **(McCluggage WG et al., 2002; Chew I et al., 2009).**

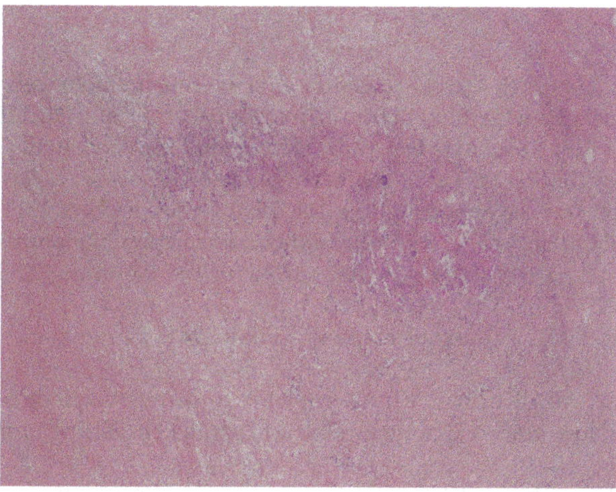

Fig. 8.a. Ovarian carcinoma after neoadjuvant therapy: The tumor presents extensive areas of fibrosis with few areas of remaining viable tumor cells.

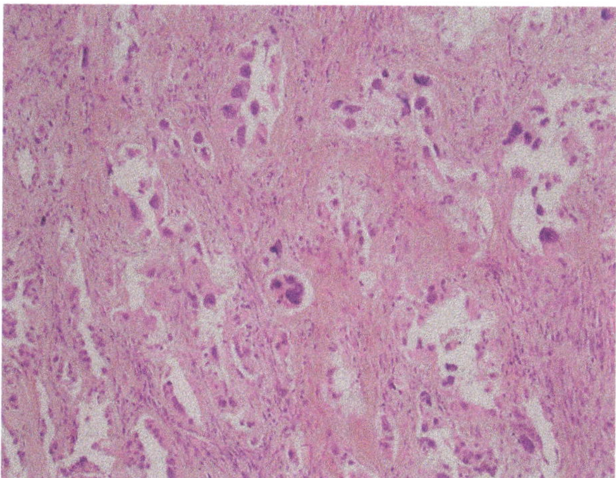

Fig. 8.b. Ovarian carcinoma after neoadjuvant therapy The nuclear changes seen including nuclear enlargement, hyperchromasia, irregular nuclear outlines and chromatin smudging.

The immunohistochemistry profile is similar to that of native untreated tumors. Ck7, CA125, WT1, ER, p53 and p16 may be of value in identifying residual tumor cells **[Miller K et al., 2008]**.

9. Conclusion

Ovarian tumors are often complex and heterogenous in nature. In this book chapter we limited our discussion to the most common ovarian tumors in adult women. This is a concise histological description of these tumors that clinicians will find useful in their daily practice.

10. References

Acien P, Abad M, Maol MJ, Garcia S, Garde J. Primary squamous cell carcinoma of the ovary associated with endometriosis. Int J Gynaecol Obstet 2010;108:16-20.

Anglesio MS, carey MS, Kobel M, Mackay H, Huntsman DG; Vancouver Ovarian Clear Cell Symposium Speakers. Clear cell carcinoma of the ovary: a report from the first ovarian clear cell symposium, June 24th, 2010. Gynecol Oncol 2011;121:407-415.

Bal A, Mohan H, Singh SB, Sehgal A. Malignant transformation in mature cystic teratoma of the ovary: report of five cases and review of the literature. Arch Gynecol Obstet 2007;275:179-182.

Bendaj A, Zaino R. GOG Pathology manual, Buffalo, NY. Gynecologic Oncologic Group 1994.

Burks RT, Sherman ME, Kurman RJ. Micropapillary serous carcinoma of the ovary: A distinctive low-grade carcinoma related to serous borderline tumors. 1996;20:1319-1330.

Chang SJ, Ryu HS, Chang KH, Yoo SC, Yoon JH. Prognostic significance of the micropapillary pattern in patients with serous borderline ovarian tumors. Acta Obstet Gynecol Scand 2008;87:476-481.

Chew I, Soslow R, Kay P. Morphologic changes in ovarian carcinoma after neoadjuvant chemotherapy: Report of a case showing extensive clear cell changes mimicking clear cell carcinoma. Int J Gynecol Pathol 2009;28:442-446.

Chu P, Wu E, Weiss LM. Cytokeratin 7 and cytokeratin 20 expression in epithelial neoplasms: A survey of 435 cases. Mod Pathol 2000;13:962-972.

DeLair D, Oliva E, Kobel M, Macias A, Gilks CB, Soslow RA. Morphologic spectrum of immunohistochemically characterized clear cell carcinoma of the ovary: a study of 155 cases. Am J Surg Pathol 2011;35:36-44.

Eichhorn JH, Young RH. Transitional cell carcinoma of the ovary: a morphologic study of 100 cases with emphasis on differential diagnosis. Am J Surg Pathol 2004;28:453-463.

Fadare O. Recent developments on the significance and pathogenesis of lymph node involvement in ovarian serous tumors of low malignant potential (borderline tumors). Int j Gynecol Cancer 2009;19:103-108.

Internatioanl Federation of Gynecology & Obstetrics. Classification and staging of malignant tumours in the female pelvis. Acta Obstet Gynecol Scand 1971;50:1-7.

Ishioka S-I, Sagae S, Terasawa K, Sugimura M, Nishioka Y, Tsukada K, Kudo R. Comparison of the usefulness between a new universal grading system for epithelial ovarian cancer and the FIGO grading system. Gynecol Oncol 2003;89:447-452.

Kaimaktchiev V, Terracciano L, Tornillo L, Spichtin H, Stoios D, Bundi M, Korcheva V, Mirlacher M, Loda M, Sauter G, Corless CL. The homeobox intestinal differentiation factor CDX2 is selectively expressed in gastrointestinal adenocarcinomas. Mod Pathol 2004;17:1392-1399.

Kurman RJ, Shih LM. Pathogenesis of ovarian cancer. Lessons from morphology and molecular biology and their clinical implications. Int J Gynecol Pathol 2008;27:151-160.

Logani S, Oliva E, Amin MB, Folpe AL, Cohen C, Young RH. Immunoprofile of ovarian tumors with putative transitional cell (urothelial) differentiation using novel urothelial markers. Histogenetic and diagnostic implications. Am J surg pathol 2003;27:1434-1441.

Malpica A, Deavers MT, Lu K, Bodurka DC, Atkinson EN, Gershenson DM, Silva EG. Grading ovarian serous carcinoma using two-tier system. Am J Surg Pathol 2004;28:496-504.

Malpica A, Deavers MT, Tornos C, Kurman RJ, Soslow R, Seidman JD, Munsell MF, Gaertner E, Frishberg D, Silva EG. Interobserver and intraobserver variability of a two-tier system for grading serous carcinoma. Am J Surg Pathol 2007; 31: 1168-1174.

May T, Virtanen C, Sharma M, Milea A, Begley H, Rosen B, Murphy KJ, Brown TJ, Shaw PA. Low malignant potential tumors with micropapillary features are moleculary similar to low-grade serous carcinoma of the ovary. Gynecol Oncol 2020;117:9-17.

McCluggage WG, Lyness RW, Atkinson RJ, Dobbs SP, Harley I, McClelland HR, Price JH. Morphological effects of chemotherapy on ovarian carcinoma. J Clin Pathol 2002;55:27-31.

McCluggage WG. The pathology of and controversial aspects of ovarian borderline tumours. Curr Opin Oncol 2010; 22:462-472.

Miller K, Price JH, Dobbs SP, McClelland RH, Kennedy K, McCluggage WG. An immunohistochemical and morphological analysis of past-chemotherapy ovarian carcinoma. J clin Pathol 2008;61:652-657.

Misdraji J. Appendiceal mucinous neoplasms. Controversial issues. Arch Pathol Lab Med 2010;134:864-870.

Mittal K, Soslow R, McCluggage WG. Application of immunohistochemistry to Gynecologic Pathology. Arch Pathol Lab Med 2008;132:402-423.

Ordonez NG. Transitional cell carcinomas of the ovary and bladder are immunophenotypically. Histopathology 2000;36:433-438.Prat J, de Nictolis M. Serous borderline tumors of the ovary. A long-term follow-up study of 137 cases, including 18 with a micropapillary pattern and 20 with microinvasion. Am J Surg Pathol 2002;26:1128-1128.

Pelkey TJ, Frierson HF, Mills SE, Stoler MH. The diagnostic utility of inhibin staining in ovarian neoplasms. Int J Gynecol Pathol 1998;17:97-105.

Ronnett BM, Zahn CM, Kurman RJ, Kass ME, Sugarbaker PH, Shmookler BM. Disseminated peritoneal adenomucinosis and peritoneal mucinous carcinomatosis; a clinicopathologic analysis of 109 caseswith emphasis on distinguishing pathologic features, site of origin, prognosis, and relationship to "pseudomyxoma peritonei". Am J Surg Pathol 1995;19:1390-1408.

Ronnett BM, Yan H, Kurman RJ, Shmookler BM, Wu L, Sugarbaker PH. Patients with pseudomyxoma peritonei associated with disseminated peritoneal adenomucinosis have a significantly more favorable prognosis than patients with peritoneal mucinous carcinomatosis. Cancer 2001;92:85-91.

Ronnett BM, Kajdacsy-Balla A, Gilks CB, Merino MJ, Silva E, Werness BA, Young RH. Mucinous borderline ovarian tumors: pints of general agreement and persistent controversies regarding nomenclature, diagnostic criteria, and behavior. Hum pathol 2004;35:949-960.

Smith Sehdev AE, Sehdev P, Kurman RJ. Noninvasive and invasive micropapillary (low-grade) serous carcinoma of the ovary: A clinicopathologic analysis of 135 cases. Am J Surg Pathol 2003;27:725-736.

Silva EG, Greshenson DM, Malpica A, Deavers M. The recurrence and the overall survival rates of ovarian serous borderline neoplasms with noninvasive implants is time dependent. Am J Surg Pathol 2006;30:1367-1371.

Silverberg SG. Histopathologic grading of ovarian carcinomas: a review and proposal. Int J Gynecol Pathol 2000;19:7-15.

Slomovitz BM, Caputo TA, Gretz HF III, Economos K, Tortoriello DV, Schlosshauer PW, Baergen RN, Isacson C, Soslow RA. A comparative analysis of 57 serous borderline tumors with and without a noninvasive micropapillary component. Am J Surg Pathol 2002;26:592-600.

Zhao C, Bratthauer GL, Barner R, Vang R. Diagnostic utility of WT1 immunostianing in ovarian Sertoli cell tumor. Am J Surg Pathol 2007;31:1378-1386.

5

Central Nervous System Involvement from Epithelial Ovarian Cancer

Gennaro Cormio, Maddalena Falagario and Luigi E. Selvaggi
University of Bari
Italy

1. Introduction

Ovarian cancer represents the leading cause of death from gynaecological cancers especially because it relapses in most of the cases.

Central nervous system and especially the encephalon are very often involved in metastatic process arising from malignancies coming from many different sites in the whole body.

The incidence of brain involvement in metastatic tumours was estimated to be around 25%, that represents a very large proportion and moreover, around 20% of the lesions found within the central nervous system are diagnosed as secondary locations of a wide spread cancer.

The most common tumours that present brain involvement are lung, breast cancers and melanomas, while the gynaecological malignancies contribute around 2% of all the brain metastases, except the trophoblastic diseases that involve the central nervous system in around 30% of the cases.

Anyway, although it was believed that central nervous system involvement from epithelial ovarian cancer was very uncommon, it is increasing of incidence.

Moreover, the comprehension of how to diagnose and treat these metastases is very important because they are usually characterized, more than the most common liver or lung metastases, by symptomatology that can severely affect the quality of life of these patients.

This new finding points out whether or not is appropriate to ask for a brain image technique in the follow up of ovarian cancer patients, and which therapy should these women receive.

Today, there are new possible therapeutic approaches including stereotactic radiosurgery, the administration of new effective and with less side effect chemotherapy agents, moreover the improvement in the neurosurgery techniques makes craniotomy from brain metastases a less riskful procedure with better outcomes.

Aim of his chapter is to analyse the clinicopathological features of these patients, the diagnosis and the different therapeutic approaches based on our experience and on all the series published in literature in the last 15 years.

2. Incidence

Central nervous system involvement from ovarian cancer is an uncommon event, but many studies published in literature agree that it is increasing in incidence. (Cormio, 2011a; Cormio 2011b; Pectasides, 2006)

The analysis of two reports present in literature about the biological behaviour of ovarian cancer in autopsied patients reveals that 1 out of 158 women with this tumour actually present a brain involvement. (Bergman, 1966; Julian, 1974)

In literature, the reported incidence ranges from 0.29 to 4.5%. (Larson, 1986; Stein, 1986; Leroux, 1991; Rodriguez, 1992; Geisler J.P. & Geisler H.E., 1995; Kaminsky-Forrett, 2000) In our recent series of 20 patients the incidence estimated was 5%. (Cormio, 2011a)

This increased incidence can be the result of three different aspects. First of all the advances in the production and management of the new chemotherapy agents have guaranteed in the last years a prolongment of life of these patients; this increased time allows the tumour to implant and grow in distant sites. Secondly, the improvement of brain image techniques allowed detecting very small lesions. Finally, the use of chemotherapy agents that seem to pass poorly the blood brain barrier results in the growth of cancer cells within the nervous tissue.

3. Ways of spread to the central nervous system

Ovarian cancer usually spreads locally into the peritoneal cavity, while the lymphatic and haematogenous route are possible but rare. Distant metastases are found in about 30% of patients and the most common localizations are liver, lungs and pleura. (Cormio, 2003a)

The dissemination of the ovarian cancer into the brain seems to occur in three possible way: via the haematogenous spread, by direct invasion of the nervous tissue after bony involvement, or in case of leptomeningeal carcinomatosis, through retrograde lymphatic spread (Pectasides, 2006)

The mechanism of meningeal dissemination is still not known, but hypothetically it should be caused by a direct invasions of the liquor through the choroid plexus, by a rupture of the brain lesions into the ventricles or subarachnoid space, or by infiltration either of the small veins in the arachnoid membrane, either of the lymphatic vessels. (Cormio, 2007).

4. Clinicopathological characteristics of the primary tumour

Different series published in literature in the last 15 years, agree that most commonly these metastases arise in patients with an advanced stage (FIGO stage III or IV), serous hystotype and poorly differentiated (G3) primary ovarian cancer (see Table 1). (Anupol, 2002; Brown III, 2005; Chen, 2009; Cohen, 2004; Cormio, 1995, 2003b, Cormio, 2011a; D'Andrea, 2005; Kastritis, 2006; Kim, 2007; Kumar, 2003; Lee, 2008; Sanderson, 2002; Sehouli, 2010; Tay & Rajesh, 2005). However Kolomainen et al. demonstrated in their series that a brain involvement could be seen quite frequently (one third of their patients) also in patients with FIGO stage I. (Kolomainen, 2002)

The median age at presentation of the ovarian cancer in patients who present brain involvement in the same series is 55,1 years, ranging from 46,7 to 60,3 years.

In most of these studies, patients were treated with the standard procedure consisting in primary optimal debulking surgery followed by platin-based chemotherapy; in particular patients of our recent study received six courses of taxol and carboplatin (Cormio, 2011a)

Clinical series (year)	No of patients	Incidence	Median age at ovarian cancer diagnosis (year)	Advanced stage disease (III-IV)	Poorly differentiated, G3 cancer	Serous hystotype
Cormio (1995)	23	-	59	20 (87%)	17 (74%)	14 (61%)
Anupol (2002)	15	1,4%	58	15 (100%)	12 (80%)	14 (93,3%)
Pothuri (2002)	14	-	59,3	13 (92,8%)	10 (71,4%)	9 (64,3%)
Sanderson (2002)	13	1,1%	55	13 (100%)	-	3 (23%)
Cormio (2003)	20	-	54	20 (92%)	12 (55%)	15 (68%)
Kumar (2003)	18	2,7%	54	16 (88,9%)	11 (55,5%)	13 (72,2%)
Cohen (2004) [1]	72	0,9%	50,4	52 (81%)	52 (83%)	14 (24%)
D'Andrea (2005)	11	-	60,3	0	-	11 (100%)
Tay & Rajesh (2005)	4	0,66%	52,5	3 (75%)	-	2 (50%)
Brown III (2005)	3	-	46,7	3 (100%)	-	2 (66,7)
Kastritis (2006) [2]	8	3%[2]	59	8 (100%)	6 (75%)	6 (75%)
Kim (2007)	13	2,7%	52	12 (92,3%)	7 (53,8%)	9 (69,2%)
Lee (2008)	15	1%	55	14 (93,3%)	-	8 (53,3%)
Sehouli (2010)	74	1,7%	53,9	62 (83,8%)	43 (58,1%)	53 (71,6%)
Chen (2011)	10	1,9%	56,6	9 (90%)	6 (60%)	7 (70%)
Cormio (2011a)	20	5%	55.5	19 (95%)	15 (75%)	14 (70%)

- data not available

[1] this study analyses all the ovarian cancer patients and not just the epithelial ones. Anyway most of patients with CNS metastases, when data were available, had a epithelial hystotype (about 93%)

[2] this study analyses only patients presented with brain involvement as isolated site of relapse, for this reason we decided not to include the incidence here calculated in the final results

Table 1. Clinicopathological characteristics of the primary ovarian cancer.

5. Clinicopathological characteristics of brain metastases

5.1 Pathology

Metastatic tumour to the brain can involve the Dura Mater and the cranial bones arising especially from breast or prostatic cancer, the leptomeninges leading to a meningeal carcinomatosis, the encephalon or the spinal cord. Metastases in the encephalon usually involve the cerebral and cerebellar hemispheres, less frequently the brainstem and the basal ganglia. Brain metastases usually arise in the zone within the cortex and the white substance that is very vascularized, only rarely they arise deeply.

Macroscopically brain metastases usually appear as grey-red nodular lesions, with or without necrotic or haemorrhagic areas. (Maiuri, 1992)

Central nervous system metastases from epithelial ovarian cancer are usually multiple and localized into the brain hemispheres, followed by the cerebellum; rarely they involve the spinal cord or a leptomeningeal dissemination is discovered. The median interval from the time of primary cancer diagnosis to the brain involvement findings is 32 months in published studies, but in some patients the brain metastases can be found as the first manifestation of the tumour, and only a deep investigation can reveal the ovarian origin. The majority of these women usually present extracranial localizations of the disease, within or not the peritoneal cavity. (See Table 2, Figures 1, 2, 3, 4)

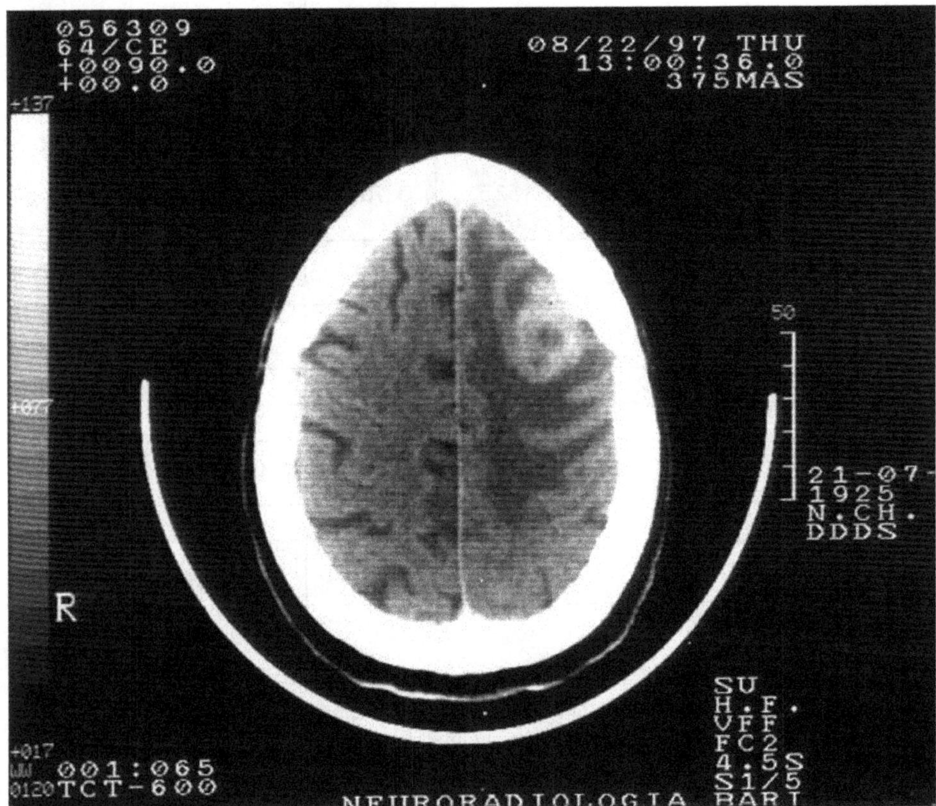

Fig. 1. Cerebral metastases from epithelial ovarian cancer.

Clinical series (year)	Mean interval to CNS metastases (months)	Patients with extracranial disease (%)	Number of CNS lesions		Localization		
			Single	Multiple	Cerebral	Cerebellar	Miscellaneous, *meningeal*
Cormio (1995)	35	14 (61%)	9 (41%)	13 (59%)	18 (78,3%)	4 (17,4%)	1 (4,3%)
Anupol (2002)	15	7 (%)	8 (53,3%)	7 (46,7%)	-	-	-
Pothuri (2002)	42	8 (57%)	12 (85,7%)	2 (14,3%)	12 (85,7%)	2 (14,3%)	0
Sanderson (2002)	36	8 (61,5%)	8 (61,5%)	5 (38,5%)	9 (69,2%)	2 (11,4%)	2 (11,4%)
Cormio (2003)	29	13 (59%)	-	-	18 (82%)	4 (18%)	0
Kumar (2003)	29	13 (72,2%)	5 (27,8%)	13 (72,2%)	13 (72,2%)	2 (11,1%)	3 (16,7%)
Cohen (2004) [1]	22	41 (57%)	25 (35%)	47 (65%)	19 (27%)	6 (8%)	47, *3* (65%)
D'Andrea (2005)	21	0	11 (100%)	0	9 (81,8%)	2 (18,2%)	0
Tay & Rajesh (2005)	16,5	4 (100%)	0	4 (100%)	1 (25%)	0	3, *1* (75%)
Brown III (2005)	19	0	1 (33,3%)	2 (66,7%)	0	1 (33,3%)	2 (66,7%)
Kastritis (2006) [2]	17,2	0	4 (50%)	4 (50%)	-	-	-
Kim (2007)	28	7 (53,8%)	2 (15,4%)	11 (84,6%)	6 (46,2%)	1 (7,7%)	6 (46,1%)
Lee (2008)	28 [3]	5 (33,3%)	5 (33,3%)	10 (66,7%)	-	-	-
Sehouli (2010)	28,8	35 (47,3%)	26 (21,4%)	48 (64,8%)	-	-	-
Chen (2011)	24,3	7 (70%)	1 (10%)	9 (90%)			
Cormio (2011a)	32,7	11 (55%)	11 (55%)	9 (45%)	9 (45%)	5 (25%)	6 (30%)

- data not available

[1] this study analyses all the ovarian cancer patients and not just the epithelial ones. Anyway most of patients with CNS metastases, when data were available, had a epithelial hystotype (about 93%)

[2] this study analyses only patients presented with brain involvement as isolated site of relapse, for this reason we decided not to include the incidence here calculated in the final results

[3] in this value are excluded two patients whose brain involvement was discovered at the same time of the ovarian cancer findings

Table 2. Clinicopathological characteristic of the brain metastases.

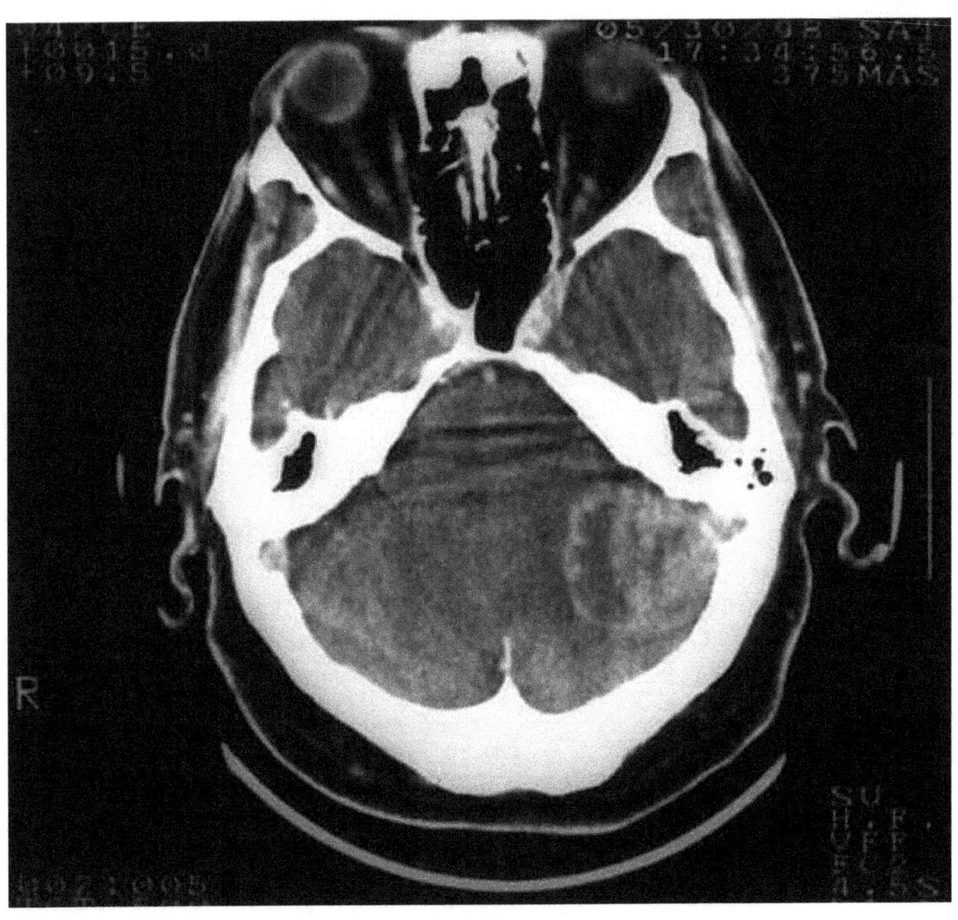

Fig. 2. Cerebellar metastases from epithelial ovarian cancer.

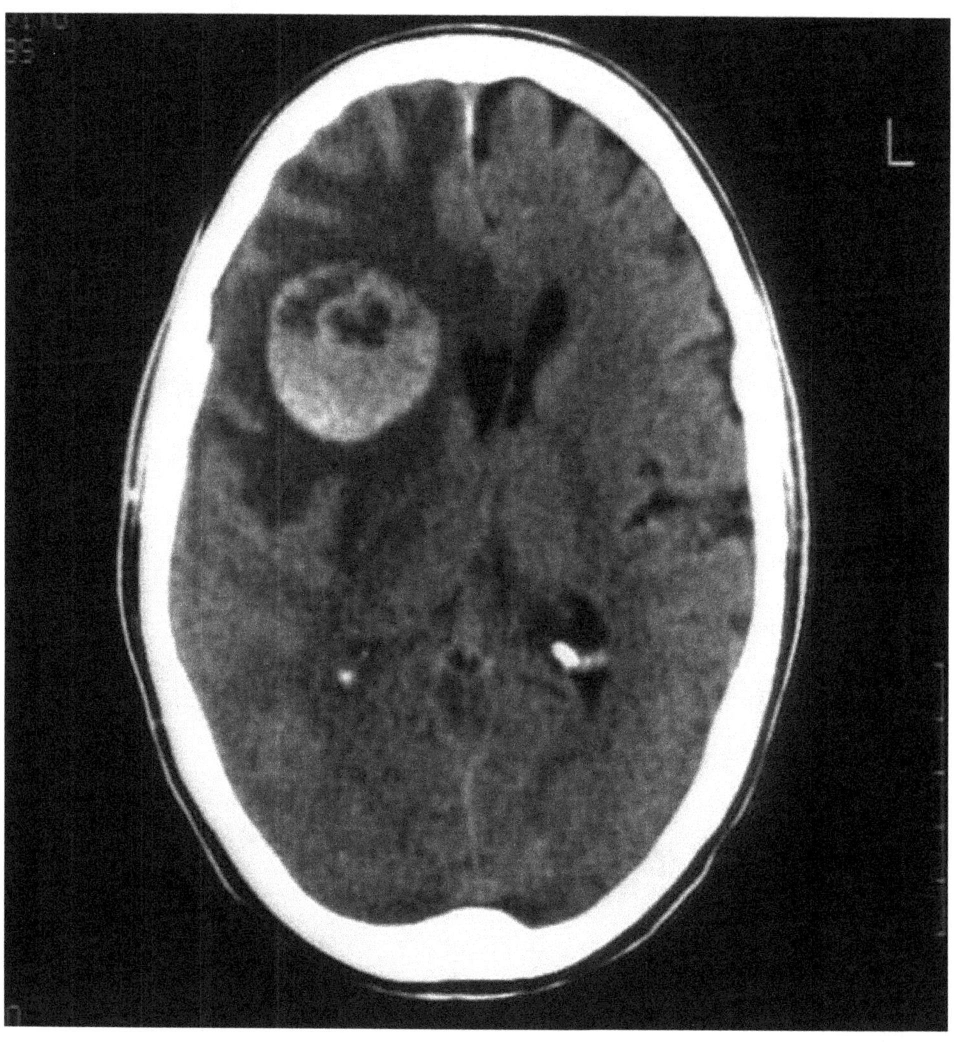

Fig. 3. Single brain metastases from epithelial ovarian cancer.

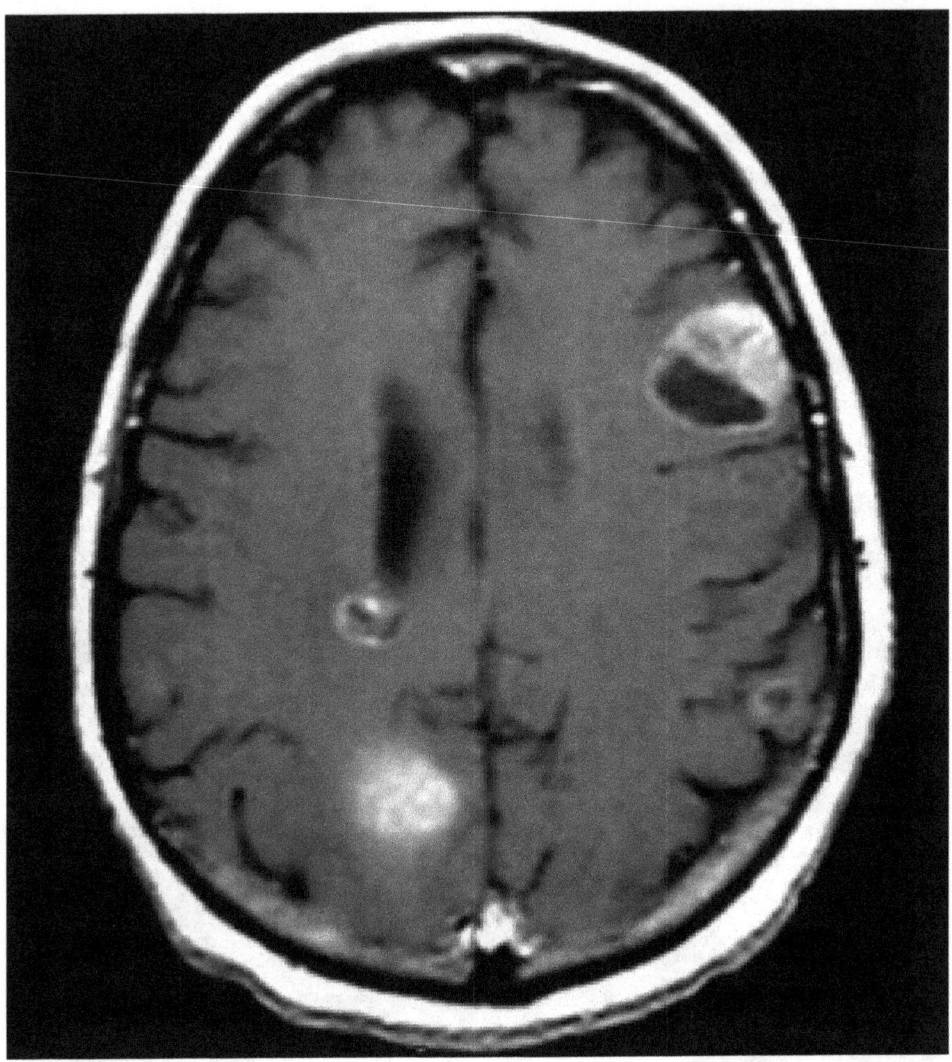

Fig. 4. Multiple brain metastases from epithelial ovarian cancer.

5.2 Clinical manifestations

The symptoms at the diagnosis of these metastases, like all central nervous system tumours, can be mild usually with an unspecific symptomatology or severe with, for example epilepsy or focal neurological deficit.

In some cases the metastases can be diagnosed after a stroke, caused by an embolism of cancer cells; in these cases usually the patients at first complain of some sort of neurological deficit that can resolve in few days, but some weeks after the clinical manifestations get quickly worse for the implant and growth of the cancer. (Maiuri, 1992)

Patients with central nervous system dissemination from ovarian cancer most commonly complain of headache, which is probably a consequence of the increased intracranial pressure caused by the oedema or the hydrocephalus, more then a consequence of the mass of the lesion itself.

Other symptoms that are often described are vomiting, confusions, visual disturbances, paresis, and weakness, loss of consciousness, seizures, and dizziness. (Cohen, 2004; Cormio, 2003; Cormio, 2011a; D'Andrea, 2005; Lee, 2008; Pectasides, 2006; Tay &Rajesh, 2005)

The leptomeningeal involvement usually causes an arise of the intracranial pressure associated with hydrocephalus; these patients more frequently than the others complain also for bowel of bladder dysfunctions, while the involvement of cranial nerves can also be possible. (Pectasides, 2006; Vitaliani R, 2009)

In our recent series of 20 patients, all patients were symptomatic at the moment of the diagnosis; most of them complain of headache, vomiting and dizziness with or without balance disturbances, less frequent symptoms were diplopia, convulsions, amnesia, confusion and pain. One patient had a left hemiparesis caused by a metastases localized in the right parietal lobe. (Cormio, 2011a)

6. Diagnosis

The diagnosis is usually suspected when a patient with ovarian cancer complains about any neurological symptoms, although asymptomatic cases are not infrequent. The symptoms themselves can already also suggest the localization of the lesions in some cases.

6.1 Imaging features

It is necessary, in our opinion, to perform either a computed tomography (CT) scan or a magnetic resonance imaging (MRI) in any patient with a history of ovarian cancer, who has any neurological defect.

Usually the first diagnosis is done both by the clinical examination that reveals neurological signs and by pre and post contrast CT scan, less commonly clinicians ask for an MRI.

The two image techniques are both effective, even if MRI seems to be the modality of choice because it has an higher resolution than CT scan, it is able to detect lesions as small as 1,9 mm; moreover MRI seems to be more effective especially for the image study of the lesions localized in the posterior fossa. (Pectasides, 2006).

In a CT scan, metastatic lesions appear as ring areas, singular or multiple, slightly hyper dense, homogeneous or not and commonly surrounded by oedema. Sometimes the metastases can have a hypo dense core for the presence of central necrosis or of a central abscess, which can sometimes simulate the diagnosis of an inflammatory abscess.

The administration of an intravenous contrast medium has been shown to enhance the sensitivity of the technique, moreover Davis et al also demonstrated that a delaying imaging after the administration and an increased volume of contrast also can increase the detection rate. (Davis, 1991)

In MRI the brain metastases appear as hypo intense nodular areas, the administration of the contrast medium (gadolinium) enhances the intensity in the image.

The most important differential diagnosis should be done with primary brain tumours, vascular conditions like strokes or haemorrhages and intracranial abscess.

Metastatic lesions, usually, can be differentiated from primary central nervous system tumours, because more frequently they are multiple and surrounded by larger areas of oedema (larger than primary tumours of the same size). Finally, the metastatic lesions
Further studies should investigate the benefits of using new image techniques as positron emission tomography or magnetic resonance spectroscopy for the diagnosis of central nervous system involvement from epithelial ovarian cancer.

6.2 Leptomenigeal carcinomatosis

The meningeal carcinomatosis from epithelial ovarian cancer is often difficult to diagnose, in fact CT scans even with contrast medium injection can be negative.
CT images usually show the presence of solid areas in the parenchyma and hydrocephalus (Chung, 2001), but not directly the presence of leptomeningeal metastases. For this reason the presence of meningeal involvement should be suspected in patient with ovarian cancer and hydrocephalus, and further investigations should be performed.
The image of choice in these patients is the contrast enhanced MRI, while the non-contrast one has been showed to be as ineffective as CT scan. (Collie, 1999)
In patients with meningeal carcinomatosis the diagnosis can be done also by the cytological analysis of the cerebrospinal fluid that reveal the presence of ovarian cancer malignant cells. (Pectasides, 2006)

6.3 The role of Ca125

The serum marker Ca125 is the strongest tumour marker for the presence of ovarian cancer. An increased value of Ca125 can be or not observed in patients with brain involvement from ovarian cancer.
In our experience we noticed that usually it arises in patients with brain involvement, who were already found to have high concentration of the tumour marker at the first diagnosis of the ovarian cancer, even if sometimes it arises also in patients without an history of increased Ca125, or it does not arise in patients for whom this lab value was used as a strong and efficient marker of the presence of the cancer during the previous therapies.
In any case, as for the primary ovarian cancer in patients with positive Ca125, this marker can be used during and after the therapy of the brain metastases in order to assess the response of the cancer to the treatment and the presence or absence of the disease during the follow up.

7. Therapy

7.1 Treatments options and clinical decisions

When it comes to decide about the different types of treatments, the first things to think about is the quality of life of these patients, in fact in very few cases limited to those patients with a good performance status, single metastases and without any sign of extracranial disease the intent of the therapy can be curative.
As already showed, a large proportion of these patients present with extracranial disease and multiple metastases, in these women it is very unlikely that any treatment of central nervous system metastases chosen can be curative, so the primary roles of the therapy must be the improvement of symptoms, the avoidance of life threatening conditions and the increase of life expectance.
Moreover, other important things to consider are the patients performance status, age, status of the disease, previous treatments and their results. All these aspects added to the

clinicopathological characteristics of the metastatic brain lesions should be strictly studied to assess the risk-benefit of each treatment modality.

Treatment options are: in emergency the therapy of the life threatening complications like increased intracranial pressure, obstructing hydrocephalus and severe epilepsy, no treatment in patients not eligible of any therapy, corticosteroids, radiotherapy administrated as whole brain radiotherapy or stereotactic radiosurgery, surgery and chemotherapy.

Due to the rarity of these metastases, this condition has not already had any guidelines that can be followed in the choice of treatment, for this reason is very important that the expert gynaecologist oncologist cooperate with the neuroradiologist and the neurosurgeon in order to decide what is best management for each patients with brain involvement from epithelial ovarian cancer.

7.2 Corticosteroids, mannitol and antiepileptic agents

The intracranial oedema is very common in women with brain metastases from epithelial ovarian cancer; it results from the damage of the blood brain barrier caused by the tumour itself that leads to an increase of the barrier permeability, with a passage of sodium and water molecules into the brain tissues.

For this reason almost all patients with this condition is eligible of receiving corticosteroids therapy just after the first diagnosis of brain involvement. In fact, corticosteroids are very effective drugs especially in reducing the surrounded oedema of these metastatic lesions, resulting in a decrease of intracranial pressure.

The mechanism of action of corticosteroids is to decrease the oedema by decreasing the permeability of the blood brain barrier and the passage of water and ions into the cerebral parenchyma. This drugs in long term administrations can lead to severe side effects like diabetes and hyperglycaemia, osteoporosis, hypertension, thyroid deficiency, hypogonadism and male impotence, cataract and several others.

The preferred molecule is the dexamethasone because of its lower mineralocorticoids effects that results in fewer side effects. The starting dose is usually 4 mg administered intravenously or orally 4 times daily, after the stabilization of the clinical manifestations the dose should be gradually decreased in a long period of few weeks, to reduce the side effects of a long corticosteroid treatment on the entire metabolism of the patients.

Corticosteroids administered in patients with metastatic brain involvement from epithelial ovarian cancer, results in few hours (usually 6- 24 hours) in the improvement of the headache and the generalized neurological symptoms, while the focal neurological deficits are less effectively improved.

The maximum result is seen usually after few days of corticosteroids treatment, but in a large number of patients their action lasts after some days from the end of the administration.

Mannitol is an osmotic diuretic that administered intravenously is effective in reducing intracranial pressure in acute cases, but with repeated administration can give a rebound effect and worsen the oedema, for this reason is used only for acutely decompensating patients in association to corticosteroids.

Some patients with brain involvement from ovarian cancer can develop convulsions and epilepsy. The prophylactic use of anticonvulsant agents is not indicated, but in patients who present epilepsy these should be administered; the most common drugs used in the clinical practice are the valproate, phenobarbital, phenytoin and carbamazepine. Phenytoin is our anticonvulsant of choice because it is usually effective, well tolerated and it can be administered both parenterally and orally.

Corticosteroids and mannitol with or without valproate or other antiepileptic drugs are usually administered in patients with multiple metastases and bad clinical conditions. Several studies present in literature demonstrated that the median survival after brain metastases involvement diagnosis in patients treated with corticosteroids alone is about 2 months, and that this value is similar to the median survival obtained in patients treated with palliative therapy with any kind of central nervous system metastatic disease. (Cohen, 2004; Kaminsky-Forrett, 2000; Pectasides, 2005; Pectasides, 2006; Markesbery, 1978; Ruderman, 1965)

7.3 Radiotherapy

The irradiation of the entire brain (whole brain radiotherapy) has been considered for years alone or after surgery, or with chemotherapy the modality of choice in the treatment of metastatic malignancies to the brain with or without extracranial disease. The standard dose for patients who are not eligible of surgery is 30 Gy administered in 10 fractions over a period of 2 weeks. Higher daily doses can be administered to reduce the duration of the treatment, but they cause more commonly a late onset encephalopathy, a severe condition that should be avoided especially in patients with a higher life expectancy. (Dropcho, 1991; Rottenberg, 1977).

This therapeutic approach can actually increase survival and relieve symptoms by reducing the oedema. It is effective in most patients on the headache, convulsions, cognitive and other neurological deficiency, moreover it also let to decrease the corticosteroids doses. Series of patients present in literature who received a uni modal treatment consisting only in whole brain radiotherapy revealed that it leads to a median survival of about 5 months, ranging from 1,5 to 27 months. (Cohen, 2004; Kaminsky-Forrett, 2000; Kumar, 2003; Pectasides, 2006; Sood, 1996)

7.4 Stereotactic radiosurgery

Stereotactic radiosurgery represents an important alternative to the surgical approach. It is a special form of radiotherapy where high doses of radiatons are delivered to the metastases using a linear accelerator or, in gamma knife radiosurgery, using a gamma knife without any surgical incision. (Edwend, 2001; Lassman, 2003; Monaco, 2008; Yo Kyung Lee, 2008)

The administered dose is inversally proportioned to the diameter of the lesion; usually for lesions smaller than 3 cm the dose is 18-20 Gy. These metastases are usually small, circular and with radiological margins well defined. More than primary brain tumours, metastatic brain tumours are suitable of being treated with stereotactic radiosurgery. (Soffietti, 2002)

Stereotactic surgery has been proven in several reports to be a good therapeutic approach for patients with brain metastases, because these cause rapid reduction of the symptomatology and of the dimensions of the lesions, with lower invasiveness.

This radiotherapy technique has a lower morbidity than surgical approach and so can be admistered also in local anesthesia in patients with systemic clinical conditions that are not suitable for general anesthesia; moreover it has also economic advantages because it does not required hospitalization.

When comparing radiosurgery with whole brain radiotherapy, it is proven that the first one has less long term side effects, such as cognitve problems.

Patients who are eligible for it are especially those with small metastases, deep seated and so surgically inaccesible lesions. (Monaco, 2008; Combs, 2004)
Anyway, there are some controversial in literature about the role of stereotactic radiosurgery, for example studies showing that these techniques does not have any impact on survival (Andrews, 2004) or that it improves outcomes only in patients with single metastases and not with multiple ones. (Pectasides, 2006)
In conclusion, for these reasons stereotactic radiosurgery is now preferred for those patients who are not eligible for surgery, with single lesions or with deep seated surgically inaccesible metastases.

7.5 Surgery

Surgical management can be used with different aims. First of all it can be used in case the diagnosis is not clear, in fact the histological examination done after surgery can clarify the diagnosis especially in those cases where the brain involvement is the first sign of the ovarian cancer and there is no clear evidence of the presence of the primary disease. Secondly, surgical approach can be also used to reduce the symptoms by removing the lesions and so the pressure that the mass causes on the brain parenchyma. Finally, surgery can be used with curative aims or in every case it is necessary to control the local intracranial disease to improve the clinical conditions and let clinicians administer other treatments for the systemic disease.
Many studies demonstrated that the surgical approach represents the best treatment modality for patients with brain involvement from epithelial cancer that are eligible for it. (Cormio, 2003; Cormio, 2011a; Cormio, 2011b; Pothuri, 2002)
For patients who are not good candidates, with extracranial sign of disease or multiple metastases, craniotomy can control symptomatology, avoid life-threatening complications; improve quality of life and also overall survival. (Buckner, 1992; Pectasides, 2006)
In a series of 56 patients, treated in our centre, with a diagnosis of central nervous system metastases from ovarian carcinoma, 22 underwent surgical resection of solitary brain metastases and survived 16 months, while the other 34 women, who were not eligible for surgery, survived only 4 months. (Cormio, 2003)
In conclusion the surgical approach should be chosen always if there are the following conditions:

- the cerebral metastases are single and superficial
- There are no radiological signs of the presence of the disease at other sites, or the activity of the primary tumour is well control
- The clinical conditions of the patients are good

7.6 Chemotherapy

The role of chemotherapy in the treatment of brain metastases from ovarian cancer is still on debate. As already précised above, the increasing rate of these metastases observed in the last few years has been attributed to chemotherapy drugs. (Lassman, 2003; Lesser, 1996).
This therapeutic approach has some advantages, such as the simple way of administration that in most cases can be done on outpatient basis or with few days hospitalization, its action on cancer cells that can be eventually presents in the whole body and the fact that it does not damage the brain tissues causing dementia or brain atrophy (Pectasides, 2006)

On the other side, the poor clinical conditions of some patients, the aggressivity of these treatments and the fact that many chemotherapy agents seem not to pass the blood brain barrier can contraindicate this procedure.

Many authors demonstrated that chemotherapy actually results in a remission of the disease and in an increased survival (Cooper, 1994; Cormio, 1995, Rodriguez, 1992; Watanabe, 2005)

An analysis conducted on 15 studies by Mc Meekin et al showed that chemotherapy has an important role because is the only therapeutic approach that, as the surgical treatment, really improves survival. (Mc Meekin, 2001).

The best choice for their ability to pass the blood brain barrier seem to be cisplatin and other platin-based drugs, etoposide, gemcitabine, docetaxel (Cormio, 1995; Melichar, 2004; Rodriguez, 1992; Vlasved, 1990; Salvati, 1994; Watanabe, 2005)

7.7 Multimodal approaches

In our experience but also in several series reported in literature the best approach for patients with brain involvement from epithelial cancer seems to be the multimodal approach; in our recent study, we demonstrated that craniotomy followed by radiotherapy and/or chemotherapy results in median survival of about 18 months. (Cormio, 2011a).

The best multimodal approach is supposed to have a double effect, on one side a local therapy such as craniotomy or stereotactic radiosurgery or whole brain radiotherapy is administered to remove and control the local spread of the cancer within the brain, on the other side the systemic treatment is able to control the wide spread of the disease.

In conclusion, the best combinations of therapies, from our experience, are surgery plus radiotherapy and eventually chemotherapy that in our opinion is the best choice for patients with extracranial disease, stereotactic radiotherapy plus whole brain radiotherapy and eventually chemotherapy.

7.8 Therapy of neoplastic meningitis

The neoplastic meningitis has been reported in very few studies, for this reason the therapeutic approach that should be chosen for this patients is currently not defined.

The therapy of neoplastic neoplastic meningitis usually consists in radiotherapy and intracerebrospinal fluid chemotherapy like intrathecal methotrexate (Chamberlain, 2005; Cormio, 2007).

Most patients who present leptomenigeal dissemination of ovarian cancer have also a wide spread dissemination of the disease, with poor clinical conditions and aggressive treatments that are usually indicated in these conditions can give more damages than benefits; for this reason plus the fact that the choice of any clinical approach must take into account first of all the improvement of the quality of life of these patients, the treatment choice is usually very difficult and must be decided for each patients.

8. Survival and prognostic factors

Although many efforts and improvements in diagnosis and treatment of central nervous system metastases from epithelial ovarian cancer have been already reached, the prognosis of this condition is still poor. In the studies present in literature the overall survivals calculated from the time of the diagnosis of the brain involvement range from 4 to 10 months. (Table 3, Figure 5)

Clinical series (year)	Survival (months) [1]
Cormio (1995)	5
Anupol (2002)	6
Pothuri (2002)	18
Sanderson (2002)	4
Cormio (2003) [2]	16
Kumar (2003)	4
Cohen (2004)	6,27
D'Andrea (2005) [3]	28
Tay & Rajesh (2005)	19,5
Brown III (2005)	-
Kastritis (2006)	-
Kim (2007)	7
Lee (2008)	14
Sehouli (2010)	6,2
Chen (2011)	3
Cormio (2011a)	17,6

- data not available
[1] the survival was calculated from the time of diagnosis of CNS metastases
[2] this study analyses only patients with solitary brain metastases who underwent surgical resection
[3] this study analyses only patients treated with surgical en bloc removal and postoperative radio-chemotherapy

Table 3. Survival in the series present in literature.

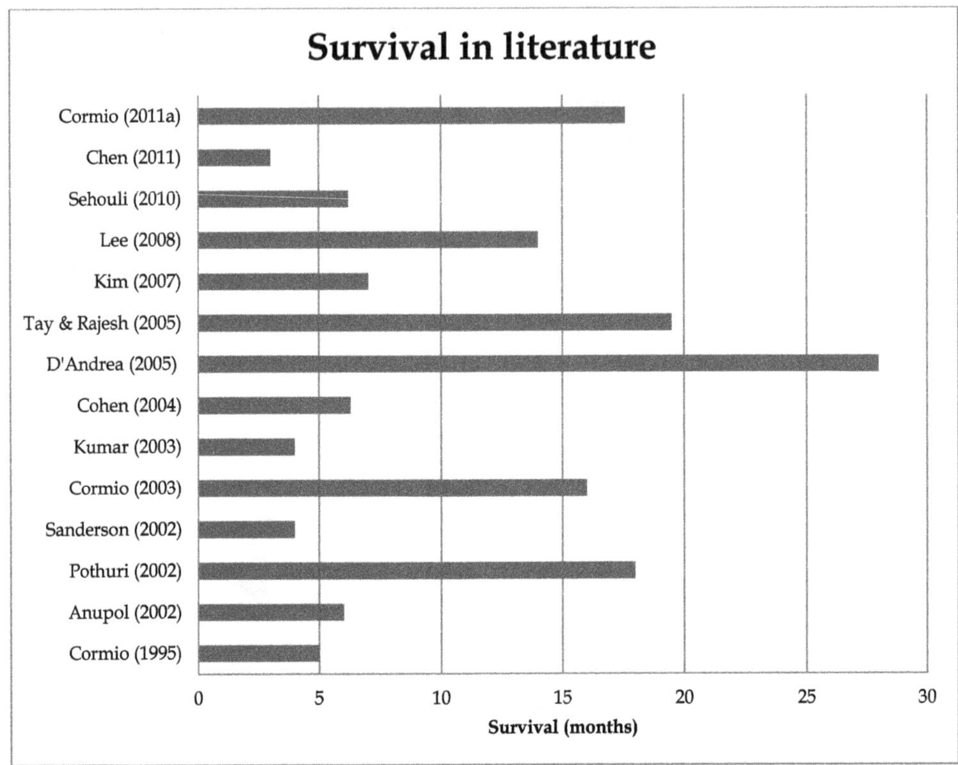

Fig. 5. Survival in the series present in literature.

Different studies present in literature demonstrated that the prognostic factors that significantly affect survival of patients with brain involvement from ovarian cancer are the presence of extracranial disease, the number of brain metastases and the treatment approaches (multi-modal therapy prolong survival in most of the studies. The prognostic factors of each study analysed are shown in Table 4.

9. Changes from the past and future prospective

In a recent study (Cormio, 2011b), we compared the a series of patients from 1995 and a series of patients from 2010 all with diagnosis of epithelial ovarian cancer and brain metastases in order to assess the difference in management and outcomes of this condition. We demonstrated that, even if the clinicopathological features both of the primary tumour and the metastases were similar in the two groups, the survival triplicate in the last 15 years going from 5 months to 18 months. This difference can be attributed to the change in the therapeutic approach. In fact, while in 1995 the therapy was given more with palliative intent, nowadays clinicians are more likely to administer more aggressive and multimodal treatments, with the intent of both improving the quality of life and the overall survival. (Anupol, 2002; Brown III, 2005; Chen, 2009; Cohen, 2004; Cormio, 1995; Cormio, 2003b; Cormio, 2011a; D'Andrea, 2005; Kastritis, 2006; Kim, 2007; Lee, 2008; Sanderson, 2002; Sehouli, 2010; Tay & Rajesh, 2005)

Study	Prognostic factors
Cormio (1995)	- number of lesions - extracranial disease - treatment (P vs RT vs O RT)
Anupol (2002)	- extracranial disease - treatment (survival with RT+O+CT > RT+O >RT+CT>RT)
Cormio (2003)	- extracranial disease - interval between ovarian cancer diagnosis and brain involvement findings - treatment (survival with O > no O)
Kumar (2003)	- serous hystotype - grade (survival in I-II > III- IV) - optimal primary surgery - extracranial disease
Cohen (2004)	*Univariate analysis* - extracranial disease - treatment (RT+O > RT or O alone> P) *Multivariate analysis* - treatment (RT+O > RT or O alone> P)
Kim (2007)	*Univariate analysis* - Karnofsky performance status > 70 better prognosis - primary lesion (controlled vs not controlled) - number of CNS metastases (single > multiple) - RPA prognostic classification (I >II>III) - extracranial disease - treatment (GKRS vs without GKRS) *Multivariate analysis* - RPA prognostic classification (I >II>III) - treatment (GKRS vs without GKRS)
Lee (2008)	- treatment (GKRS > WBRT)
Sehouli (2010)	- number of CNS metastases (single > multiple) - Karnofsky performance status > 60 better prognosis - platinum sensitive diseases have better survival - grading - FIGO stage NB: no multimodal therapy and extracranial metastases
Cormio (2011a)	- FIGO stage - extracranial disease - treatment (O >no O; multimodal>unimodal treatment) - response after brain metastases therapy (complete > incomplete or absent)

Table 4. Prognostic factors in the studies present in literature.

Future efforts can be put on one side, on the improvement of early diagnosis by the investigation of the role of new imaging techniques such as positron emission tomography and magnetic resonance spectroscopy in the detection of brain metastases, and on the other side on the improvement of treatment modality with higher efficacy and lower morbidity like the new radio surgical techniques. Although many authors agree that a multimodal approach results in better prognosis, further studies should be done to fix some guidelines for the treatment of these patients.

Finally, further studies are also needed to investigate the role of chemotherapy especially in patients with both brain metastases and extracranial metastases from ovarian cancer, in order to find a therapy that can control both the local and systematic manifestations of these cancer.

10. Conclusions

In conclusion, even if brain metastases from ovarian cancer have always been considered an uncommon event, they are increasing of incidence. All patients with ovarian cancer who present neurological symptoms must undergo a CT or MRI scan of the brain.

The treatment choice must take into account the clinicopathological characteristics of the metastases and of primary cancer, the presence of extracranial disease and obviously the performance status of the patients. Moreover the therapy should be aim both to have a remission of the disease and to improve the quality of life.

Patients with poor performance status and/or multiple and not isolated metastases usually undergo palliative therapy consisting in mannitol, corticosteroids and anticonvulsant. In patients who are eligible for therapy the possibilities include: craniotomy, stereotactic radiosurgery (including the new gamma knife one), whole brain radiotherapy and chemotherapy. These approaches can be combined in multi-modal treatments.

Although older studies suggested that these patients should undergone only palliative management, in the last 15 year's published studies many authors agree that a multi-modal treatment is the modality of choice in selected patients and can achieve a long-term remission and a better quality of life. (Anupol, 2002; Brown III, 2005; Chen, 2009; Cohen, 2004; Cormio, 1995; Cormio, 2003b; Cormio, 2011a; D'Andrea, 2005; Kastritis, 2006; Kim, 2007; Lee, 2008; Sanderson, 2002; Sehouli, 2010; Tay & Rajesh, 2005).

An aggressive multimodal approach should be aimed both to cure local and systemic disease and leads to an improvement in duration and quality of life.

Multi centre studies should investigate the better combination of surgery, radiotherapy and chemotherapy giving particular attention to the role of different antineoplastic drugs in order to find a standard treatment for these patients.

11. References

Andrews, D. W.; Scott, C. B.; Sperduto P. W.; Flanders, A. E.; Gaspar, L. E.; Schell, M. C.; Werner-Wasik, M.; Demas, W.; Ryu, J.; Bahary, J. P.; Souhami, L.; Rotman, M.; Mehta, M. P.; Curran, W. J. Jr (2004) Whole brain radiation therapy with or without stereotactic radiosurgery boost for patients with one to three brain metastases: phase III results of the RTOG 9508 randomised trial. *Lancet*. 363:1665–1672.

Anupol, N.; Ghamande, S.; Odunsi, K.; Driscoll, D.; Lele, S. (2002) Evaluation of prognostic factors and treatment modalities in ovarian cancer patients with brain metastases. *Gynecologic Oncology.* Jun;85(3):487-92.

Bergman, F. (1966) Carcinoma of the ovary: a clinicopathological study of 86 autopsied cases with special reference to mode of spread. *Acta Obstetricia et Gynecologica Scandinavica.* 45:211-231

Brown, J.V. 3rd; Goldstein, B.H.; Duma, C.M.; Rettenmaier, M.A., Micha J.P. (2005) Gamma-knife radiosurgery for the treatment of ovarian cancer metastatic to the brain. *Gynecologic Oncology* 97:858–861.

Chamberlain, M. C. (2005) Neoplastic meningitis. *Journal of Clinical Oncology.* 23:3605-3613

Chen, Y.L.; Cheng, W.; Hsieh, C.; Chen, C. (2011)Brain metastasis as a late manifestation of ovarian carcinoma. *European Journal of Cancer Care.* 20: 44-49

Chung, P.; Allerton, R. (2001) Malignant meningitis secondary to ovarian carcinoma: an unusual occurrence. *Clinical Oncology (The Royal College of Radiologists).* 13:112 - 113.

Cohen, Z.R.; Suki, D.; Weinberg, J.S.; Marmor, E.; Lang, F.F.; Gershenson, D.M.; Sawaya, R. (2004) Brain metastases in patients with ovarian carcinoma: prognostic factors and outcome. Journal of Neurooncology. Feb; 66(3):313-25.

Collie, D. A.; Brush, J. P.; Lammie, G. A.; Grant, R.; Kunkler, I.; Leonard, R.; Gregor, A.; Sellar, R. J. (1999) Imaging features of leptomeningeal metastases. *Clinical Radiology,* 54:765 - 771.

Cooper, K. G.; Kitchener, H. C.; Parkin, D. E. (1994) Cerebral metastases from epithelial ovarian carcinoma treated with carboplatin. *Gynecologic Oncology.* 55:318–323.

Cormio, G.; Maneo, A.; Parma, G.; Pittelli, M.R.; Miceli, M.D.; Bonazzi, C. (1995) Central nervous system metastases in patients with ovarian carcinoma. *Annals of Oncology* 6:571-574.

Cormio, G.; Loizzi, V.; Selvaggi, L.E. (2007) Leptomeningeal involvement after remission of brain metastases from ovarian cancer. *International Journal of Gynaecology & Obstetrics.* Nov;99(2):139.

Cormio, G.; Rossi, C.; Cazzolla, A.; Resta, L.; Loverro, G.; Greco, P.; Selvaggi, L.E. (2003) Distant metastases in ovarian carcinoma. *International Journal of Gynecological Cancer.* 13(2): 125-9

Cormio, G.; Maneo, A.; Colamaria, A.; Loverro, G.; Lissoni, A.; Selvaggi, L. (2003) Surgical resection of solitary brain metastasis from ovarian carcinoma. An analysis of 22 cases. *Gynecologic Oncology* 89: 116-119

Cormio, G.; Loizzi, V.; Falagario, M.; Calace, A.; Colamaria, A.; De Tommasi, A.; Selvaggi, L.E. (2011) Central nervous system metastases from epithelial ovarian cancer: prognostic factors and outcomes. *International Journal of Gynecological Cancer* 21(5):816-21

Cormio, G.; Loizzi, V.; Falagario, M.; Lissoni, A.A.; Resta, L.; Selvaggi, L.E. (2011) Changes in the management and outcome of central nervous system involvement from ovarian cancer since 1994. *International Journal of Gynecology and Obstetric* 114(2):133-6

D'Andrea, G.; Roperto, R.; Dinia, L.; Caroli, E.; Salvati, M.; Ferrante, L. (2005) Solitary cerebral metastases from ovarian epithelial carcinoma: 11 cases. *Neurosurgical Review.* Apr;28(2):120-3.

Davis, P. C.; Hudgins, P. A.; Peterman, S. B.; Hoffman, J. C. Jr. (1991) Diagnosis of cerebral metastases: double-dose delayed CT vs contrast-enhanced MR imaging. *American Journal of Neuroradiology* Mar-Apr;12(2):293-300

Dropcho, E.J. (1991) Central nervous system injury by therapeutic irradiation. *Neurologic Clinics* 9:969-988

Ewend, M. G.; Carey, L. A.; Morris D. E.; Harvey, R. D.; Hensing, T. A. (2001) Brain metastases. *Current Treatment Options in Oncology.* 2:537–547.

Geisler, J.P. & Geisler, H.E. (1995) Brain metastases in epithelial ovarian carcinoma. *Gynecologic Oncology.* May;57:246-9.

Julian, C. G.; Goss, J.; Blanchard, K.; Woodruff, J. D.(1974) Biologic behavior of primary ovarian malignancy. *Obstetrics & Gynecology.* 44:873-884

Kaminsky-Forrett, M.C.; Weber, B.; Conroy, T.; & Spaeth, D. (2000) Brain metastases from epithelial ovarian carcinoma. *International Journal of Gynecological Cancer* **10**, 366–371.

Kastritis, E.; Efstathiou, E.; Gika, D.; Bozas, G.; Koutsoukou, V.; Papadimitriou, C.; Pissakas, G.; Dimopoulos, M.A.; Bamias, A. (2006) Brain metastases as isolated site of relapse in patients with epithelial ovarian cancer previously treated with platinum and paclitaxel-based chemotherapy. *International Journal of Gynecological Cancer.* May-Jun;16(3):994-9.

Kim, T.J.; Song, S.; Kim, C.K.; Kim, W.Y.; Choi, C.H.; Lee, J.H.; Lee, J.W.; Bae, D.S.; Kim, B.G. (2007)Prognostic factors associated with brain metastases from epithelial ovarian carcinoma. *International Journal of Gynecological Cancer.* Nov-Dec;17(6):1252-7.

Kolomainen, D.F.; Larkin, J.M; Badran, M.; A'Hern, R.P.; King, D.M.; Fisher, C.; Bridges, J.E.; Blake, P.R.; Barton, D.P.; Shepherd, J.H.; Kaye, S.B.; Gore, M.E. (2002) Epithelial ovarian cancer metastazing to the brain: a late manifestation of the disease with an increasing incidence. *Journal of Clinical Oncology* **20**, 982-986.

Kumar, L.; Barge, S.; Mahapatra, A. K.; Thulkar, S.; Rath, G. K.; Kumar, S.; Mishra, R.; Dawar, R.; Singh, R. (2003) Central nervous system metastases from primary epithelial ovarian cancer. *Cancer Control.* May-Jun;10(3):244-53.

Lassman, A. B.; DeAngelis, L. M. (2003) Brain metastases. *Neurologic Clinics.* 21: 1-23.

Larson, D.M.; Copeland, L.J.; Moser, R.P.; Malone, J.M.; Gershenson, D.M.; Wharton, J.T. (1986) Central nervous system metastases in epithelial ovarian carcinoma. *Obstetrics and Gynecology* 68, 746–750.

Lee, Y.K.; Park, N.H.; Kim, J.W.; Song, Y.S.; Kang, S.B.; Lee, H.P. (2008) Gamma-knife radiosurgery as an optimal treatment modality for brain metastases from epithelial ovarian cancer. *Gynecologic Oncology.* Mar;108(3):505-9.

Leroux, P.D.; Berger, M.S.; Elliot, P.; Tamimi, H. (1991) Cerebral metastases from ovarian carcinoma. *Cancer* 67, 2194–2199.

Lesser, G. J. (1996) Chemotherapy of cerebral metastases from solid tumors. *Neurosurgery Clinics of North America.* 7:527–536.

Maiuri, F.; D'Andrea, F. (1992) Neurochirurgia (second edition), Editoriale Bios s.a.s., Cosenza, Italy.

Markesbery W. R.; Brooks W. H.; Gupta G. D.; Young A. B. (1978) Treatment for patients with cerebral metastases. *Archives of Neurology.* 35:754–756.

McMeekin, D. S.; Kamelle, S. A.; Vasilev, S. A.; Tillmanns, T. D.; Gould, N. S.; Scribner, D. R.; Gold, M. A.; Guruswamy, S.; Mannel, R. S. (2001) Ovarian cancer metastatic to the brain: what is the optimal management. *Journal of Surgical Oncology.* 78:194200; discussion 200–201.

Melichar, B.; Urminská, H.; Kohlová, T.; Nová, M.; Cesák, T. (2004) Brain metastases of epithelial ovarian carcinoma responding to cisplatin and gemcitabine combination chemotherapy: a case report and review of the literature. *Gynecologic Oncology.* Aug;94(2):267-76.

Monaco III, E.; Kondziolka, D.; Mongia, S.; Niranjan, A.; Flickinger, J. C.; Dade Lunsford, L. (2008) Management of brain metastases from ovarian and endometrial carcinoma with stereotactic radiosurgery. *Cancer.* 113, 9:2610-14.

Pectasides, D.; Aravantinos, G.; Fountzilas, G.; Kalofonos, C.; Efstathiou, E.; Karina, M.; Pavlidis, N.; Farmarkis, D.; Economopoulos, T.; Dimopoulos, M. A. (2005) Brain metastases from epithelial ovarian cancer. The Hellenic Cooperative Oncology Group (HeCOG) experience and review of the literature. *Anticancer Research.* 25:3553–3558.

Pectasides, D.; Pectasides, M.; Economopoulos, T. (2006) Brain metastases from epithelial ovarian cancer: a review of the literature. *The Oncologist.* 11:252-260.

Pothuri, B.; Chi, D.S.; Reid, T.; Aghajanian, C.; Venkatraman, E.; Alektiar, K.; Bilsky, M.; Barakat, R.R. (2002) Craniotomy for central nervous system metastases in epithelial ovarian carcinoma. *Gynecologic Oncology.* Oct;87(1):133-7.

Rodriguez, G.C.; Soper, J.T.; Berchuck, A.; Oleson, J.; Dodge, R.; Montana, G.; Clarke-Pearson, D.L. (1992) Improved palliation of cerebral metastases in epithelial ovarian cancer using combined modality approach including radiation therapy, chemotherapy and surgery. *Journal of Clinical Oncology* **10**, 1553–1560

Rottenberg, D.A.; Chernik, N.L.; Deck, M.D.; Ellis, F.; Posner, J.B. (1077) Cerebral necrosis following radiotherapy of external neoplasm. *Annals of Neurology* 1:339-357

Ruderman, N. B.; Hall, T. C. (1965) Use of glucocorticoids in the palliative treatment of metastatic brain tumors. *Cancer.* 18:298–306.

Salvati, M.; Cervoni, L. (1994) Solitary cerebral metastasis from ovarian carcinoma: report of 4 cases. *The Journal of Neuro-Oncology.* 19:75–77.

Sanderson, A.; Bonington, S.C.; Carrington, I.M.; Alison, D.L.; Spencer, J.A. (2002) Cerebral metastasis and cerebral events in women with ovarian cancer. *Clinical Radiology* 57:815-819.

Sehouli, J.; Pietzner, K.; Harter, P.; Münstedt, K.; Mahner, S.; Hasenburg, A.; Camara, O.; Wimberger, P.; Boehmer, D.; Buehling, K.J.; Richter, R.; El Khalfaoui, K.; Oskay-Ozcelik, G. (2010) Prognostic role of platinum sensitivity in patients with brain metastases from ovarian cancer: results of a German multicenter study. *Annals of Oncology.* Nov;21(11):2201-5

Sood A.; Kumar L.; Sood R.; Sandhu M. S.(1996) Epithelial ovarian carcinoma metastatic to the central nervous system: a report on two cases with review of literature. *Gynecologic Oncology.* 62:113–118.

Soffietti, R.; Ruda, R.; Mutani, R. (2002) Management of brain metastes. *Journal of Neurology* 249:1357-1369

Stein, M.; Steiner, M.; Ben-Schachar, M.; Kuten, A.; Malberger, E.; Goldsher, D.; Robinson, E. (1987) Leptomeningeal involvement by epithelial ovarian cancer: a case report. Stein, M.; Steiner, M.; Ben-Schachar, M.; Kuten, A.; Malberger, E.; Goldsher, D.;

Robinson, E. (1987) Leptomeningeal involvement by epithelial ovarian cancer: a case report. *Gynecologic Oncology.* Jun;27(2):241-5.Jun;27(2):241-5.

Tay, S.K. & Rajesh, H. (2005) Brain metastases from epithelial ovarian cancer. *International Journal of Gynecological Cancer.* Sep-Oct;15(5):824-9.

Vitaliani, R.; Spinazzi, M.; Del Mistro, A. R.; Manara, R.; Tavolato, B; Bonifati, D. M. (2009) Subacute onset of deafness and vertigo in a patient with leptomenigeal metastasis from ovarian cancer. *Neurological Science.* Feb; 30(1):65-7.

Vlasveld, L. T.; Beynen, J. H.; Boogerd, W.; Ten Bokkel Huinink, W. W.; Rodenhuis, S. (1990) Complete remission of brain metastases of ovarian cancer following high-dose carboplatin: a case report and pharmacokinetic study. *Cancer Chemotherapy and Pharmacology.* 25:382–383.

Watanabe, A.; Shimada, M.; Kigawa, J.; Iba, T.; Oishi, T.; Kanamori, Y.; Terakawa, N. (2005) The benefit of chemotherapy in a patient with multiple brain metastases and meningitis carcinomatosa from ovarian cancer. *International Journal of Clinical Oncology.* 10:69–71.

Yoo-Kyung, L. ; Noh-Hyun, P. ; Jae Weon, K. ; Yong-Sang, S. ; Soon-Beom, K. ; Hyo-Pyo, L. (2008) Gamma-knife radiosurgery as an optimal treatment modality for brain metastases from epithelial ovarian cancer. *Gynecologic Oncology* 108 :505-509.

6

Therapeutic Strategies in Ovarian Cancer

Dan Ancuşa, Octavian Neagoe, Răzvan Ilina,
Adrian Carabineanu, Corina Şerban and Marius Craina
University of Medicine and Pharmacy „Victor Babeş" Timişoara
Romania

1. Introduction

Therapeutic management for ovarian cancer (OC) requires effective treatment methods such as optimization in terms of technical variability, dosage, or administration period and the introduction of new therapeutic methods in the existing protocols, all in order to improve immediate results, especially of the long term. Establishing therapeutic strategies are based on the main factors that influence cancer development and prognosis of primary starting point of the ovary. Studies have established even a prognostic profile of OC and a profile of the degree of response to chemotherapy [Spentzos, 2005].

Complex treatment should involve the main therapeutic methods to combat both the primary ovarian tumor and secondary determinations:

- Surgery
- Chemotherapy
- Radiation therapy and recently
- Biological therapy and
- Hormone

The main prognostic factor and therapeutic attitude that divides into two different directions is the set of FIGO stage of disease. With FIGO, a number of other factors require the combination of several methods of therapeutic treatment in the same direction.

2. Therapeutic strategies in early ovarian cancer

OC is confined to early stages I-IIa FIGO. In this stage of OC, therapeutic strategies differ depending on the presence of several prognostic factors, according to which natural evolution of the disease progresses differently. They are represented mainly by:

- FIGO stage
- Grading
- Histology
- Increased amount of ascites
- Preoperative or intraoperative tumor intrusion
- Development of the primary extracapsular tumor
- Patient age

For early stages of OC, Vasey established in 2008 a range of risk depending on the therapeutic attitude that fits (Table 1) [Vasey, 2008].

Good prognosis	Medium prognosis	Poor prognosis
Stage Ia Grade 1 Optimal Staging CA125 ≤ 130	Stage Ib Grade 2 Suboptimal staging	Stage Ic Grade 3 Biopsy only Pre-op rupture Aneuploidy

Table 1. Range in early OC [Vasey-2008].

However, Virgote considered the main prognostic factor tumor grading in tumor recurrence risk, followed in order by preoperative tumor, intraoperative tumor rupture, namely age [Vergote, 2001].

2.1 Radiation

Radiotherapy, either whole abdomen teletherapy or intraperitoneal with 32P brachytherapy is a method that initially had similar results with combined-modality therapy (CMT), when it was not done with chemotherapy based on platinum ions. Lately it was abandoned due to inferior results and increased risk to platinum-based CMT, in which the rate of major complications locally was increased. Thus, these procedures are currently strict historical interest method [Vergote, 1992; Young, 2003].

2.2 Surgery

OC surgery for early stages follow both the primary tumor, complete excision to the limits cancer and dissemination in the main sires, to their excision or biopsy of their evaluation by sampling [Zoung, 1983; Cass, 2001].

Surgery methods are the following:

- Abdominal hysterectomy with bilateral anexectomy by median approach
- Total omentectomy
- Biopsy pelvic peritoneum (a Pap smear test form the peritoneum fragments from diaphragm is accepted as an alternative method) [Chhieng, 2011].
- Sampling bilateral pelvic and paraaortic lymph nodes
- Lavage cytology of peritoneal cavity
- Appendectomy in all patients with OC epithelial origin, especially if they have mucinous histology or clear cell [Ozols, 2005].

Controversy and debate regarding surgery has occurred for the patients came seeking preservation of reproductive function in these stages. Conservative surgery consisting of unilateral anexectomy is accepted as a therapeutic method in young patients with OC in first stage, with favorable histological structure (low malignant potential, stromal tumors, germinomas) and seeking fertility preservation [Ozols, 2005]. Literature data for carefully and properly selected cases, do not report an increased risk of relapse, or a lower survival rate in patients treated conservatively compared to those treated aggressively [Young, 2003].

If the inspection is suspecting lesion on contralateral ovary in patients treated conservatively, surgical treatment, in addition to unilateral anexectomy should be supplemented by targeted biopsy of suspicious areas [Ozols, 2005]. The presence of tight adhesions between adjacent organs and regional annexes requires the overstaging and the right therapy approach by aggressive surgery and the introduction of adjuvant chemotherapy [Ozols, 2005]. Minimally invasive approach to OC (laparoscopic or robotic) is a therapeutic method that tends to win ever more ground in early stages of OC. Larger studies are needed to analyze the laparoscopic approach compared to the staging and treatment of early OC [Medeiros, 2011]. For patients with favorable prognostic factors (std. Ia, Ib, G1) surgery is considered sufficient as the only therapeutic approach without requiring the association of adjuvant chemotherapy [Young, 2003]. For patients with moderate (std. Ib, G2, suboptimal staging), or with poor prognostic factors (std. Ic, IIa, G3, clear cell carcinoma, close adhesions, break tumor near the operation) surgery is insufficient, requiring adjuvant CMT compulsory association as a therapy method complementary to the management of these cases [Trimbos, 2003].

2.3 Chemotherapy

Chemotherapy as an adjuvant in the treatment protocol of early OC has always been an issue that concerns the role and selection of cases where its use proves its real efficiency in terms of median progression-free survival (PFS) and especially overall survival (OS). The controversies about the application of OC in the early stages CMT year refer specifically to:

- The group of patients to be associated
- Type of CMT and the timing
- Regimens (monotherapy/polytherapy)
- The administration (number of series)

Initially addressed to the patients with the increased prognostic risk groups of early OC, the indication of the application of CMT was extended to patients with moderate risk group due to significant differences in overall survival and median progression-free survival [Young, 2003]. Regarding the timing of CMT in patients with early OC, both technically and as a result, CMT is totally adjuvant; its administration is in fact a therapy nonsense, which would require an initial biopsy laparatomy for a resectable case in radical limits. As an extrapolation of the results obtained with different regimens applied to patients with advanced OC, it was concluded that the most effective combination therapy is the combined protocol Carboplatin AUC 5 to 7.5 mg/ml/min + Paclitaxel 175mg/m^2/3h [Kyrgiou, 2006].

Some studies that compared adjuvant CMT versus "watchful waiting", established that the use of adjuvant CMT improves OS and PFS in high-risk patients with early stages of OC. This was confirmed recently by a metanalysis comprising five prospective randomized studies. Its final conclusion was that the patients who received platinum-based adjuvant chemotherapy had better OS [hazard ratio (HR) 0.71, 95% confidence interval (CI) 0.53-0.93] and PFS (HR 0.67, 95% CI 0.53- 0.84) than patients who did not receive treatment adjuvant [Colombo, 2010]. One of the conclusions of mentioned metanalysis surprised by considering early adjuvant CMT as a factor influencing the final results in OC, but was very important in the further development of specific cases and suboptimal staging. Later was observed that two thirds of the studies that classified patients of having early stages OC, could classified that patients in higher stages. In these cases there was a significant difference in OS and PFS terms considering association or not adjuvant CMT at initial surgery resection. However, in suboptimal staged group with unfavorable prognostic factors, adjuvant CMT could address and properly stage the group of patients [Trimbos, 2003]. The controversy regarding the duration of the adjuvant CMT tried to be clarified in GOG-157 study which demonstrated that 6 cycles of Carboplatin + Paclitaxel have the same therapeutic effect (OS and PFS) with only 3 cycles with the same combination, but only with an increased cumulative toxicity [Bell, 2003]. A 33 percent reduction in the risk of loco-regional relapse, demonstrated using the same 6-cycle regimens, compared with 3 cycles, led to the routine use of CMT under standard adjuvant 6 cycles [Bell, 2003].

3. Therapeutic strategies in advanced ovarian cancer

There is a significant difference between the management of early stages and advanced stages of OC management and the latter, there is a difference between stages II B - III C, respectively, stage IV. The inclusion of stage II was made considering prognosis of patients with OC at this stage, and data showed that are closer to those of stage III. For stage II B - III C of OC, therapeutic methods are represented by chemotherapy and surgery, radiotherapy with more historical significance and biological therapy.

3.1 Radiation

Radiotherapy (either WAR or intraperitoneal brachytherapy) was analyzed in several studies, the last completed in 2003. The studies have underlined the utility of this method but also the increased risks of major complications [Verheijen, 2006].

3.2 Surgery

In the early stages of OC, surgery proposed a radical intervention intended to remove the entire tumor, on the one hand, and to estimate the peritoneal dissemination of cancer in any sites for a more accurate staging, on the other hand. In advanced stages, cytoreductive surgery (CRS) has the main purpose not to excise the whole tumor, but to obtain a small volume of residue lesions. Direct proportionality between the individual and the extent of cytoreduction evolution was demonstrated by multiple studies. In 2002, Bristov even proposed a mathematical model, showing that the ultimate goal of surgery is to obtain under 1 cm of residual tumor, which can involve, if feasible, multivisceral resections, peritonectomy, stripping diaphragm, pelvic radical dissection, splenectomy [Marszalek, 2010]. A review on the subject showed an increased OS from 17 to 39 months [Bristow, 2002]. Discussions regarding aggressive surgical risk refer to the degree that is vital for the patient. Thus, if the patient is suitable for CRS at primary laparatomy, then the biopsy is followed by neoadjuvant CMT and subsequently secondary CRS [Tangjitgamol, 2010]. It is preferable that secondary CRS be performed after three cycles of CMT and be followed by three cycles of adjuvant with the same regimen CMT. In patients with complete response to treatment, a second look surgery has not proven be beneficial of the OS. Secondary CRS scheduled after neoadjuvant CMT does not show a clear increased of OS [Winter, 2008].

3.3 Chemotherapy

Chemotherapy is a mandatory means in the treatment of advanced OC. Over time there have been many controversies concerning:

- When administered CMT
- Therapeutic regimes
- Simultaneous therapy versus sequential therapy
- Duration of therapy (no. of cycles)
- Route of administration
- Tumor residue

3.3.1 Timing CMT

The debate is limited not only about using CMT as adjuvant, but also about the possibility of its association as neoadjuvant therapy. Administration of preoperative CMT (preferably 3 cycles) has proven useful only in cases where primary optimal CRS surgery was impossible to perform, and response to treatment favorable, allowing a secondary CRS [Vergote, 2010]. Survival, however, in these cases proved to be a less than optimal in primary CRS cases followed by adjuvant CMT [Kumar, 2010]. The remaining cases that could benefit from primary CRS will receive mandatory six cycles of adjuvant CMT 3 weeks each.

3.3.2 Regimens

Since 1996 it was formulated the standard scheme for CMT in advanced OC, combination of platinum and taxane ions, causing abandonment included Cyclofosfamide regimens, doxorubicin or 5-fluorouracil [McGuire, 1996]. The response rates to this combination in patients with advanced OC were different, depending on the degree of primary CRS: 70% for suboptimal CRS and over 80% for primary optimal CRS [Ozols, 2003].

Usefulness of paclitaxel-based chemotherapy potentiation of platinum ions was demonstrated in Gynecologic Oncology Group (GOG) 111 study and European-Canadian (OV-10) trial, but it has not been confirmed by following studies: The Third International Collaborative Ovarian Neoplasm Study (ICON-3) and GOG 132 [McGuire, 1996; Stuart, 1998; Muggia, 2000]. GOG 114 study underlines the effectiveness of carboplatin and cisplatin same regimes combined with a top low toxicity for carboplatin [Ozols, 2003]. In combination with paclitaxel chemotherapy comparing the study above demonstrates increased efficiency of carboplatin in terms of OS and PFS. This is another argument in favor of regime 7.5 Carboplatin/Paclitaxel 175 mg/m^2/3h, as concluded in GOG 158 study [Ozols, 2003].

3.3.3 Simultaneous versus sequential therapy

Sequential administration of cytostatics in combination regimens is also an important controversy in the treatment of advanced OC. In GOG-132 study and The European-Canadian study, one of the conclusions was that the benefit of platinum ions taxane association is found both in the system simultaneously, and in the sequence [Vermorken, 2000, Piccart, 2000]. In GOG 132 study was also demonstrated that OS was similar in regimens combined platinum + taxane type ions, regardless of the combination simultaneously, or sequentially, resulting less encouraging for monotherapy (regimes based exclusively platinum ions showing a 5-year OS 67%). The weakest cytostatic agent used as monotherapy was paclitaxel (exclusive regimes showing a 5-year OS 42%) [Vermorken, 2000; Muggia, 2000].

Trial and Randomization	Patient Number	Stage	CCR (%)	Median PFS (months)	Median OS (months)
GOG-111	386	III, IV			
Paclitaxel (135 mg/m2)			51	18	38
Cisplatin (75 mg/m2)				P = .0002	P = .0001
Cyclosphosphamide (750 mg/m2)			31	13	24
Cisplatin (75 mg/m2)					
OV10	668	IIB IV			
Paclitaxel (175 mg/m2)			50	16	35
Cisplatin (75 mg/m2)				P = .0005	P = .0016
Cyclophosphamide (750 mg/m2)			36	12	25
Cisplatin (75 mg/m2)					
ICON-3	2074	Ia IV			
Paclitaxel (175 mg/m2)			NA	17.3	36.1
Carboplatin (AUC 5 to 6)				P = .19	P = .74
Carboplatin (AUC 5 to 6)			NA	16.1	35.4a
Cisplatin (50 mg/m2)					
Doxorubicin (50 mg/m2)					
Cyclophosphamide (500 mg/m2)					
GOG-132	614	III IV			
Paclitaxel (135 mg/m2)			NA	16	35b
Cisplatin (75 mg/m2)					
Cisplatin (100 mg/m2)			NA	16.4	30.2
Paclitaxel (200 mg/m2)			NA	11.4	26

Table 2. Randomized Trials of Paclitaxel versus Non-Paclitaxel First-Line Therapy in Advanced Epithelial Ovarian Cancer [De Vita, 2008].

3.3.4 Duration of therapy (number of cycles)

Three randomized trials that analyzed the effectiveness of increasing the number of cycles of CMT on the OS have concluded unanimously that the results are similar, but increased the frequency of complications (especially neurological). The cumulative toxicity was directly proportional with the number of cycles. It was established that the optimal number of cycles is 6, each separated by 3 weeks of rest between them [Colombo, 2010].

3.3.5 Route of administration

Until recently, the route of administration of the CMT was systemic intravenous peripheral or central. Increasing concentration in the peritoneal cavity of CMT after primary CRS, without causing systemic side effects, is believed to be a result of the ratio of cisplatin, paclitaxel, respectively, between the peritoneum and systemic circulation central. Since then, it appeared the idea of intraperitoneal CMT [Rothenberg, 2003]. Since 1980 analyzed in numerous randomized trials, intraperitoneal administration of CMT was shown to improve OS and PFS in optimal cytoreduced patients and in terms of pathological complete remission in patients in whom cytoreduction was actually, suboptimal (residual tumor < 2 cm was accepted as optimal at that time), compared with only intravenous administration of

CMT [Alberts, 1987]. GOG-172 (Armstrong, 2006) study pointed out that the combination of CMT to the intravenous intraperitoneal resulting OS rise from 49.7 to 65.6 months (35%) and PFS from 19 to 24 months (with 26%), but with a greatly increased associated toxicity. In 58% of cases resulted the abandonment of intraperitoneal administration of CMT, making only 42% complete the 6 cycles (given on day 2 and day 8). Cochrane's metanalysis, balancing risks and benefits, reported in eight randomized trials of systemic administration of CMT (intraperitoneal association and administration) concluded that effect is beneficial in terms of OS (hazard ratio 0.799) and PFS (hazard ratio 0.792) [Jaaback, 2006]. Despite these favorable results, many authors have remained skeptical about this therapy, which was still considered at an experimental level [Gore, 2006; Ozols, 2006]. Since 1994, the efficiency of intraperitoneal CMT is questioned, by administering in hyperthermia. In this respect, there were a lot series of studies that examined the usefulness of this method in the management of OC. CMT administration at 39 to 44,5 degrees Celsius, in addition to increased locoregional and systemic toxic effect, translated into a major complication rate of 28.3% [Ryu, 2004] and a perioperative mortality of 3.7% [Gori, 2005].

HIPEC indications can be summarized in:

- Recurrent or persistent disease: the use of intraperitoneal CMT extended the period of progression of OC lesion from 10 to 21.8 months [Zanon, 2004; Helm, 2007].
- As first-line therapy: although logical, it is recommended an aggressive approach of OC, but when it was applied, the number of cases was too small for a conclusion [Piso, 2004].
- When CRS is scheduled after neoadjuvant CMT, it is preferably an optimal cytoreduction followed by HIPEC. The number of cases remained was insufficient to have a clear conclusion [Reichman, 2005; Yoshida, 2005].
- CMT as consolidation therapy, when it is applicable second look surgery or after a partial response in these cases.

One study observed an improvement from 19.8 to 48.7 months and OS of 52, 8 to 63.4 months (Ryu - cisplatin + interferon treatment) [Ryu, 2004]. These results are relative, since, although in large numbers, the patients from this study were not homogeneous in terms of progress including early cases. Another study obtained a recurrence rate of 69.9% for HIPEC compared with 63.1% in the control group, a difference of OS from 64.4 to 46.4 months, but proved to be insignificant ($p = 0.29$), due to lots of inhomogeneity [Gori, 2005].

Several ways to amend the standard treatment protocols were tried in order that adjuvant CMT to increase:

- Addition of the third chemotherapy
- Management of locoregional chemotherapy
- Maintenance Chemotherapy
- Increasing doses
- The combination of biological therapy

GOG-111 and OV-10 studies identified the need to improve therapeutic strategies considering long-term adverse outcomes [McGuire, 1996; Stuart, 1998].

Combination of the third drug

The combination of the third drug joins the regimen used to treat OC (Carboplatin - Paclitacsel). Other chemotherapy gemcitabine Dacsil, topotecan achieved an improvement of the OS or PFS, but with a toxicity increased as studies ICON-5 and GOG 182 have shown. The role of the third combination chemotherapy was relevant for mucinous adenocarcinoma OC type or clear cell [Bookman, 2006].

Locoregional administration of CMT

Results of studies on intraperitoneal chemotherapy have been mentioned previously.

Increasing doses of CMT

The concept of increasing doses of CMT has been divided in two: on the one hand, the concept of increasing the dose (increasing the effective dose per chemotherapy cures the same secventiality) and, on the other hand, the concept of dose densification (the same dose in more frequent cycles). Increasing the desired effect by increasing the dose of chemotherapy was ruled out by the study AGO-Ovar/AIO and EBMT in 2007. The study showed that there were no significant differences in OS and PFS terms [Mobus, 2007]. In 2008, Isonishi and collaborators demonstrated, however, through a study on 631 patients randomized, that in the second year, OS and PFS are significantly influenced (77.7 versus 83.6, respectively 17.1 versus 27.9) after the densification of Carboplatin dosage scheme - Paclitaxel, when these were administered weekly [Ionishi, 2008].

Maintenance therapy

The maintenance therapy requires long term administration, after six cycles of combined CMT or variable number of cycles of CMT administered as monotherapy. Most studies that examined the maintenance therapy with ions of platinum, taxanes, topotecan, epirubicin, surprised no significant differences in OS and PFS terms. One study reported that maintenance therapy for 12 months with Paclitaxel 7 months improved PFS [Markman, 2003; Markman, 2009].

4. Therapeutic strategies in recurrent ovarian cancer

Patients that experienced disease relapse or are refractory to first-line treatment are candidates for second-line chemotherapy. An ideal agent will provide broad antitumor activity, demonstrate a favorable toxicity profile, and have generally convenient administration, among other factors. Additionally, many of the more active agents used in second-line treatment (e.g., gemcitabine, liposomal doxorubicin, and topotecan) are non-cross-resistant to first-line therapies. They exhibit novel mechanisms of action relative to cisplatin/carboplatin and paclitaxel, thereby targeting a different aspect of cell division. The agents include members of the platinum and taxane families, such as carboplatin and paclitaxel (every 3 weeks and weekly schedules), respectively; the topoisomerase I inhibitor topotecan; the liposome-encapsulated anthracycline doxorubicin (liposomal doxorubicin); and the novel antimetabolite gemcitabine. The clinical utility (benefit-risk ratio) of these agents in the recurrent ovarian cancer setting will be reviewed briefly below.

Hexamethylmelamine

Hexamethylmelamine (altretamine; Hexalen; MGI Pharma, Bloomington, MN) is an approved single-agent therapy for ovarian cancer. It has the advantage of oral administration, which may be preferable for some patients. However, it has been demonstrated only limited activity in patients with relapsed platinum-refractory ovarian cancer [Markman, 2003].

Platinum

Patients that were found to be platinum sensitive at first-line therapy are likely to benefit from reintroduction of platinum on disease recurrence. Both cisplatin (Platinol; Bristol-Myers Squibb, Princeton, NJ) and carboplatin (Paraplatin; Bristol-Myers Squibb) are FDA-approved for the treatment of recurrent ovarian cancer and are often used as monotherapy or in combination with paclitaxel. Carboplatin is considerably less nephrotoxic than cisplatin; however, because the primary route of clearance is renal, the potential for acute renal toxicity should be monitored when it is established the dosage. In clinical trials of single-agent carboplatin, overall tumor response rates ranged from 21% to 30% in platinum-resistant or platinum-refractory patients and from 27% to 53% in platinum-sensitive patients [Williams, 1992; Kavanagh J, 1995; Bolis G, 2001]. Furthermore, the proportion of patients with stable disease was approximately 18% to 33%.

Gemcitabine plus Platinum

Gemcitabine (Gemzar; Eli Lilly and Co., Indianapolis, IN) has received approval in other indications but is still investigational in the treatment of ovarian cancer. Gemcitabine can be safely combined with carboplatin for the treatment of patients with relapsed ovarian cancer [du Bois, 1995]. The gemcitabine plus carboplatin regimen recently compared favorably with carboplatin alone in a randomized trial in patients with relapsed platinum-sensitive ovarian cancer, producing significant improvements in quality of life, significantly faster palliation of abdominal symptoms, significant improvements in response rate, and a significant increase in progression-free survival.

Paqclitaxel

- Every three weeks

Paclitaxel (Taxol; Bristol-Myers Squibb) is indicated as first-line (with cisplatin or carboplatin) and subsequent therapy for the treatment of ovarian cancer. The taxane is administered in two different schedules; however, the FDA-approved dosing is intravenous administration over 3 or 24 hours once every 3 weeks. In studies of paclitaxel administered on this schedule, overall tumor response rates were approximately 22% in platinum-resistant or platinum-refractory patients and 45% in platinum-sensitive patients [Cantu 2002; Gore, 1995; Trimble, 1993]. Median survival in platinum-resistant or refractory patients ranged from 6 to 9 months and was 26 months in 47 evaluable platinum-sensitive patients is generally less favorable than it is when the agent is administered weekly; therefore, partly because of the sometimes debilitating toxicity associated with the approved schedule, investigators have developed interest in evaluating the antitumor activity and tolerability of weekly schedules.

- Weekly

Although weekly paclitaxel is not an approved regimen in ovarian cancer therapy, overall tumor responses were at least comparable and potentially higher than those achieved with the every-3-week's schedule in preliminary studies in patients with recurrent disease [Rosenberg, 2002].

Platinum plus paclitaxel

Patients who responded to combination first-line therapy may benefit from reintroduction of platinum and paclitaxel on disease recurrence. In the largest study to date conducted in collaboration with the International Collaborative Ovarian Neoplasm (ICON4) and three cooperative groups, 802 relapsed patients with ovarian cancer were randomized to treatment with platinum plus a taxane or single-agent platinum [Parmar, 2003] . Overall tumor response rate in the combination group was 66% compared with 54% in the platinum treatment group (P = 0.06). Notably, the hazard ratios for progression-free survival and overall survival were 0.76 and 0.82, respectively, favoring platinum plus paclitaxel over single-agent platinum in both cases. Thus, there was a statistically significant difference in survival favoring the platinum plus paclitaxel combination compared with single-agent platinum (P = 0.023) [Parmar, 2003].

Topotecan

Topotecan (Hycamtin; GlaxoSmithKline, Philadelphia, PA) is an active and well-established agent currently indicated [topotecan (1.5 mg/m^2) on days 1 through 5 of a 21-day cycle] for the treatment of relapsed metastatic ovarian cancer after failure of initial or subsequent chemotherapy.

Docetaxel

Although docetaxel (Taxotere; Aventis Pharmaceuticals Inc., Bridgewater, NJ) is more commonly used in the treatment of non–small-cell lung cancer and breast cancer, recent studies have been conducted in patients with relapsed ovarian cancer [Rose, 2003; Markman, 2003]. In the largest study, with 60 paclitaxel-resistant ovarian cancer patients receiving docetaxel (100 mg/m^2) every 21 days, Rose and collaborators reported a response rate of 22%, including 5% and 17% complete and partial response rates, respectively [Rose, 2003].

Gemcitabine

Although is not currently FDA-approved for the treatment of ovarian cancer, gemcitabine (Gemzar; Eli Lilly and Co.) has typically been administered as monotherapy in pretreated patients with ovarian cancer.

Etoposide

Etoposide (VePesid; Bristol-Myers Squibb) inhibits topoisomerase II and thus inhibits DNA synthesis. In a phase II study in patients with recurrent ovarian cancer investigated etoposide (150 mg/m^2) on days 1 through 3 of a 28-day cycle [Eckhardt, 1990]. Of the 71 patients evaluable for response, 1 achieved a complete response, and 5 achieved a partial response. An additional 48 patients had stable disease.

5. Conclusions

The questions of optimal treatment duration and whether patients should receive treatment to disease progression remain unanswered. However, in the absence of definitive evidence addressing optimal treatment duration in patients with relapsed disease, it should be recognized and appreciated that a number of agents are available that offer a level of flexibility and treatment customization heretofore unseen in the management of recurrent ovarian cancer in this generally poor-prognosis patient population. These agents should be wielded with the critical goal of balancing the efficacy and toxicity of particular agents and schedules with their effect on symptoms and quality of life.

6. References

Alberts, D.S.; Liu, P.Y.; Hannigan, E.V. et al. (1996). Intraperitoneal cisplatin plus intravenous cyclophosphamide versus intravenous cisplatin plus intravenous cyclophosphamide for stage III ovarian cancer. *New England Journal of Medicine* Vol. 335, No.26, (December, 1996), pp. 1950-1955.

Bell, J.; Brady, M.; Lage, J.M. et al. (2006). A randomized phase III trial of three versus six cycles of carboplatin and paclitaxel as adjuvant treatment in early stage ovarian epithelial carcinoma: a Gynecologic Oncology Group study. *Gynecologic Oncology,* Vol. 102, No.3, (September, 2006), pp. 432-439.

Bookman, M.A. (2006). GOG0182-ICON5: 5-arm phase III randomized trial of paclitaxel (P) and carboplatin (C) vs combinations with gemcitabine (G), PEG-lipososomal doxorubicin (D), or topotecan (T) in patients (pts) with advanced-stage epithelial ovarian (EOC) or primary peritoneal (PPC) carcinoma. [Abstract] *Journal of Clinical Oncology,* Vol. 24 (Suppl 18): A-5002, 256s.

Bristow, R.E.; Tomacruz, R.S.; Armstrong, D.K.; Trimble, E.L.; Montz, F.J. (2002). Survival effect of maximal cytoreductive surgery for advanced ovarian carcinoma during the platinum era: a meta-analysis. *Journal of Clinical Oncology,* Vol. 20, No.5, (March, 2002), 1248-1259.

Cass, I.; Li, A.J.; Runowicz, C.D.; Fields, A.L. et al. (2001). Pattern of lymph node metastases in clinically unilateral stage I invasive epithelial ovarian carcinomas. *Gynecologic Oncology,* Vol. 80, No.1, (January, 2001), pp. 56–61.

Chhieng, D.; Hui, P. (2011). Cytology and surgical pathology of gynecologic neoplasms, *Current Clinical Pathology,* 193-207.

Colombo, N.; Peiretti, M.; Parma, G.; Lapresa, M.; Mancar, R. (2010). Newly diagnosed and relapsed epithelial ovarian carcinoma: ESMO Clinical Practice Guidelines for diagnosis, treatment and follow-up, *Annals of Oncology,* Vol. 21, (May, 2010), pp. v23–v30.

Gore, M.; du Bois, A.; Vergote, I. (2006). Intraperitoneal chemotherapy in ovarian cancer remains experimental. *Journal of Clinical Oncology,* Vol. 24, No. 28, (October, 2006), 4528-4530.

Gori, J.; Castano, R.; Toziano M. et al. (2005). Intraperitoneal hyperthermic chemotherapy in ovarian cancer. *International Journal of Gynecological Cancer,* 15(2):233–239

Helm, C.W.; Eduards, R.P. (2007). Intraperitoneal Cancer Therapy, Humana Press, Totowa, New Jersey.

Helm, C.W.; Randall-Whitis, L.; Martin, R.S.; Metzinger, D.S.; Gordinier, M.E.; Parker, L.P.; Edwards, R.P. (2007). Hyperthermic intraperitoneal chemotherapy in conjunction with surgery for the treatment of recurrent ovarian carcinoma. *Gynecologic Oncology* Vol. 105, No. 1, (April, 2007), pp. 90–96.

Isonishi, S.; Yasuda, Takahashi, F.; Katsumata, N.; Kimura, E. Randomized phase III trial of conventional paclitaxel and carboplatin (c-TC) versus dose dense weekly paclitaxel and carboplatin (dd-TC) in women with advanced epithelial ovarian, fallopian tube, or primary peritoneal cancer: Japanese Gynecologic Oncology, *Journal of Clinical Oncology,* 26: 2008 (May 20 suppl; abstr 5506).

Jaaback, K. Johnson, N. (2006). Intraperitoneal chemotherapy for the initial management of primary epithelial ovarian cancer. *Cochrane Database Systematic Reviews,* Vol.25, No.1, (January, 2006), CD005340.

Kumar, L.; Hariprasad, R.; Kumar, S. et al. (2010). Upfront surgery versus neoadjuvant chemotherapy in advanced epithelial ovarian carcinoma (EOC): a randomized study. IGCS 13. Prague 2010 (A824).

Kyrgiou, M.; Salanti, G.; Pavlidis, N.; Paraskevaidis, E.; John, P.A. Survival benefits with diverse chemotherapy regimens for ovarian cancer: Meta-analysis of Multiple Treatments, *Journal of the National Cancer Institute,* Vol. 98, No. 22, (November 2006), pp. 1655-1663.

Markman, M.; Liu, P.Y. Moon, J. et al. (2009). Impact on survival of 12 versus 3 monthly cycles of paclitaxel (175 mg/m2) administered to patients with advanced ovarian cancer who attained a complete response to primary platinum-paclitaxel: follow-up of a Southwest Oncology Group and Gynecologic Oncology Group phase 3 trial. *Gynecologic Oncology,* Vol. 114, No.2, (August, 2009), pp. 195-198.

Markman, M.; Liu, P.Y.; Wilczynski, S.; Monk, B.; Copeland, L.J. Alvarez, R.D. et al. (2003). Phase III randomized trial of 12 versus 3 months of maintenance paclitaxel in patients with advanced ovarian cancer after complete response to platinum and paclitaxel-based chemotherapy: a Southwest Oncology Group and Gynecologic Oncology Group trial., *Journal of Clinic Oncology,* Vol. 21, No.13, (July, 2003), pp. 2460-2465.

Marszalek, A.; Alran, S.; Scholl, S.; Fourchotte, V.; Plancher, C. et al. (2010). Outcome in Advanced Ovarian Cancer following an Appropriate and Comprehensive Effort at Upfront Cytoreduction: A Twenty-Year Experience in a Single Cancer Institute, *International Journal of Surgical Oncology,* vol. 2010.

McGuire, W.P.; Hoskins, W.J.; Brady, M.F.; et al. (1996). Cyclophosphamide and cisplatin compared with paclitaxel and cisplatin in patients with stage III and stage IV ovarian cancer. *New England Journal of Medicine,* Vol. 334, No.1, (January, 1996), pp. 1-6.

Medeiros, L.R.F.; Rosa, D.D.; Bozzetti, M.C.; Rosa, M.; Edelweiss, M.I. et al. (2008). Laparoscopy versus laparotomy for FIGO Stage I ovarian cancer, *The Cochrane Database of Systematic Reviews,* Vol. 8, No. 4: CD005344.

Mobus, V.; Wandt, H.; Frickhofen, N. et al. (2007). Phase III trial of high dose sequential chemotherapy with peripheral blood stem cell support compared with standard dose chemotherapy for first-line treatment of advanced ovarian cancer: intergroup trial of the AGO-Ovar AIO and EBMT. *Journal of Clinical Oncology,* Vol.25, No.27, (September, 2007), pp. 4187–4193.

Muggia, F.M.; Braly, P.S.; Brady, M.F.; et al. (2000). Phase III randomized study of cisplatin versus paclitaxel versus cisplatin and paclitaxel in patients with suboptimal stage III or IV ovarian cancer: a gynecologic oncology group study. *Journal of Clinical Oncology,* Vol. 18, No.1, (January, 2000), pp. 106-115.

Ozols, R.F.; Bookman MA, du Bois A, et al. (2006). Intraperitoneal cisplatin therapy in ovarian cancer: comparison with standard intravenous carboplatin and paclitaxel. *Gynecologic Oncology,* Vol. 103, No.1, (October, 2006), pp. 1-6.

Ozols, R.F.; Bundy, B.N.; Greer, B.E. et al. (2003). Phase III trial of carboplatin and paclitaxel compared with cisplatin and paclitaxel in patients with optimally resected stage III ovarian cancer: a Gynecologic Oncology Group study. *Journal of Clinical Oncology,* Vol. 21:3194.

Ozols RF, Rubin SC, Thomas G, et al. (2005). Epithelial ovarian cancer, in Hoskins WJ, Perez CA, Young RC (eds): *Principles and Practice of Gynecologic Oncology,* 4th ed, Philadelphia, Lippincott Williams & Wilkins, pp. 919-922.

Piccart, M.J.; Bertelsen, K.; James, K. et al. (2000). Randomized intergroup trial of cisplatin-paclitaxel versus cisplatin-cyclophosphamide in women with advanced epithelial ovarian cancer: three-year results. *The Journal of National Cancer Institute*, Vol. 92, No. 9, (May, 2000), pp.699-708.

Piso, P.; Dahlke, M-H.; Loss, M, et al. (2004). Cytoreductive surgery and hyperthermic intraperitoneal chemotherapy in peritoneal carcinomatosis from ovarian cancer. *World Journal of Surgical Oncology,* Vol. 2, pp. 21–27.

Reichman, T.W.; Cracchiolo B, Sama J, et al. (2005). Cytoreductive surgery and intraoperative hyperthermic chemoperfusion for advanced ovarian carcinoma. *Journal of Surgical Oncology,* Vol. 90, No.2, (May, 2005), pp. 51–56.

Rothenberg ML, Liu PY, Braly PS, et al. (2003). Combined intraperitoneal and intravenous chemotherapy for women with optimally debulked ovarian cancer: results from an intergroup phase II trial. *Journal of Clinical Oncology,* Vol. 21:1313

Ryu, K.S.; Kim, J.H.; Ko, H.S. et al. (2004). Effects of intraperitoneal hyperthermic chemotherapy in ovarian cancer. *Gynecologic Oncology,* Vol. 94, No.2, pp. 325–332.

Spentzos, D.; Levine, D.A.; Kolia, S.; et al. (2005). Unique gene expression profile based on pathologic response in epithelial ovarian cancer, *Journal of Clinical Oncology,* Vol. 23, No.31, pp. 7911-7918.

Spentzos, D.; Levine, D.A.; Ramoni, M.F. et al. (2004). Gene expression signature with independent prognostic significance in epithelial ovarian cancer. *Journal of Clinical Oncology,* Vol. 22, No.23, (December, 2004), pp. 4700-4710.

Stuart G, Bertelsen K, Mangioni C, et al: Updated analysis shows a highly significant overall survival for cisplatin-paclitaxel as first-line treatment of advanced ovarian cancer: Mature results of the EORTC-NOCOVA-NCI-C and Scottish intergroup trial. *Proceedings of the American Society of Clinical Oncology,* 17:361A, (abstr 1394).

Tangjitgamol, S.; Manusirivithaya, S.; Laopaiboon, M.; Lumbiganon, P.; Bryant, A. (2010). Interval debulking surgery for advanced epithelial ovarian cancer. *The Cochrane Database of Systematic Reviews,* Vol. (10):CD006014.

Trimbos, J.B.; Parmar, M.; Vergote, I. et al. (2003). International collaborative ovarian neoplasm trial 1 and adjuvant chemotherapy in ovarian neoplasm trial: two parallel randomized phase III trials of adjuvant chemotherapy in early-stage ovarian carcinoma. *The Journal of National Cancer Institute,* Vol. 95, No. 2, pp. 105–112.

Vasey, P.A.; Gore, M.; Wilson, R.; Rustin, G.; Gabra H. (2008). A phase Ib trial of docetaxel, carboplatin and erlotinib in ovarian, fallopian tube and primary peritoneal cancers, *British Journal of Cancer,* Vol. 98, pp. 1774–1780.

Vergote, I.; Brabanter, J.; Fyles, A.; Bertelsen, K.; Einhorn, N.; Sevelda, P.; Gore, ME, at al. Prognostic importance of degree of differentiation and cyst rupture in stage I invasive epithelial ovarian carcinoma, *Lancet,* Vol. 357, Issue 9251, (January 2001), pp. 176- 182.

Vergote, I.; Trope, C.G.; Amant, F. et al. (2010). Neoadjuvant chemotherapy or primary surgery in stage IIIC or IV ovarian cancer. *New England Journal of Medicine,* Vol. 363, No.10, (September, 2010), pp. 043-953.

Vergote, I.B.; Vergote-De Vos, L.N. Abeler, V.M. et al. (1992). Randomized trial comparing cisplatin with radioactive phosphorus or whole-abdomen irradiation as adjuvant treatment of ovarian cancer. *Cancer,* Vol. 69, No.3, (February, 1992), pp. 741-749.

Verheijen, R.H.; Massuger, L.F.; Benigno, B.B. et al. (2006). Phase III trial of intraperitoneal therapy with yttrium-90-labeled HMFG1 murine monoclonal antibody in patients with epithelial ovarian cancer after a surgically defined complete remission. *Journal of Clinical Oncology,* Vol. 24, No.4, (February, 2006), pp. 571-578.

Vermorken, J.B. (2000). Optimal treatment for ovarian cancer: taxoids and beyond, *Annals of Oncology,* Vol. 11, Suppl 3, pp. 131-139.

Winter, W.E. 3rd, Maxwell, G.L. Tian, C. et al. (2008). Tumor residual after surgical cytoreduction in prediction of clinical outcome in stage IV epithelial ovarian cancer: a Gynecologic Oncology Group Study. *Journal of Clinical Oncology,* Vol. 26, No.1, (January, 2008), pp. 83–89.

Yoshida, Y.; Sasaki, H.; Kurokawa, T.; et al. (2005). Efficacy of intraperitoneal continuous hyperthermic chemotherapy as consolidation therapy in patients with advanced epithelial ovarian cancer: a long-term follow-up. *Oncology Reports,* Vol.13, No.1, (January, 2005), pp. 121–125.

Young, R.C.; Brady, M.F.; Nieberg, R.K. et al. (2003). Adjuvant treatment for early ovarian cancer: a randomized phase iii trial of intraperitoneal 32P or intravenous cyclophosphamide and cisplatin a Gynecologic Oncology Group Study. *Journal of Clinical Oncology,* Vol.21, No.23, (December, 2003), pp. 4350-5355.

Young, R.C.; Decker, D.G.; Wharton, J.T.; Piver, M.S. et al. (1983). Staging laparotomy in early ovarian cancer. *The Journal of American Medical Association,* Vol. 250, No. 22, 3072–3076.

Young, R.C. (2003). Early-stage ovarian cancer: to treat or not to treat. *Journal of National Cancer Institute,* Vol. 95, No.2, (January, 2003), pp. 94-95.

Zanon, C.; Clara, R.; Chiappino, I. et al. (2004). Cytoreductive surgery and intraperitoneal chemohyperthermia for recurrent peritoneal carcinomatosis from ovarian cancer. *World Journal of Surgery,* Vol. 28, No.10, (October, 2004), pp. 1040–1045.

7

Peripheral Neuropathy in Ovarian Cancer

Yi Pan
Department of Neurology & Psychiatry, Saint Louis University
USA

1. Introduction

Peripheral neuropathy is not uncommon in ovarian cancer. The incidence density of peripheral neuropathy was 21.5 per 1000 person-years in ovarian cancer, 15.3 per 1000 person-years in breast cancer and 18.3 per 1000 person-years in lung cancer for patients who received platinum-taxane combination chemotherapy (Nurgalieva et al., 2010). Carboplatin/paclitaxel is the chemotherapy of choice for advanced ovarian cancer, which has been reported to associate with chemotherapy induced neurotoxicity in as high as 54% of patients after their first-line 6 cycles of treatment and with 23% of patients with residual neuropathy after a median follow up of 18 months (Pignata et al., 2006). However, peripheral neuropathy in ovarian cancer is not always due to chemotherapeutic agents. Other etiologies of neuropathy in ovarian cancer patients are focal compression, nutritional deficiency, metabolic abnormalities, endocrine disorders, and paraneoplastic neurological syndromes.

A detailed medical history is most important for the diagnosis of neuropathy including symptoms, distribution, duration and course of the neuropathy. The past medical and social history may reveal a possible cause such as diabetes, inflammation, or a toxic or nutritional etiology. A positive family history may suggest a hereditary neuropathy. A neurologic examination is required to confirm the presence of neuropathy. Electrodiagnostic studies, including nerve conduction study and electromyography, are used to reveal the severity and its distribution pattern; underlying process demyelination or axonal loss; sensory, motor or a combination. One limitation of nerve conduction study is that it assess the function of only the large diameter nerve fibers, and not small fibers. Quantitative sensory testing, epidermal nerve fiber density, or autonomic function testing are used to evaluate small fiber neuropathy. Blood tests may reveal the etiology of nutritional, metabolic, endocrine, inflammatory, paraneoplastic, infectious, toxic, or hereditary neuropathies.

2. Chemotherapy-induced neuropathy

Seven cytotoxic chemotherapy agents have been approved by the FDA for advanced ovarian cancer since 1978. They are cisplatin, carboplatin, altretamine, paclitaxel, topotecan, liposomal doxorubicin and gemcitabine. Among them, cisplatin, caboplatin, altretamine, and paclitaxel have significant neurotoxicity. Although bone marrow suppression and neurotoxicity are the major side-effects related to chemotherapy, neurotoxicity is often the decisive factor limiting the dose of chemotherapy agent since bone marrow suppression can be overcome with growth factors, blood transfusion, or bone marrow transplantation. Chemotherapy-induced peripheral neuropathy is clearly related to the dose per cycle, as well as the cumulative dose. However, pre-existing nerve abnormalities (debates mellitus, hereditary neuropathies, alcoholism, previous neurotoxic treatments, or malnutrition) make nerves more susceptible to chemotherapy-induced neuropathy. The incidence of chemotherapy-induced neuropathy varies in the literature due to a wide range of individual drug doses, cumulative doses, treatment schedules, and the combined use with other drugs. The other challenge is different grading systems that have been utilized, including Eastern Cooperative Oncology Group (ECOG), National Cancer Institute–Common Toxicity Criteria (NCI-CTC), and World Health Organization (WHO) toxicity criteria. The common toxicity scales are designed to allow a rapid examination of the patients with peripheral neurotoxicity by oncologists based on clinical symptoms and signs. Total Neuropathy Score (TNS) also includes neurological examination and nerve conduction study, which grade accurately and correlated well with NCI-CTC and ECOG scores (Cavaletti et al., 2006). The Functional Assessment of Cancer Therapy/Gynecologic Oncology Group-Neurotoxicity (FACT/GOG-Ntx) questionnaire is used to evaluate symptoms and concerns associated specifically with chemotherapy-induced neuropathy, which was found to be reliable for assessing quality of life in ovarian cancer patient with neuropathy (Calhoun et al., 2003).

2.1 Platinum agents

Platinum agents cisplatin, carboplatin, and oxaliplatin have been used for the treatment of ovarian cancer. Cisplatin was approved for the treatment of ovarian cancer in 1978, and is currently administered for advanced ovarian cancer intravenously and intraperitoneally (Armstrong et al., 2006, Markman et al., 2001). Carboplatin was approved in 1989, and subsequently became a part of the first-line therapy for ovarian cancer in combination with a taxane. It was found to be less neurotoxicity than cisplatin (du Bois et al., 2003). In 2002, a third-generation platinum drug, oxaliplatin, was approved for treatment of metastatic colorectal cancer; however, 70% of the patients receiving oxaliplatin were affected by some degree of sensory neuropathy (McWhinny et al., 2009). Oxaliplatin in combination with variety of chemotherapy agents (cyclophosphamide, gemcitabine, paclitaxel and pegylated liposomal doxorubicin) has been reported in phase II clinical trials of ovarian cancer (Harnett et al., 2007, Misset et al., 2001, Nicoletto, 2006, Recchia et al., 2007, Viens et al., 2006).

Platinum-induced peripheral neuropathy has elements common to all three agents with some distinctive patterns. The severity of neurotoxicity in platinum agents from greatest to least is cisplatin, oxaliplatin, and carboplatin (McWhinny et al., 2009). Cisplatin produces a predominantly sensory neuropathy characterized by painful paresthesia, numbness, and diminished vibratory sense. Symptoms often begin in the feet, and typically occur during the first few cycles of treatment. When severe, gait ataxia may appear. Lhermitte sign may occur. Large fiber function is more affected than small fiber function. Autonomic neuropathy in general is not prominent. Weakness and motor neuropathy are less common. Sensory disturbance is typical in a symmetrical stocking and glove distribution, with decreasing proprioception and vibratory sensation. Deep tendon reflexes are reduced or absent. Peripheral neuropathy is often not completely reversible. Symptoms may be worse transiently after therapy is discontinued (coasting effect). Neurotoxicity has been reported in 47% of the patients treated with cisplatin compared with 25% of those treated with the non-cisplatin regimen in 387 patients with ovarian cancer. The severity was much higher at cumulative doses of cisplatin between 500 and 600 mg/m^2 (Van Der Hoop et al., 1990). Carboplatin induced neuropathy has similar symptoms to those of cisplatin, but absent Lhermitte sign. The neurotoxicity of carboplatin is generally considered to be less frequent, and less severe than cisplatin. Grade 3/4 sensory neuropathy was 13.5% in the cisplatin regimen versus 7.2% in the carboplatin regimen (du Bois et al., 2003). In addition to chronic sensory neuropathy similar to cisplatin, oxaliplatin also causes acute cold-aggravated transient painful paresthesia, which occurs within hours of each infusion, and typically resolves within hours to days. These symptoms can be accompanied by jaw and eye pain, possibly due to muscle cramps.

Cisplatin and oxaliplatin undergo hydrolysis to a greater extent than carboplatin, and may associate with more severe patterns of neurotoxicity (McWhinny et al., 2009). In addition, cisplatin produces about three times more platinum-DNA adducts in the dorsal root ganglion than does oxaliplatin and with greater neurotoxicity (Ta et al., 2006). The neurotoxicity is the result of platinum compounds accumulating in the dorsal root ganglia, leading to shrinking or loss of dorsal root ganglia neurons and a resultant sensory neuronopathy (Krarup-Hansen et al., 1999), which is likely why the motor fibers are primarily spared. Platinum-DNA-protein cross-links have been proposed as a mechanism for the platinum antitumor activities (Chválová et al., 2007). Platinum compounds interfere with DNA replication and metabolic function of the dorsal root ganglia. The "coasting" phenomenon may result from platinum accumulation in the dorsal root ganglia over a long period time. Cisplatin also induces apoptosis in dorsal root ganglion by binding to nuclear DNA and mitochondrial DNA (Podratz et al., 2011). There is also the secondary degeneration of the posterior columns, which likely accounts for the Lhermitte sign. Oxaliplatin affects nerve excitability through voltage-dependent mechanisms, with specific effects mediated through axonal Na+ channel inactivation. It may be the cause of the acute neurotoxicity of oxaliplatin (Park et al., 2011a).

2.2 Taxanes (paclilaxel / Docetaxel)

Paclitaxel and docetaxel are frequently used taxanes in ovarian cancer. Paclitaxel combined with carboplatin is now considered as a standard first-line therapy for advanced ovarian cancer, but neurological toxicity is a clinically significant adverse effect (Mayerhofer et al., 2000). Docetaxel combined with carboplatin has been suggested to be a promising alternative, particularly in terms of minimizing the incidence and severity of peripheral neuropathy (Pfisterer et al., 2004 and Vasey et al., 2004). Nab-paclitaxel is an albumin-bound paclitaxel that has lesser hypersensitivity reactions, but seems to be similar to paclitaxel for inducing neuropathy.

Paclitaxel induces a progressive, predominantly sensory neuropathy. Symptoms can occur after the first dose, and include painful paresthesia as well as numbness of the hands and feet. Transient myalgia is common after each dose, which usually resolves within days. Sensory loss presents in a stocking-glove distribution. Ankle jerks and other reflexes may be diminished or absent, which progresses with cumulative doses. Both small and large fiber sensory functions are affected. Muscle strength is frequently preserved or only minimally affected. Docetaxel presents similar clinical manifestations as paclitaxel, but with different toxicity profiles. Docetaxel/carboplatin was associated with 11% grade 2 or higher sensory neuropathy compared with 30% in paclitaxel/carboplatin. Motor neuropathy grade 2 or higher was 3% in Docetaxel/carboplatin versus 7% in paclitaxel/carboplatin. However, docetaxel/carboplatin was associated with significantly more grade 3-4 neutropenia as 94% versus 84% (Vasey et al., 2004). Docetaxel was tolerated better by patients because of less neuropathic pain and myalgia (Pan & Kao 2007). Overall, either single or cumulative dose is the most important factor to consider in taxanes-induced neuropathy. Most symptoms usually improve or resolve after discontinuation of treatment, however, severe symptoms may persist for a long period of time (Argyriou et al., 2008).

The taxanes block tubulin depolymerisation, leading to the inhibition of microtubule dynamics and cell cycle arrest. Paclitaxel and docetaxel accumulate microtubules in axon, dorsal root ganglia, and Schwann cells. These defective microtubules inhibit axonal transport, axonal sprouting, or nerve regeneration (Manfredi & Horwitz 1984, Rowinsky and Donehower 1995). In rat model, both paclitaxel and docetaxel equally induced severe and dose-dependent neuropathy measured with neurophysiological methods, however, the morphometric examination demonstrated more detrimental effect of paclitaxel on nerve fibers (Persohn et al., 2005). In patients, paclitaxel produced early sensory dysfunction in 4 weeks as increasing in stimulus threshold and reduction in sensory amplitudes on neurophysiological and nerve excitability studies; 71% of patients developed symptoms by 6 weeks after administration of about 500 mg/m^2 (Park et al., 2011b). Reduced sensory amplitudes or abolishment of sensory responses on neurophysiology studies were also found in patients treated with docetaxel (New et al., 1996, Pan & Kao 2007). Taxanes-induced peripheral neuropathy is a predominant axonal sensory neuropathy.

2.3 Altretamine

Altretamine was approved by the FDA to treat refractory ovarian cancer in 1990. It is an alkylating agent, binding to and cross-linking of nucleic acid chains. Altretamine induces a mild sensorimotor axonal polyneuropathy that is reversible on cessation of the drug. The neuropathy consists of paresthesia, decreased position and vibrating sense, hyporeftexia, and motor weakness. The incidence of neuropathy (primarily sensory) was between 5-10%(Manetta et al., 1990, Olver et al., 2001, Vergote et al., 1992). Prognosis is usually good with the reversal of the neuropathy upon discontinuation of treatment.

2.4 Neuroprotection

There is currently no standard treatment for the prevention of chemotherapy induced neuropathy. However, neuroprotection studies revealed some potential agents although none of them are commonly employed at present. The ideal candidate for neuroprotection should be safe, well-tolerated, and effective. Most importantly it should not interfere with the cytotoxic activity of chemotherapy.

2.4.1 Acetyl-L-carnitine

Acetyl-L-carnitine, the acetyl ester of L-carnitine, naturally occurs in plants and animals. Acetyl-L-carnitine plays an essential role in metabolism to facilitation of fatty acid utilization. Acetyl-L-carnitine has demonstrated neuroprotective and neurotrophic actions in other neuropathies. In a multicenter, randomized, double-blind, placebo-controlled, diabetic neuropathy study with 333 patients, acetyl-L-carnitine or placebo was administered intramuscularly at a dosage of 1000 mg/day for 10 days and continued orally at a dosage of 2000 mg/day for 355 days (De Grandis & Minardi 2002). Acetyl-L-carnitine showed a statistically significant improvement in mean nerve conduction velocity and amplitude compared with placebo. The greatest changes were observed in sural and ulnar sensory nerves, and the peroneal motor nerve. After 12 months of treatment, pain was reduced 39% from baseline in the acetyl-L-carnitine group, but only 8% in the placebo group (De Grandis & Minardi 2002). Acetyl-L-carnitine also showed significant improvements in sural nerve fiber numbers and regenerating nerve fiber clusters in two 52-week randomized placebo-controlled clinical diabetic neuropathy trials (Sima et al., 2005). Low levels of serum acetyl-L-carnitine were found in patients with antiretroviral toxic neuropathy (James 1997). After 6 months of acetyl-L-carnitine (1500 mg twice daily, oral), small sensory fibers increased from skin biopsy in HIV-positive patients with antiretroviral toxic neuropathy. Improvement of innervation continued in the epidermis and dermis after 24 months of treatment (Hart et al., 2004). In a randomized study, acetyl-L-carnitine treatment produced a significantly greater reduction in pain compared with placebo (P=0.022) when administered 500 mg intramuscularly twice daily for 14 days, followed by orally 1000 mg twice daily for 42 days in patients with antiretroviral toxic neuropathy (Youle et al., 2007).

Acetyl-L-carnitine was found to be able to reduce the neurotoxicity of cisplatin and paclitaxel without interfering with antineoplastic effects of either medication (Pisano et al., 2003) as well as the neurotoxicity of oxaliplatin in rat models (Ghirardi et al., 2005). It was also confirmed that acetyl-L-carnitine does not affect the cytotoxicity of paclitaxel or carboplatin on ovarian cancer cells (Engle et al., 2009). In rats, acetyl-L-carnitine prevented paclitaxel-induced neuropathic pain, the swollen and vacuolated mitochondria caused by paclitaxel in C-fibers, but not in A-fibers (Jin et al., 2008). In addition, acetyl-L-carnitine decreased the spontaneous discharge of A-fibers and C-fibers, and blocked the development of the paclitaxel-evoked pain in the sural nerve of rats (Xiao and Bennett 2008). Acetyl-L-carnitine has been investigated in 2 open label clinical trials in chemotherapy-induced neuropathy. Acetyl-L-carnitine was administrated orally 1g 3 times a day for 8 weeks in 25 patients with neuropathy during paclitaxel or cisplatin therapy (Bianchi et al. 2005). All patients except one reported symptomatic relief, and only two reported nausea. Sensory neuropathy improved in 15 of 25 patients, and motor neuropathy improved in 11 of 14 patients. Total neuropathy score that included neurophysiological studies improved in 23 (92%) patients. Symptomatic improvement persisted in 12 of 13 evaluable patients at median 13 months. Acetyl-L-carnitine (1 g intravenous infusion over 1-2 hours) was also investigated in 26 patients with paclitaxel and/or cisplatin-induced neuropathy (Maestri et al. 2005). At least one WHO grade improvement in the peripheral neuropathy severity was shown in 73% of the patients. Insomnia related to acetyl-L-carnitine was reported in one patient. At present, there is no double-blind, placebo controlled studies to confirm the effect of acetyl-L-carnitine in chemotherapy-induced neuropathy.

2.4.2 Amifostine

Amifostine is approved as a cytoprotective adjuvant for use in cancer chemotherapy and radiotherapy involving DNA-binding chemotherapeutic agents including platinum and alkylating agents. The cytoprotective activity of amifostine is proposed to decrease DNA interstrand crosslinks of platinum and alkylating agents, and to scavenge free radicals. Common side effects are hypotension, nausea and vomiting.

Amifostine cytoprotection was investigated in a multicenter randomized controlled trial in 242 advanced ovarian carcinoma patients with the first-line treatment of cisplatin and cyclophosphamide. The study demonstrated a significant reduction in hematologic, renal, and neurologic toxicities with equivalent therapeutic response and survival (Rose 1996). Later, a phase II study was conducted by the Gynecologic Oncology Group. Twenty-seven patients received intravenous paclitaxel (175 mg/m^2) followed by amifostine (740 mg/m^2) and cisplatin (75 mg/m^2). Four of 27 patients developed grade 2 to 4 neurotoxicity based on clinical assessments, Cancer Institute-Common Toxicity Criteria and the Functional Assessment of Cancer Therapy/Gynecologic Oncology Group-Neurotoxicity. The neuropathic events exceeded the predetermined threshold level, and the study was closed (Moore et al., 2003). In a double-blind randomized placebo-controlled amifostine study of 72 patients in first-line treatment of advanced ovarian cancer with carboplatin/paclitaxel with or without epirubicin, amifostine improved sensory neuropathy according to Cancer Institute-Common Toxicity Criteria with objective neurological assessment. The improvement included two-point discrimination, vibration perception and tendon reflex, but there were almost no differences in self-estimated specific sensory or motor symptoms comparing with placebo. In addition, amifostine failed to improve the global health status quality of life score, and worsened nausea and vomiting (Hilpert et al., 2005). The other randomized study in 90 ovarian cancer patients treated with standard carboplatin/paclitaxel with or without amifostine reported no symptoms of neurotoxicity in 40% of the carboplatin/paclitaxel group versus 49% of the carboplatin/paclitaxel/amifostine group. Grad II sensory neuropathy was in 12% of the carboplatin/paclitaxel group versus 2% of the carboplatin/paclitaxel/amifostine group. Amifostine was temporarily interrupted in five patients due to hypotension. Quality of life questionnaires showed no difference in neurotoxicity scores between both study arms (De Vos et al., 2005).

American Society of Clinical Oncology published 2008 clinical practice guideline. Amifostine may be considered for prevention of cisplatin-associated nephrotoxicity, reduction of grade 3 to 4 neutropenia. It is not recommended for protection against platinum or paclitaxel associated neuropathy (Hensley et al., 2009).

2.4.3 Glutamate

The amino acid glutamate is naturally in many foods. Glutamate is the most abundant excitatory neurotransmitter in the vertebrate nervous system. Like the closely related amino acid glutamine, glutamate was investigated in a randomized, placebo-controlled, double-blinded clinical and electrodiagnostic study. Forty-three ovarian cancer patients were available for analysis following six cycles of paclitaxel treatment. Twenty-three patients were supplemented by glutamate at a daily dose of 500 mg three times, while 20 patients received a placebo. The only statistical difference was found in lower pain scores in the glutamate group. There was no significant difference in neurological examinations, questionnaires and sensory-motor nerve conduction studies between the two groups (Loven et al., 2009). Therefore, based on limited study, glutamate has not demonstrated neuroprotective properties against peripheral neurotoxicity.

2.4.4 Glutamine

Glutamine is a neutral amino acid that plays a critical role in protein synthesis, as a source of cellular energy, and nitrogen donation. The neuroprotective role in chemotherapy induced neuropathy has not been reported in ovarian cancer. Two non-randomized, controlled studies investigated the effect of glutamine (10 g orally three times a day) in single high-dose paclitaxel (825 mg/m^2) induced peripheral neuropathy in breast cancer with a total of 91 patients (Stubblefield et al., 2005, Vahdat et al., 2001). Both paired pre- and post-paclitaxel evaluations shown that the glutamine group had a statistically significant reduction in the incidence and severity of peripheral neuropathy, reduced symptoms and sign in dysesthesias, numbness, weakness and abnormal vibration sense. There were significant reductions in the amplitude and conduction velocity of the motor and sensory nerves from the baseline in both groups, and glutamine did not appear to exert a protective effect (Stubblefield et al., 2005, Vahdat et al., 2001). The role of oral glutamine in preventing oxaliplatin-induced neuropathy was evaluated in 86 patients with colorectal cancer (wang et al., 2007). Patients were randomized to receive or not receive glutamine (15 g twice a day). Glutamine had significantly lower incidence of grade 1-2 peripheral neuropathy, reduced interference with activities of daily living, and did not result in a need for oxaliplatin dose reduction. There were no significant differences between groups in electrophysiological abnormalities, or survival (wang et al., 2007). All 3 clinical trials found that oral glutamine reduces the symptoms of chemotherapy-induced neuropathy, but it does not prevent declining nerve function as measured by nerve conduction study. In addition, none of these studies was randomized, or placebo-controlled. There is a lack of sufficient evidence to recommend oral glutamine for the prevention of chemotherapy induced neuropathy.

2.4.5 Glutathione

Glutathione is a tripeptide. It is an antioxidant to prevent cellular damage by reactive oxygen species such as free radicals. Glutathione was postulated to reduced the toxicity of cisplatin, and a multi-center, double-blind, randomized, placebo controlled phase III trial was conducted in 151 ovarian cancer patients with 74 patients in cisplatin/glutathione group, and 77 patients in cisplatin/placebo group (Smyth et al.,1997). The objective was to determine whether glutathione would enhance the feasibility of giving six cycles of cisplatin at 100 mg/m^2. Glutathione (3 g/m^2) or placebo was given with cisplatin every 3 weeks. Fifty-eight percent of patients completed 6 cycles of treatment in the glutathione group versus 39% of patients in the control group ($P = 0.04$). The glutathione group also showed significantly less nephrotoxicity, and better quality of life scores. Glutathione only suggested a trend towards less neurotoxicity. Sensory neuropathy was 39% in the glutathione group versus 49% in the control group. Motor neuropathy was 9% in the glutathione group versus 12% in the control group measured with common toxicity criteria.

Shortly before the clinical trial for ovarian cancer, glutathione showed efficacy in the prevention of cisplatin induced neurotoxicity, and did not reduce the clinical activity of cisplatin in a randomized double-blind placebo-controlled trial with 50 gastric cancer patients (Cascinu et al., 1995). Glutathione was given intravenously at a dose of 1.5 g/m^2 immediately before cisplatin administration, and at a dose of 600 mg by intramuscular injection on days 2 to 5. Normal saline was administered to patients in the placebo group. Clinical neurologic evaluation and electrophysiologic investigations were performed at baseline, after 9 (cisplatin cumulative dose, 360 mg/m2) and 15 (cisplatin cumulative dose, 600 mg/m2) weeks of treatment. At the 9th week, no patients showed clinically evident neuropathy in the glutathione group, compared to 16 patients in the placebo group. After the 15th week, 4 of 24 patients in the glutathione group suffered from neurotoxicity versus 16 of 18 in the placebo group (P = .0001). Neurophisiologic studies showed a significant reduction of sensory nerve amplitude in the placebo group but not in the glutathione group (Cascinu et al., 1995). Later, glutathione in oxaliplatin-induced neurotoxicity was also demonstrated in a randomized, double-blind, placebo-controlled trial by the same authors with a similar study design (Cascinu et al., 2002). After 12 cycles (oxaliplatin cumulative dose 1,200 mg/m^2), grade 2 to 4 neurotoxicity was observed in 3 of 21 patients in the glutathione group, and in 8 of 19 patients in the placebo group (P=.004). Sural sensory nerve conduction study showed a statistically significant reduction in the placebo group but not in the glutathione group. This study provides evidence that glutathione is a promising drug for the prevention of oxaliplatin induced neuropathy without a reduction of the clinical activity of oxaliplatin. The results from above clinical trials on the efficacy of glutathione are encouraging, but it should be further confirmed in large scale randomized, double-blind, placebo-controlled trials.

2.4.6 Vitamin E

Vitamin E is a fat soluble vitamin with antioxidant property. Low plasmatic levels of vitamin E had been found in patients with severe cisplatin induced neurotoxicity (Bove et al., 2001). Supplementation of vitamin E has shown neuroprotection in patients receiving cisplatin, paclitaxel, or their combination.

Pace and colleagues performed both preclinical study and a pilot clinical trial to evaluate the neuroprotective effect of vitamin E in cisplatin induced neuropathy (Pace et al., 2003). In preclinical studies, nude mice carrying the human melanoma tumor were treated with cisplatin alone or in combination with vitamin E. Cisplatin combined with vitamin E showed no differences in tumor growth, tumor weight, or life span of nude mice as compared to treatment with cisplatin alone. Forty-seven patients were randomly assigned to the vitamin E group during cisplatin chemotherapy, or the control group with cisplatin chemotherapy alone. Vitamin E 300 mg daily was administered orally before cisplatin chemotherapy and continued for 3 months after the suspension of treatment in the vitamin E group. Twenty-seven patients completed six cycles of cisplatin chemotherapy: 13 patients in the vitamin E group and 14 patients in the control group. The incidence of neurotoxicity was significantly lower in the vitamin E group (30.7%) than it was in the control group (85.7%). The severity of neurotoxicity, measured with a comprehensive neurotoxicity score based on clinical and neurophysiological parameters, was significantly lower in patients of the vitamin E group than in patients in the control group (2 versus 4.7) (Pace et al., 2003). Later, Pace and colleagues performed a 2 center, double-blind, randomized, placebo controlled study of cisplatin induced neuropathy in solid tumor patients (Pace et al., 2010). A total of 108 patients treated with cisplatin chemotherapy were randomly assigned to receive vitamin E (400 mg/day) or placebo orally. Only 41 patients who received a cumulative dose of cisplatin higher than 300 mg/m^2 were eligible for statistical analysis with 17 in the vitamin E group and 24 in the placebo group. The incidence of neurotoxicity was significantly lower in the vitamin E group (5.9%) than in the placebo group (41.7%) ($p< 0.01$). Neurotoxicity was measured with Total Neuropathy Score, and revealed a mean score of 1.4 in the vitamin E group versus 4.1 in the placebo group ($p < 0.01$). On sensory nerve conduction study, mean sural and median sensory amplitudes were both significantly reduced in the control group, while only mildly reduced in the sural nerve and unchanged in the median nerve in the vitamin E group (Pace et al., 2010).

Argyriou and colleagues conducted 3 randomized, open label with blind assessment, controlled trials to determine whether vitamin E has a neuroprotective effect in chemotherapy-induced peripheral nerve damage. In 3 trials, a total 93 patients treated with six cycles of cisplatin, paclitaxel, or their combination were randomly assigned to a vitamin E group or a control group. Patients were followed by neurologic examination and electrophysiologic study. Patients assigned to the vitamin E group received oral vitamin E at a daily dose of 600 mg/day during chemotherapy and 3 months after its cessation were compared to patients of the control group. The incidence of neurotoxicity differed significantly between the two groups. The percentage of patients with neurotoxicity was 18.7-25% in the vitamin E group and in 62.5-73.3% in the control group. Mean peripheral neuropathy scores were 2.25-4.99 for patients of the vitamin E group and 10.62-11.5 for patients of the control group (Argyriou et al., 2005, 2006a, 2006b). Their studies showed that vitamin E effectively protects patients with cisplatin/paclitaxel induced peripheral neuropathy. Interestingly, vitamin E supplement at dose from 300 mg to 600 mg daily in all above clinical trials seems to have a similar range of reduction of the incidence of peripheral neurotoxicity. The promising results warrant additional double-blind, randomized, placebo controlled trials in ovarian cancer with carboplatin/paclitaxel treatment for the safety, and efficacy.

Acetyl-L-carnitine, amifostine, glutamate, glutamine, glutathione and vitamin E, reviewed here, are only some of the possible neuroprotective agents investigated for chemotherapy induced neuropathy. Other agents, such as acetylcysteine, calcium and magnesium, diethyldithiocarbamate, and Org 2766 have been investigated , but only limited data is available. At present, the neuroprotection data is insufficient to conclude that any of these agents prevent or limit the neurotoxicity in chemotherapy-induced neuropathy (Albers et al., 2011).

Future research for neuroprotective agents needs well designed clinical trials in chemotherapy-induced neuropathy with a validated grading system, quality of life measurement and evidence of improvement in nerve structure or function, such as epidermal nerve fiber density or electrophysiology study. Otherwise, clinical measurement alone may be symptomatic treatment instead of neuroprotection.

2.4.7 Symptomatic treatment of neuropathic pain

Chemotherapy induced sensory neuropathy may cause neuropathic pain reported as burning, tingling, pins and needles sensation, shooting, cramping, and deep aching. Neuropathic pain is frequently treated with antidepressants, anticonvulsants, topical agents, and analgesics. This treatment must be individualized. Combinations of different agents should be considered in some patients. Slow dose escalation may improve drug tolerability (Pan and Thomas 2001). A new evidence-based guideline for treating painful diabetic neuropathy was issued by the American Academy of Neurology, the American Association of Neuromuscular and Electrodiagnostic Medicine, and the American Academy of Physical Medicine and Rehabilitation based on a systematic review of literature from 1960 to 2008 (Bril et al., 2011). This guideline recommends using pregabalin for painful diabetic neuropathy if clinically appropriate; venlafaxine, duloxetine, amitriptyline, gabapentin, valproate, opioids, capsaicine and percutaneous electrical nerve stimulation are probably effective and should be considered. This guideline can be used for the treatment of chemotherapy induced neuropathic pain.

Pregabalin is an anticonvulsant, which does not bind to plasma proteins or interact with other drugs. It has demonstrated efficacy in 4 randomized, double-blind, multicenter studies of painful diabetic neuropathy (Frampton & Scott 2004, Satoh et al., 2011). Pregabalin is given 2 to 3 times daily. From an initial dose of 50 or 75 mg/day, may be increased to 300 mg/day gradually, and later, to 600 mg/day as needed. Adverse effects of pregabalin include dizziness, somnolence, peripheral edema, headache, blurred vision, and constipation.

Venlafaxine is an antidepressant. It is a serotonin, norepinephrine, and dopamine reuptake inhibitor. A moderate effect of pain relief was found compared with placebo (Rowbotham et al., 2004). Venlafaxine XR 75 mg daily may be increased to 150 mg daily. Venlafaxine is well tolerated; the adverse events are nausea, headache, somnolence, dry mouth, and dizziness.

Duloxetine is an antidepressant, a reuptake inhibitor of serotonin and norepinephrine. Duloxetine at doses of 60 and 120 mg a day improved neuropathic pain in several randomized, double-blind studies of diabetic neuropathy and was rather well tolerated (Goldstein et al., 2005). A more common initial side effect, nausea, can be curtailed if the drug is started at a low dose of 20 or 30 mg during the first week.

Amitriptyline has been investigated in several double-blind, randomized trials. Amitriptyline, desipramine, and fluoxetine were compared at a mean daily dose of 105, 111, and 40 mg respectively in 2 randomized, double-blind, crossover studies of painful diabetic neuropathy. Amitriptyline and desipramine relieved pain in 74% and 61% of 38 patients respectively, whereas fluoxetine showed no difference compared with placebo in 46 patients (Max et al., 1992). Amitriptyline should be started at a dosage of 10 to 25 mg/day and increased by 10 to 25 mg/week to the maximum effect or tolerated dosage. Bedtime administration may help to reduce day time sedation. The adverse events most commonly reported are dry mouth, sedation, constipation, nausea, and urinary retention as well as orthostatic hypotension and tachycardia in elderly patients. Amitriptyline should be administrated with caution in patients with urinary retention, glaucoma, constipation, impaired liver function, or cardiovascular disease.

Gabapentin is currently the most frequently used anticonvulsant for painful neuropathy, and also does not bind to plasma proteins or interact with other drugs. A double-blind, placebo-controlled trial demonstrated pain reduction with gabapentin at 900 to 3600 mg/day in 165 patients with diabetic neuropathy (Backonja et al., 1998). Gabapentin can reduce chemotherapy-induced neuropathic pain at a low dose of 800 mg/day (Tsavaris et al., 2008). Adverse events may include fatigue, dizziness, somnolence, and weight gain. Gabapentin should be started at a dose of 100 to 300 mg/day and slowly increased to the maximum effect or tolerated dosage. Occasionally, a previously effective dose needs to be increased to maintain pain control in the absence of objective evidence of disease progression, possibly due to habituation.

3. Entrapment neuropathy

Entrapment neuropathy is caused by focal compression, restriction, or mechanical distortion of a nerve in a fibrous or fibro-osseous tunnel. Chemotherapy-induced peripheral neuropathy can make nerves more vulnerable to compression or to stretching nerve injury. Minor compression may lead to focal demyelination or axonal injury. Entrapment neuropathy should be suspected if symptoms are focal or unilateral instead of symmetrical, length dependent or generalized. Positive Tinel's sing may be found at the entrapment site. Nerve conduction study and electromyography can localize the abnormality and reveal the severity. Several common entrapment neuropathies should be recognized as below.

Median nerve entrapment at the wrist is the most common entrapment neuropathy as median nerve passes the carpal tunnel. Symptoms involve the thumb, index and middle fingers with numbness, tingling and burning, but referred pain can radiate to forearm or arm. Symptoms may be worse at night, or after using of the hand. Examination may reveal sensory deficit for light touch in the median nerve distribution distal to carpal tunnel. Thenar weakness and atrophy are seen in the severe entrapment cases. Nerve conduction study frequently demonstrates prolonged sensory nerve latency, reduced amplitude, and prolonged distal motor latency. The initial treatment is wrist splint in neutral position. Severe entrapment needs surgical carpal tunnel release.

Ulnar nerve entrapment at the elbow is the second most common entrapment neuropathy. The ulnar nerve may be directly compressed in the retrocondylar grove or entrapped through cubital tunnel. Symptoms present as tingling or numbness in the fifth and part of the fourth fingers, hypothenar eminence and the dorsum of the hand. Weakness or atrophy of the interossei muscles causes clawing of the fourth and fifth fingers in severe entrapment. Nerve conduction study reveals slow conduction velocity across the elbow segment. Electromyography may reveal acute and chronic denervation in ulnar nerve innervated muscles. Elbow protector, avoidance of repetitive elbow flexion and extension, and direct pressure from excessive elbow leaning may resolve the symptoms. Surgical release of compression or anterior translocation may be considered if symptoms persist after conservative treatment.

Common peroneal nerve entrapment at the fibular head is the most common entrapment neuropathy in the leg. Direct pressure to the fibular head, or habitual leg crossing can result foot drop, inversion, and sensory deficits at the lateral lower leg. Nerve conduction study may reveal slow motor conduction velocity across the fibular head. Electromyography may reveal acute and chronic denervation in common peroneal or deep nerve innervated muscles. Ankle-foot orthosis can improve the gait when foot drop is present.

Posterior tibial nerve is more frequently entraped distally at the tarsal tunnel instead of the proximal segment. The most common pathology relates to external compression from shoes that are too tight or to plaster casts. Others include posttraumatic fibrosis, tendon sheath cysts, and rheumatoid arthritis. The plantar nerves may be damaged within the tarsal tunnel or more distally as they course through the arch and sole of the foot. The medial plantar nerve is injured more commonly than the lateral, and may cause burning pain in the toes and the sole of the foot, which is difficult to deferential from chemotherapy-induced neuropathy if it involves both feet. Nerve conduction study may confirm entrapment at the tarsal tunnel, however, planter nerve sensory response is not easy to elicit, may be absent even without tarsal tunnel syndrome. If the sural sensory study is abnormal, absent planter nerve sensory response may be due to generalized peripheral neuropathy. Tarsal tunnel syndrome treatment, at least initially, should be conservative to remove possible outside compression, such as shoes. When conservative measures fail, surgical release may be considered.

Lateral femoral cutaneous nerve entrapment is usually entrapped at the inguinal ligament with obesity, direct compression by a belt, but rarely in the proximal segment of femoral nerve by retroperitoneal tumor, hematoma, ascites or other conditions with increased intra-abdominal pressure. This nerve is a pure sensory nerve and entrapment causes numbness, burning, and/or pain on the anteriorlateral thigh. Most patients with lateral femoral cutaneous nerve neuropathy, except for those with iliacus or retroperitoneal hematoma that might require surgical intervention, are treated conservatively, while waiting for spontaneous remyelination or reinnervation.

Dellon and colleagues reported clinical success of surgical decompression in 80 percent of their patients, including chemotherapy-induced neuropathy if patients had positive Tinel's sign on the known anatomic compression sites. Five of 9 in the report were ovarian cancer patients treated with cisplatin or paclitaxel or both. Three patients had complaints of pain localized in a single extremity with single nerve compression. Single nerve decompression was successful for those patients. The other 2 ovarian cancer patients had multiple decompression in lower extremities. Surgical decompression has resulted in restoration of sensation and relief of pain. (Dellon et al., 2004).

4. Neurologic paraneoplastic syndromes

Paraneoplastic syndromes are rare, and occur as a remote effect of tumor, not by mass lesions, metastases, or anti-tumor treatment. The prevalence of paraneoplastic syndromes is very low, as only one patient was found with neurological paraneoplastic syndrome as cerebellar degeneration in 908 patients with primary ovarian malignancy (Hudson et al., 1993). Neurologic paraneoplastic disorders are autoimmune diseases, and can affect any part of the central (cerebellar degeneration, limbic encephalitis, opsoclonus-myoclonus, and brainstem encephalitis), or peripheral nervous system (subacute sensory neuronopathy, and autonomic insufficiency). Unlike chemotherapy-induced neuropathy, subacute sensory neuronopathy can begin in arm, legs, or face, and spread proximally to trunk, with progressively loss all sensations. Neurological paraneoplastic syndromes are caused by an autoimmune response to proteins (onconeural antigents) that are shared by the cancer and the peripheral or central nerve systems. They are Hu, Yo, Ri, CV2, amphiphysin, Ma, Ta, Tr, NMDA. Ovarian cancer patients may express proteins Hu, Yo, Ri and anti-amphiphysin (Titulaer et al., 2011). Therefore, test antibodies for Hu, Yo, Ri and anti-amphiphysin can help to diagnose neurological paraneoplastic syndrome in ovarian cancer. In a retrospective study of 73 Hu-antibody positive patients, neurological paraneoplastic syndromes are 55% sensory neuropathy, 22% cerebellar degeneration, 15% limbic encephalitis, and 16% brainstem encephalitis (Sillevis Smitt et al., 2002).

Treatment of paraneoplastic syndromes in ovarian cancer should primarily treat the malignancy. Corticosteroids, cyclophosphamide and other immunosuppressant may be used. Intravenous immune globulin or plasma exchange can be tried. However, all treatment may not be beneficial to subacute sensory neuronopathy.

5. Conclusion

Peripheral neuropathy in ovarian cancer is complex. When patients develop neuropathy symptoms in ovarian cancer, we cannot simply conclude that it is chemotherapy-induce neuropathy. It is a challenge to treat this condition. Diagnosis of the etiology of the neuropathy, treating the underlying disease, correction of metabolic, nutritional, and endocrine abnormalities, and decompression of the nerve entrapment will preserve nerve function. The goals of treatment are reduction of symptoms, improvement of function and patient's quality of life.

6. Reference

Albers, J.W.; Chaudhry, V.; Cavaletti, G. and Donehower, R.C. (2011) Interventions for preventing neuropathy caused by cisplatin and related compounds. *Cochrane Database Syst Rev.* Vol.16, No.2, (February 2011), pp. CD005228.

Argyriou, A.A.; Chroni, E.; Koutras, A.; Ellul, J.; Papapetropoulos, S.; Katsoulas, G.; Iconomou, G. and Kalofonos, H.P. (2005) Vitamin E for prophylaxis against chemotherapy-induced neuropathy: a randomized controlled trial. *Neurology,* Vol.64, No.1, (Jan 11, 2005), pp.26-31.

Argyriou, A.A.; Chroni, E.; Koutras, A.; Iconomou, G.; Papapetropoulos, S.; Polychronopoulos, P. and Kalofonos, H.P. (2006a) Preventing paclitaxel-induced peripheral neuropathy: a phase II trial of vitamin E supplementation. *J Pain Symptom Manage.* Vol.32, No.3, (September 2006), pp. 237-244.

Argyriou, A.A.; Chroni, E.; Koutras, A.; Iconomou, G.; Papapetropoulos, S.; Polychronopoulos, P. and Kalofonos, H.P. (2006b) A randomized controlled trial evaluating the efficacy and safety of vitamin E supplementation for protection against cisplatin-induced peripheral neuropathy: final results. *Support Care Cancer,* Vol.14, No.11, (November, 2006), pp.1134-1140.

Argyriou, A.; Koltzenburg, M.; Polychronopoulos, P.; Papapetropoulos, S. and Kalofonos, H.P. (2008) Peripheral nerve damage associated with administration of taxanes in patients with cancer. *Crit Rev Oncol Hematol,* Vol.66, No.3, (June 2008), pp.218-228.

Armstrong, D.K.; Bundy, B.; Wenzel, L.; Huang, H.Q.; Baergen, R.; Lele, S.; Copeland, L.J. Walker, J.L.; Burger, R.A. and Gynecologic Oncology Group. (2006) Intraperitoneal cisplatin and paclitaxel in ovarian cancer. *N Engl J Med,* Vol.354, No.1, (Janary 5, 2006), pp. 34-43.

Backonja, M.; Beydoun, A.; Edwards, K.R.; Schwartz, S.L.; Fonseca, V.; Hes, M.; LaMoreaux, L. and Garofalo, E. (1998) Gabapentin for the symptomatic treatment of painful neuropathy in patients with diabetes mellitus: a randomized controlled trial. *JAMA,* Vol.280, No.21, (December 2, 1998), pp.1831-1836.

Bianchi, G.; Vitali, G.; Caraceni, A.; Ravaglia, S.; Capri, G.; Cundari, S.; Zanna C.; and Gianni, L. (2005) Symptomatic and neurophysiological responses of paclitaxel- or cisplatin-induced neuropathy to oral acetyl-L-carnitine. *Eur J Cancer,* Vol.41, No.12, (August 2005), pp. 1746-1750.

du Bois, A.; Lück, H.J.; Meier, W.; Adams, H.P.; Möbus, V.; Costa, S.; Bauknecht, T.; Richter, B.; Warm, M.; Schröder, W.; Olbricht, S.; Nitz, U.; Jackisch, C.; Emons, G.; Wagner, U.; Kuhn, W.; Pfisterer, J. and Arbeitsgemeinschaft Gynäkologische Onkologie Ovarian Cancer Study Group. (2003) A randomized clinical trial of cisplatin/paclitaxel versus carboplatin/paclitaxel as first-line treatment of ovarian cancer. *J Natl Cancer Inst.,*Vol.95, No.17, (September 3, 2003), pp.1320-1329.

Bove, L.; Picardo, M.; Maresca, V.; Jandolo, B. and Pace, A. (2001) A pilot study on the relation between cisplatin neuropathy and vitamin E. *J Exp Clin Cancer Res.* Vol.20, No.2, (June 2001), pp. 277-280.

Bril, V.; England, J.; Franklin, G.M.; Backonja, M.; Cohen, J.; Del Toro, D.; Feldman, E.; Iverson, D.J.; Perkins, B.; Russell, J.W. and Zochodne, D. (2011) Evidence-based Guideline: Treatment of Painful Diabetic Neuropathy: Report of the American Academy of Neurology, the American Association of Neuromuscular and Electrodiagnostic Medicine, and the American Academy of Physical Medicine and Rehabilitation. *Neurology,* Vol.76, No.20, (March 17, 2011), pp. 1758-1765.

Calhoun, E.A.; Welshman, E.E.; Chang, C.H.; Lurain, J.R.; Fishman, D.A.; Hunt, T.L. and Cella, D.(2003) Psychometric evaluation of the Functional Assessment of Cancer Therapy/Gynecologic Oncology Group-Neurotoxicity (Fact/GOG-Ntx) questionnaire for patients receiving systemic chemotherapy. *Int J Gynecol Cancer,* Vol.13, No.6, (November-December 2003), pp.741-748.

Cascinu, S.; Cordella, L.; Del Ferro, E.; Fronzoni, M. and Catalano, G. (1995) Neuroprotective effect of reduced glutathione on cisplatin-based chemotherapy in advanced gastric cancer: a randomized double-blind placebo-controlled trial. *J Clin Oncol,* Vol.13, No.1, (Janury 1995), pp.26-32.

Cascinu S Catalano V Cordella L Labianca R Giordani P Baldelli AM Beretta GD Ubiali E Catalano G. (2002) Neuroprotective effect of reduced glutathione on oxaliplatin-based chemotherapy in advanced colorectal cancer: a randomized, double-blind, placebo-controlled trial. *J Clin Oncol,* Vol.20, No.16, (August 15, 2002), pp.3478-3483.

Cavaletti, G.; Jann, S.; Pace, A.; Plasmati, R.; Siciliano, G.; Briani, C.; Cocito, D.; Padua, L.; Ghiglione, E.; Manicone, M.; Giussani, G and Italian NETox Group. (2006) Multi-center assessment of the Total Neuropathy Score for chemotherapy-induced peripheral neurotoxicity. *J Peripher Nerv Syst,* Vol.11, No.2, (June 2006), pp. 135-141.

Chválová, K.; Brabec, V. and Kaspárková, J. (2007) Mechanism of the formation of DNA-protein cross-links by antitumor cisplatin. *Nucleic Acids Res,* Vol.35, No.6 (February 28, 2007), pp. 1812-1821.

Dellon, A.L; Swier, P.; Maloney, C.T. Jr.; Livengood, M.S. & Werter, S (2004) Chemotherapy-induced neuropathy: treatment by decompression of peripheral nerves. , Vol.114, No.2, (August 2004), pp.478-483.

Engle, D.B.; Belisle, J.A.; Gubbels, J.A.; Petrie, S.E.; Hutson, P.R.; Kushner, D.M. and Patankar. M.S. (2009) Effect of acetyl-l-carnitine on ovarian cancer cells' proliferation, nerve growth factor receptor (Trk-A and p75) expression, and the cytotoxic potential of paclitaxel and carboplatin. *Gynecol Oncol,* Vol.112, No.3, (March 2009), pp.631-636.

Frampton, J.E. and Scott, L.J. (2004) Pregabalin: in the treatment of painful diabetic peripheral neuropathy. Drug Vol.64, No.24, (2004): pp. 2813-2820

Ghirardi, O.; Lo Giudice, P.; Pisano, C.; Vertechy, M.; Bellucci, A.; Vesci, L.; Cundari, S.; Miloso, M.; Rigamonti, L.M.; Nicolini, G.; Zanna, C. and Carminati, P. (2005) Acetyl-L-Carnitine prevents and reverts experimental chronic neurotoxicity induced by oxaliplatin, without altering its antitumor properties. *Anticancer Res,* Vol.25, No.4, (July-August 2005), pp.2681-2687.

Goldstein, D.J; Lu, Y.; Detke, M.J.; Lee, T.C. and Iyengar, S. (2005) Duloxetine vs. placebo in patients with painful diabetic neuropathy. *Pain,* Vol.116, No.1-2, (July 2005), pp. 109-118.

De Grandis, D. and Minardi, C. (2002) Acetyl-L-carnitine (levacecarnine) in the treatment of diabetic neuropathy. A long-term, randomised, double-blind, placebo-controlled study. *Drugs R D,* Vol.3, No.4, (2002), pp. 223-231.

Harnett, P.; Buck, M.; Beale, P.; Goldrick, A.; Allan, S.; Fitzharris, B.; De Souza, P.; Links, M.; Kalimi, G.; Davies, T. and Stuart-Harris, R. (2007) Phase II study of gemcitabine and oxaliplatin in patients with recurrent ovarian cancer: an Australian and New Zealand Gynaecological Oncology Group study. *Int J Gynecol Cancer,* Vol.17, No.2, (March-April 2007), pp.359-366.

Hart, A.M.; Wilson, A.D.; Montovani, C.; Smith, C.; Johnson, M.; Terenghi, G. and Youle, M. (2004) Acetyl-l-carnitine: a pathogenesis based treatment for HIV-associated antiretroviral toxic neuropathy. *AIDS,* Vol.18, No.11, (July 23, 2004), pp. 1549-1560.

Hensley, M.L.; Hagerty, K.L.; Kewalramani, T.; Green, D.M.; Meropol, N.J.; Wasserman, T.H.; Cohen, G.I.; Emami, B.; Gradishar, W.J.; Mitchell, R.B.; Thigpen, J.T.; Trotti, A. 3rd; von Hoff, D. and Schuchter, L.M. (2009) American Society of Clinical Oncology 2008 clinical practice guideline update: use of chemotherapy and radiation therapy protectants. *J Clin Oncol,* Vol.27, No.1, (January 1, 2009), pp. 127-145.

Hilpert, F.; Stähle, A.; Tomé, O.; Burges, A.; Rossner, D.; Späthe, K.; Heilmann, V.; Richter, B.; du Bois, A . and Arbeitsgemeinschaft Gynäkologische Onkologoie (AGO) Ovarian Cancer Study Group (2005) Neuroprotection with amifostine in the first-line treatment of advanced ovarian cancer with carboplatin/paclitaxel-based chemotherapy--a double-blind, placebo-controlled, randomized phase II study from the Arbeitsgemeinschaft Gynäkologische Onkologoie (AGO) Ovarian Cancer Study Group. *Support Care Cancer,* Vol.13, No.10, (October 2005), pp. 797-805.

Hudson, C.N.; Curling, M.; Potsides, P. and Lowe, D.G. (1993) Paraneoplastic syndromes in patients with ovarian neoplasia. *J R Soc Med,* Vol.86, No. 4, (April 1993), pp. 202-204.

James, J.S. (1997) Drug-related neuropathy: low acetylcarnitine levels found. *AIDS Treat News,* Vol.21, No.265, (February 1997), pp. 6-7.

Jin, H.W.; Flatters, S.J.; Xiao, W.H.; Mulhern, H.L. and Bennett, G.J. (2008) Prevention of paclitaxel-evoked painful peripheral neuropathy by acetyl-L-carnitine: effects on axonal mitochondria, sensory nerve fiber terminal arbors, and cutaneous Langerhans cells. *Exp Neurol,* Vol.210, No.1, (March 2008), pp.229-237.

Krarup-Hansen, A.; Rietz, B.; Krarup, C.; Heydorn, K.; Rørth, M. and Schmalbruch, H. (1999) Histology and platinum content of sensory ganglia and sural nerves in patients treated with cisplatin and carboplatin: an autopsy study. *Neuropathol Appl Neurobiol,* Vol.25, No.1, (Febuary 1999), pp. 29-40.

Loven, D.; Levavi, H.; Sabach, G.; Zart, R.; Andras, M.; Fishman, A.; Karmon, Y.; Levi, T.; Dabby, R. and Gadoth, N. (2009) Long-term glutamate supplementation failed to protect against peripheral neurotoxicity of paclitaxel. *Eur J Cancer Care,* Vol.18, No.1, (January 2009), pp.78-83.

Maestri, A.; De Pasquale Ceratti, A.; Cundari, S.; Zanna, C.; Cortesi, E. and Crinò, L. (2005) A pilot study on the effect of acetyl-L-carnitine in paclitaxel- and cisplatin-induced peripheral neuropathy. Tumori, Vol.91, No.2, (March-April 2005), pp.135-138.

Manetta, A.; Colin MacNeill, C.; Judith A. Lyter, J.A.; Scheffler. B.; Podczaski, E.S.; James E. Larson, J.E. and Philip Schein, P. (1990) Hexamethylmelamine as a single second-line agent in ovarian cancer. Gynecologic Oncology, Vol.36, No.1, (January 1990), pp. 93-96.

Markman, M.; Bundy, B.N.; Alberts, D.S.; Fowler, J.M.; Clark-Pearson, D.L.; Carson, L.F.; Wadler, S. and Sickel, J. (2001) Phase III trial of standard-dose intravenous cisplatin plus paclitaxel versus moderately high-dose carboplatin followed by intravenous paclitaxel and intraperitoneal cisplatin in small-volume stage III ovarian carcinoma: an intergroup study of the Gynecologic Oncology Group, Southwestern Oncology Group, and Eastern Cooperative Oncology Group. *J Clin Oncol,* Vol.19, No.4 (February 15, 2001), pp. 1001-1007.

Max, M.B.; Lynch, S.A.; Muir, J.; Shoaf, S.E.; Smoller, B. and Dubner, R. (1992) Effects of desipramine, amitriptyline, and fluoxetine on pain in diabetic neuropathy. *N Engl J Med,* Vol.326, No.19, (May 7, 1992), pp.1250-1256.

Mayerhofer, K.; Bodner-Adler, B.; Bodner, K. Leodolter, S. and Kainz, C. (2000) Paclitaxel/carboplatin as first-line chemotherapy in advanced ovarian cancer: efficacy and adverse effects with special consideration of peripheral neurotoxicity. *Anticancer Res,* Vol.20, No.5C, (September-October 2000), pp. 4047-4050.

McWhinny, S.R.; Goldberg, R.M. and McLeod, H.L. (2009) Platinum neurotoxicity pharmacogenetics. *Mol Cancer Ther.* Vol.8, No.1. (January 2009), pp.10-16.

Misset, J.L.; Vennin, P.; Chollet, P.H.; Pouillart, P.; Laplaige. P.H.; Frobert, J.L.; Castera, D.; Fabro, M.; Langlois, D.; Cortesi, E.; Lucas, V.; Gamelin, E.; Laadem, A. and Otero, J. (2001) Multicenter phase II-III study of oxaliplatin plus cyclophosphamide vs. cisplatin plus cyclophosphamide in chemonaive advanced ovarian cancer patients. *Ann Oncol,* Vol.12, No.10. (Oct. 2001), pp. 1411-1415.

Moore, D.H.; Donnelly, J.; McGuire, W.P.; Almadrones, L.; Cella, D.F.; Herzog, T.J.; Waggoner, S.E. and Gynecologic Oncology Group. (2003) Limited access trial using amifostine for protection against cisplatin- and three-hour paclitaxel-induced neurotoxicity: a phase II study of the Gynecologic Oncology Group. *J Clin Oncol,* Vol.21, No.22(November 15, 2003), pp. 4207-4213.

New, P.Z.; Jackson, C.E.; Rinaldi, D.; Burris, H. and Barohn, R.J. (1996) Peripheral neuropathy secondary to docetaxel (Taxotere). *Neurology,* Vol.46, No.1, (January 1996), pp. 108-111.

Nicoletto, M.O.; Falci, C.; Pianalto, D.; Artioli, G.; Azzoni, P.; De Masi, G.; Ferrazzi, E.; Perin, A.; Donach, M. and Zoli, W. (2006) Phase II study of pegylated liposomal doxorubicin and oxaliplatin in relapsed advanced ovarian cancer. *Gynecol Oncol,* Vol.100, No.2, (Feb. 2006), pp. 318-323.

Nurgalieva, Z.; Xia, R.; Liu, C.C.; Burau, K.; Hardy, D. & Du, X.L. (2010) Risk of chemotherapy-induced peripheral neuropathy in large population-based cohorts of elderly patients with breast, ovarian, and lung cancer. *Am J Ther,* Vol.17, No.2, (March-April 2010), pp.148-158.

Olver, I.; Davy, M.; Lüftner, D.; Park, S.H.; Egorin, M.; Ellis, A. and Webster, L. (2001) A phase I study of paclitaxel and altretamine as second-line therapy to cisplatin regimens for ovarian cancer. *Cancer Chemother Pharmacol,* Vol.48, No.2, (August 2001), pp.109-114.

Pace, A.; Savarese, A.; Picardo, M.; Maresca, V.; Pacetti, U.; Del Monte, G.; Biroccio, A.; Leonetti, C.; Jandolo, B.; Cognetti, F. and Bove, L. (2003) Neuroprotective effect of vitamin E supplementation in patients treated with cisplatin chemotherapy. *J Clin Oncol,* Vol.21, No.5, (Mar 1, 2003), pp. 927-931.

Pace, A.; Giannarelli, D.; Galiè, E.; Savarese, A.; Carpano, S.; Della Giulia, M.; Pozzi, A.; Silvani, A.; Gaviani, P.; Scaioli, V.; Jandolo, B.; Bove, L.; Cognetti, F. (2010) Vitamin E neuroprotection for cisplatin neuropathy: a randomized, placebo-controlled trial. *Neurology,* Vol.74, No.9, March 2, 2010), pp.762-766.

Pan, Y. and Thomas, F. (2001) Neuropathic pain: treatment. In: *Medlink Neurology,* Weimer, L.H. ed. MedLink Corporation. http://www.medlink.com/medlinkcontent.asp

Pan, Y. and Kao, M.S. (2007) Discordance of clinical symptoms and electrophysiologic findings in taxane plus platinum-induced neuropathy. *Int J Gyneocol Cancer,* Vol.17, No.2, (March-April 2007), pp.394-397.

Park, S.B.; Lin, C.S.; Krishnan, A.V.; Goldstein, D.; Friedlander, M.L. and Kiernan, M.C. (2011a) Utilizing natural activity to dissect the pathophysiology of acute oxaliplatin-induced neuropathy. *Exp Neurol,* Vol.227, No.1, (January 2011), pp.120-127.

Park, S.B.; Lin, C.S.; Krishnan, A.V.; Friedlander, M.L.; Lewis, C.R. and Kiernan, M.C. (2011b) Early, progressive, and sustained dysfunction of sensory axons underlies paclitaxel-induced neuropathy. *Muscle Nerve,* Vol.43, No.3, (March 2011), pp.367-374.

Pfisterer, J.; du Bois, A.; Wagner, U.; Quaas, J.; Blohmer, J.U.; Wallwiener, D. and Hilpert, F. (2004) Docetaxel and carboplatin as first-line chemotherapy in patients with advanced gynecological tumors. A phase I/II trial of the Arbeitsgemeinschaft Gynakologische Onkologie (AGO-OVAR) Ovarian Cancer Study Group. *Gynecol Oncol,* Vol.92, No.3, (March 2004), pp. 949-956.

Pignata, S.; De Placido, S.; Biamonte, R.; Scambia, G.; Di Vagno, G.; Colucci, G.; Febbraro, A.; Marinaccio, M.; Lombardi, A.V.; Manzione, L.; Cartenì, G.; Nardi, M.; Danese, S.; Valerio, M.R.; de Matteis, A.; Massidda, B.; Gasparini, G.; Di Maio, M.; Pisano, C.& Perrone, F. (2006) Residual neurotoxicity in ovarian cancer patients in clinical remission after first-line chemotherapy with carboplatin and paclitaxel: the Multicenter Italian Trial in Ovarian cancer (MITO-4) retrospective study. *BMC Cancer,* Vol.6, No.5, (January 2006), pp.1-7.

Pisano, C.; Pratesi, G.; Laccabue, D.; Zunino, F.; Lo Giudice, P.; Bellucci, A.; Pacifici, L.; Camerini, B.; Vesci, L.; Castorina, M.; Cicuzza, S.; Tredici, G.; Marmiroli, P.; Nicolini, G.; Galbiati, S.; Calvani, M.; Carminati, P . and Cavaletti, G. (2003)

Paclitaxel and Cisplatin-induced neurotoxicity: a protective role of acetyl-L-carnitine. *Clin Cancer Res,* Vol.9, No.15, (Nov 15, 2003), pp. 5756-5767.

Podratz, J.L.; Knight, A.M.; Ta, L.E.; Staff, N.P.; Gass, J.M.; Genelin, K.; Schlattau, A.; Lathroum, L. and Windebank, A.J. (2011) Cisplatin induced Mitochondrial DNA damage in dorsal root ganglion neurons. *Neurobiol Dis,* Vol.41, No.3, (March 2011), pp.661-668.

Persohn, E.; Canta, A.; Schoepfer, S.; Traebert, M.; Mueller, L.; Gilardini, A.; Galbiati, S.; Nicolini, G.; Scuteri, A.; Lanzani, F.; Giussani, G. and Cavaletti, G. (2005) Morphological and morphometric analysis of paclitaxel and docetaxel-induced peripheral neuropathy in rats. *Eur J Cancer,* Vol.41, No.10, (July 2005), pp.1460-1466.

Recchia, F.; Saggio, G.; Amiconi, G.; Di Blasio, A.; Cesta, A.; Candeloro, G.; Carta, G.; Necozione, S.; Mantovani, G. and Rea, S. (2007) A multicenter phase II study of pegylated liposomal doxorubicin and oxaliplatin in recurrent ovarian cancer. *Gynecol Onco,* Vol.106, No.1, (July 2007), pp.164-169.

Rose, P.G. (1996) Amifostine cytoprotection with chemotherapy for advanced ovarian carcinoma. *Semin Oncol,* Vol.23, No.4 Suppl 8, (August 1996), pp.83-89.

Rowbotham, M.C.; Goli, V.; Kunz, N.R. and Lei, D. (2004) Venlafaxine extended release in the treatment of painful diabetic neuropathy: a double-blind, placebo-controlled study. *Pain,* Vol.110, No.3, (August 2004), pp. 697-706.

Rowinsky, E.K., and Donehower, R.C. Paclitaxel (Taxol) (1995) *N Engl J Med,* Vol.332, No.15, (April 13, 1995), pp.1004-1014

Satoh, J.; Yagihashi, S.; Baba, M. Suzuki, M.; Arakawa, A.; Yoshiyama, T. and Shoji, S.(2011) Efficacy and safety of pregabalin for treating neuropathic pain associated with diabetic peripheral neuropathy: a 14 week, randomized, double-blind, placebo-controlled trial. *Diabet Med,* Vel.28, No.1, (January 2011) pp. 109-116.

Sillevis Smitt, P.; Grefkens, J.; de Leeuw, B.; van den Bent, M.; van Putten, W.; Hooijkaas, H. and Vecht, C. (2002) Survival and outcome in 73 anti-Hu positive patients with paraneoplastic encephalomyelitis/sensory neuronopathy. *J Neurol,* Vol.249, No.6(June 2002), pp. 745-753.

Sima, A.A.; Calvani, M.; Mehra, M.; Amato, A. and Acetyl-L-Carnitine Study Group. (2005) Acetyl-L-carnitine improves pain, nerve regeneration, and vibratory perception in patients with chronic diabetic neuropathy: an analysis of two randomized placebo-controlled trials. *Diabetes Care,* Vol.28, No.1, (January 2005), pp. 89-94.

Stubblefield, M.D.; Vahdat, L.T.; Balmaceda, C.M.; Troxel, A.B.; Hesdorffer, C.S. and Gooch, C.L. (2005) Glutamine as a neuroprotective agent in high-dose paclitaxel-induced peripheral neuropathy: a clinical and electrophysiologic study. *Clin Oncol,* Vol.17, No.4, (June 2005), pp. 271-276.

Smyth, J.F.; Bowman, A.; Perren, T.; Wilkinson, P.; Prescott, R.J.; Quinn, K.J. and Tedeschi, M. (1997) Glutathione reduces the toxicity and improves quality of life of women diagnosed with ovarian cancer treated with cisplatin: results of a double-blind, randomised trial. *Ann Oncol,* Vol.8, No.6, (June 1997), pp. 569-73.

Ta, L.E.; Espeset, L.; Podratz, L. and Windebank, A.J. (2006) Neurotoxicity of oxaliplatin and cisplatin for dorsal root ganglion neurons correlates with platinum-DNA binding. *Neurotoxicology,* Vol.27, No.6, (December 2006), pp.992-1002.

Titulaer, M.J.; Soffietti, R.; Dalmau, J.; Gilhus, N.E.; Giometto, B.; Graus, F.; Grisold, W.; Honnorat, J.; Sillevis Smitt, P.A.; Tanasescu, R.; Vedeler, C.A.; Voltz, R.; Verschuuren, J.J. and European Federation of Neurological Societies (2011) Screening for tumours in paraneoplastic syndromes: report of an EFNS task force. ***Eur J Neurol***, Vol.18, No.1, (January 2011), pp. 19-e3.

Tsavaris, N. ; Kopterides, P. ; Kosmas, C. ; Efthymiou, A. ; Skopelitis, H. ; Dimitrakopoulos, A. ; Pagouni, E.; Pikazis, D.; Zis, P.V. amd Koufos, C. (2008) Gabapentin monotherapy for the treatment of chemotherapy-induced neuropathic pain: a pilot study. *Pain Med*, Vol.9, No.8, (November 2008), pp. 1209-1216.

Vahdat, L.; Papadopoulos, K.; Lange, D.; Leuin, S.; Kaufman, E.; Donovan, D.; Frederick, D.; Bagiella, E.; Tiersten, A.; Nichols, G.; Garrett, T.; Savage, D.; Antman, K.; Hesdorffer, C.S. and Balmaceda, C. (2001) Reduction of paclitaxel-induced peripheral neuropathy with glutamine. *Clin Cancer Res*, Vol.7, No.5, (May 2001), pp. 1192-1197.

Van Der Hoop, R. G., Van Der Burg, M. E. L., Ten Huinink, W. W. B., Van Houwelingen, J. C. and Neijt, J. P. (1990), Incidence of neuropathy in 395 patients with ovarian cancer treated with or without cisplatin. *Cancer* Vol.66, No.8, (October 1990), pp. 1697–1702.

Vasey, P.A.; Jayson, G.C.; Gordon, A.; Gabra, H.; Coleman, R.; Atkinson, R.; Parkin, D.; Paul, J.; Hay, A.; Kaye, S.B. and Scottish Gynaecological Cancer Trials Group. Phase III randomized trial of docetaxel-carboplatin versus paclitaxel-carboplatin as first-line chemotherapy for ovarian carcinoma. *J Natl Cancer Inst*, Vol.96, No.22. (Nov 17, 2004), pp.1682-1691.

Vergote, I.; Himmelmann, A.; Frankendal, B.; Scheistrøen, M.; Vlachos, K.' and Tropé, C. (1992) Hexamethylmelamine as second-line therapy in platin-resistant ovarian cancer. *Gynecol Onco*,. Vol. 47, NO. 3, (December 1992), pp.282-286.

Viens, P.; Petit, T.; Yovine, A.; Bougnoux, P.; Deplanque, G.; Cottu, P.H.; Delva, R.; Lotz, J.P.; Belle, S.V.; Extra, J.M. and Cvitkovic, E. (2006) A phase II study of a paclitaxel and oxaliplatin combination in platinum-sensitive recurrent advanced ovarian cancer patients. *Ann Oncol*, Vol.17, No.3, (March 2006), pp.429-436.

De Vos, F.Y.; Bos, A.M.; Schaapveld, M.; de Swart, C.A.; de Graaf, H.; van der Zee, A.G. Boezen, H.M.; de Vries, E.G. and Willemse, P.H. (2005) A randomized phase II study of paclitaxel with carboplatin +/- amifostine as first line treatment in advanced ovarian carcinoma. *Gynecol Oncol*, Vol.97, No.1, (April 2005), pp. 60-67.

Wang, W.S.; Lin, J.K.; Lin, T.C.; Chen, W.S.; Jiang, J.K.; Wang, H.S.; Chiou, T.J.; Liu, J.H.; Yen, C.C. and Chen, P.M. (2007) Oral glutamine is effective for preventing oxaliplatin-induced neuropathy in colorectal cancer patients. *Oncologist*, Vol.12, No.3, (March 2007), pp. 312-319.

Wolf, S.; Barton, D.; Kottschade, L.; Grothey, A. and Loprinzi, C. (2008) Chemotherapy-induced peripheral neuropathy: prevention and treatment strategies. *Eur J Cancer*, Vol.44, No.11, (July 2008), pp.1507-1515.

Xiao, W.H. and Bennett, G.J. (2008) Chemotherapy-evoked neuropathic pain: Abnormal spontaneous discharge in A-fiber and C-fiber primary afferent neurons and its suppression by acetyl-L-carnitine. *Pain*, Vol.135, No.3, (April 2008), pp. 262-70.

Youle, M.; Osio, M. and ALCAR Study Group. (2007) A double-blind, parallel-group, placebo-controlled, multicentre study of acetyl L-carnitine in the symptomatic treatment of antiretroviral toxic neuropathy in patients with HIV-1 infection. *HIV Med*, Vol.8, No.4, (May 2007), pp.241-250.

8

Combined Cytoreductive Surgery and Perioperative Intraperitoneal Chemotherapy for the Treatment of Advanced Ovarian Cancer

Antonios-Apostolos K. Tentes[1],
Nicolaos Courcoutsakis[2] and Panos Prasopoulos[2]
[1]*Didimotichon General Hospital,*
[2]*Alexandroupolis University Hospital*
Greece

1. Introduction

Ovarian cancer is the leading cause of death from gynecologic cancer and the fifth cause of cancer deaths in women in developed countries (Yancik, 1993; Cannistra, 1993). The number of deaths seems to increase the last few years. More than 70% of the patients with ovarian cancer have advanced disease at the time of initial diagnosis because they remain asymptomatic in early stages (Roberts, 1996). Ovarian cancer is the most frequent intraceolomic malignancy presenting with peritoneal spread. In the past debulking surgery combined with systemic chemotherapy offered long-term survival in less than 10% of the patients (Smith & Day, 1979). The standard treatment of advanced ovarian cancer is cytoreductive surgery followed by systemic chemotherapy (Hacker et al, 1983; Neijt et al, 1991; Hoskins et al, 1992). Despite systemic chemotherapy based on platinum and taxanes 5 and 10-year survival rate do not exceed 20% and 10% respectively because the majority of the patients develop recurrence (Mc Guire & Ozols, 1998; Piccart et al, 2000). The disease remains characteristically confined to the peritoneal surfaces for most of its natural course (Bergmann, 1996). Surgical resection of the tumor may not be complete and microscopic or even macroscopic residual tumor may be left behind. In these situations the intraperitoneal route of administration of cytostatic drugs is a logical approach.

Patients with diseases that have similar biological behavior to ovarian cancer are offered significant survival benefit when they are treated with perioperative intraperitoneal chemotherapy integrated in cytoreductive surgery. In pseudomyxoma peritonei (Sugarbaker, 2006), peritoneal sarcomatosis (Rossi et al, 2004), peritoneal mesothelioma (Yan et al, 2007), colorectal cancer with peritoneal dissemination (Elias et al, 2009; Mahteme et al, 2004; Verwaal et al, 2008), as well as in gastric cancer with peritoneal carcinomatosis (Yonemura et al, 1996; Yu et al, 1998) survival is improved with this treatment strategy. The last two decades the method has been used in ovarian cancer with promising results.

2. Prognostic indicators of advanced ovarian cancer

2.1 Peritoneal Cancer Index (PCI)

The clinical utility of the FIGO staging system has been well established since its first report in 1964 (Odicino et al, 2001) but does not provide clear details about the extent and distribution of the peritoneal spread.

In contrast the peritoneal cancer index is a useful clinical variable by which the evaluation of the extent and distribution of the peritoneal malignancy is clear and accurate and has been continuously used in pseudomyxoma peritonei (Sugarbaker, 2006), peritoneal mesothelioma (Yan et al, 2007), colorectal cancer with peritoneal dissemination (Elias, 2001; Sugarbaker, 1999; Gomez-Portilla et al, 1999), and peritoneal sarcomatosis (Rossi et al, 2004; Esquivel & Sugarbaker, 1998).

The calculation of the peritoneal cancer index is possible with the division of the abdomen and pelvis in 13 different regions (Figure 1). Two transverse and two sagittal planes are used to divide the abdomen and pelvis in nine regions. The upper transverse plane is the lowest part of the costal margin and the lower plane is the anterior superior iliac spine. The sagittal planes divide the abdomen in three equal sectors. The abdominopelvic region 0 (AR-0) includes the midline incision, the greater omentum and the transverse colon. The abdominopelvic region 1 (AR-1) includes the superior surface of the right lobe of the liver, the undersurface of the right hemidiaphragm, and the right retrohepatic space. The epigastric fat, the left lobe of the liver, the lesser omentum and the falciform ligament are included in the abdominopelvic region 2 (AR-2). The abdominopelvic region 3 (AR-3) includes the undersurface of the left hemidiaphragm, the spleen, the tail of the pancreas, as well as the anterior and posterior surface of the stomach. The descending colon and the left abdominal gutter are included in abdominopelvic region 4 (AR-4). The left pelvic side wall and the sigmoid colon are included in the abdominopelvic region 5 (AR-5). The abdominopelvic region 6 (AR-6) includes the internal female genitalia, the cul-de-sac of Douglas, and the rectosigmoid colon. The abdominopelvic region 7 (AR-7) includes the right pelvic side wall, the base of the cecum, and the appendix. The abdominopelvic region 8 (AR-8) includes the ascending colon and the right paracolic gutter. The small bowel and its mesentery are divided in four additional regions in upper jejunum (AR-9), lower jejunum (AR-10), upper ileum (AR-11), and lower ileum (AR-12). The peritoneal cancer index is the summation of the tumor volume in each one of the 13 different regions in which the abdomen and the pelvis are divided.

Although the inclusion of the anatomic structures in the abdominopelvic regions is arbitrary the assessment of the distribution and extent of the peritoneal dissemination is detailed.

2.2 Tumor volume

The tumor volume is assessed as LS-0 (lesion size) when no visible tumor is detected, as LS-1 when tumor nodules are < 0.5 cm in their largest diameter, as LS-2 when tumor nodules are 0.5-5 cm in their largest diameter, and as LS-3 when tumor nodules are > 5 cm in their largest diameter, or there are confluent any size nodules. LS-0, LS-1, and LS-2 are considered small volume tumors, and LS-3 large volume tumors (Figure 1) (Jacquet & Sugarbaker, 1996).

The tumor volume is a significant prognostic indicator of survival in advanced ovarian cancer (Tentes et al, 2003; Piso et al, 2004; Raspagliesi et al; 2006, Di Giorgio et al, 2008).

The extent of peritoneal dissemination in ovarian cancer may also be assessed with the use of the Lyon staging system, and the Dutch simplified peritoneal carcinomatosis index (SPCI) (Gilly et al, 2006). The assessment of the extent and distribution of peritoneal carcinomatosis using anyone of the above staging systems is helpful in excluding from surgery those patients who are not expected to be offered any benefit from cytoreductive surgery.

In patients with high-grade tumors and high PCI complete cytoreduction is not feasible. In contrast, patients with low-grade tumors such as pseudomyxoma peritonei, grade I sarcoma and cystic peritoneal mesothelioma may easily undergo complete cytoreduction even if they have very high PCI. Therefore, in these situations the prognosis is related only to the completeness of cytoreduction. In addition, in very aggressive high grade tumors such as unresectable common bile duct cancer or unresectable cancer of the head of the pancreas the peritoneal cancer index is of no prognostic significance, even if it is low. In addition, the lymph node involvement in groups of lymph nodes that have no anatomic relation to the primary tumor the prognosis is poor despite a low PCI, because the favorable PCI is overridden by the systemic disease.

Peritoneal Cancer Index

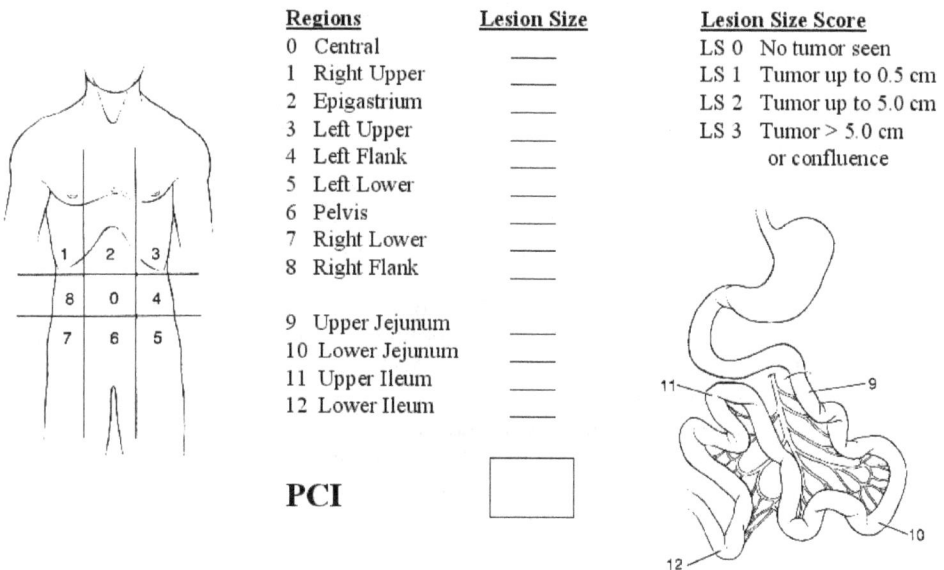

Regions	Lesion Size
0 Central	____
1 Right Upper	____
2 Epigastrium	____
3 Left Upper	____
4 Left Flank	____
5 Left Lower	____
6 Pelvis	____
7 Right Lower	____
8 Right Flank	____
9 Upper Jejunum	____
10 Lower Jejunum	____
11 Upper Ileum	____
12 Lower Ileum	____
PCI	

Lesion Size Score	
LS 0	No tumor seen
LS 1	Tumor up to 0.5 cm
LS 2	Tumor up to 5.0 cm
LS 3	Tumor > 5.0 cm or confluence

Fig. 1. Assessment of PCI by summation of the lesion size in the 13 regions in which the abdomen and pelvis are divided.

2.3 Prior Surgical Score (PSS)

Prior surgical score is a useful prognostic indicator of survival for patients with peritoneal malignancy. If surgery has not been performed or only biopsy or laparoscopy has been performed then the score is 0 (PSS-0). In patients that have undergone surgery in one abdominopelvic region the score is 1 (PSS-1). For those patients that have undergone surgery in 2-5 abdominopelvic regions the score is 2 (PSS-2) and for those patients that have undergone surgery in > 5 abdominopelvic regions the score is 3 (PSS-3) (Jacquet & Sugarbaker, 1996).

Prior surgical score is a significant prognostic indicator of survival in peritoneal sarcomatosis, appendiceal cancer, and peritoneal mesothelioma (Rossi et al, 2004; Jacquet & Sugarbaker, 1996; Sebbag et al, 2000). The significance of PSS has been questioned by other studies for pseudomyxoma peritonei and peritoneal mesothelioma (Brigand et al, 2006; Deraco et al, 2006; Miner et al, 2005; Baratti et al, 2007). In ovarian cancer PSS has been identified as a significant prognostic indicator of survival in one study (Look et al, 2004). The value of PSS in ovarian cancer is currently under investigation.

2.4 Completeness of cytoreduction score

In ovarian cancer the residual tumor is the most significant indicator for long-term survival (Hacker et al, 1983; Neijt et al, 1991; Hoskins et al, 1992; Eisenkop et al, 2003; Hunter et al, 1992; Bristow et al, 2002; Tentes et al, 2006; Piso et al, 2004; Raspagliesi et al, 2006; Di Giorgio et al, 2008; Look et al, 2004). Gynecologists oncologists use the terms optimal and suboptimal cytoreduction to define the quality of the surgical result. The level of optimal cytoreduction has been arbitrarily set from 5 mm to 3 cm. The Gynecologic Oncology Group has shown that survival progressively decreases as the residual tumor increases from microscopic to 2 cm (Hoskins et al, 1994). As a consequence optimal cytoreduction is defined as the operation with no macroscopic residual disease. Survival is not improved if the residual tumor is more than 2 cm in its largest diameter and these patients do not survive longer than patients with 10 cm residual disease, which means that aggressive surgery such as bowel resection is not indicated if the residual tumor can not be less than 2 cm (Hoskins et al, 1994).

The completeness of cytoreduction is a different approach to residual disease. For gastrointestinal cancer the completeness of cytoreduction score is defined as CC-0 if no macroscopically tumor is left after cytoreductive surgery, as CC-1 if nodules less than 2.5 mm are left after surgery, as CC-2 if the residual nodules are > 2.5 mm and < 2.5 cm, and as CC-3 if tumor nodules > 2.5 cm or a confluence of tumor nodules in the abdomen or in the pelvis are left behind after cytoreductive surgery. For high-grade tumors only CC-0 surgery is considered to be complete cytoreductive surgery. For low-grade tumors CC-0 and CC-1 cytoreductions are considered complete cytoreductive operations.

The completeness of cytoreduction score is the most significant prognostic indicator of survival in patients with pseudomyxoma peritonei (Sugarbaker, 2006; Miner et al, 2005; Baratti et al, 2007) peritoneal mesothelioma (Yan et al 2007; Sebbag et al, 2000; Brigand et al, 2006; Deraco et al, 2006), colorectal cancer with peritoneal carcinomatosis (Sugarbaker, 1999; Gomez-Portilla et al, 1999) gastric cancer with peritoneal carcinomatosis (Yonemura et al, 2003), and peritoneal sarcomatosis (Rossi et al, 2004; Berthet et al, 1999).

The completeness of cytoreduction score in advanced ovarian cancer has been demonstrated to be a significant prognostic indicator of survival (Tentes et al, 2003; Tentes et al, 2006; Piso et al, 2004; Raspagliesi et al, 2006; Di Giorgio et al, 2008).

2.5 Performance status

Long-term survival in ovarian cancer is related to patient's performance status (Tentes et al, 2006). Patients with poor performance status can not tolerate extensive surgery such as cytoreductive surgery because of increased morbidity and hospital mortality. The preoperative performance status and the extent of the peritoneal carcinomatosis are prognostic indicators of hospital morbidity (Reuter et al, 2008)

3. Treatment of advanced ovarian cancer

3.1 Cytoreductive surgery-standard peritonectomy procedures

The most powerful tool in the treatment of the diseases that have already disseminated at the peritoneal surfaces is surgical resection of the macroscopically visible tumor. For this purpose standard peritonectomy procedures have been used. The initially described six peritonectomy procedures (Sugarbaker, 1995) have recently been modified to the: 1) epigastric peritonectomy, 2) right subdiaphragmatic peritonectomy, 3)) left subdiaphragmatic peritonectomy, 4) greater omentectomy ± splenectomy 5) lesser omentectomy, 6) pelvic peritonectomy, 7) cholecystectomy and resection of the omental bursa, 8) right parietal peritonectomy, 9) left parietal peritonectomy, and 10) resection of other organs (antrectomy, colectomy other than low anterior, subtotal colectomy, total gastrectomy, segmental intestinal resection) (Sugarbaker, 1999).

In retrospective studies the residual tumor has been identified as the most significant prognostic indicator of survival (Hacker et al, 1983; Neijt et al, 1991; Hoskins et al, 1992; Eisenkop, 2003). Meta-analyses have documented the same finding (Hunter et al, 1992; Bristow et al, 2002) but no prospective trial has been performed. The feasibility of complete cytoreduction using standard peritonectomy procedures in ovarian cancer is 78.4% (Tentes et al, 2006; Chi et al, 2004).

3.1.1 Patient's position

The patient is placed in modified lithotomy position. This place provides access to the perineum. A hyperthermia blanket is placed on the operating table to warm the patient during surgery. A midline incision from xyphoid process to the symphysis pubis is used for maximal exposure of the abdominal cavity.

3.1.2 Epigastric peritonectomy procedure

Epigastric peritonectomy procedure is used in re-operations and includes wide resection of the old scar with the round and the falciform ligament of the liver. Sometimes resection of the xyphoid process is required for maximal exposure of the subdiaphragmatic areas.

3.1.3 Right subdiaphragmatic peritonectomy procedure

The peritoneum beneath the right hemidiaphragm is stripped until the bare area of the liver is encountered. If tumor has seeded the anterior surface of the liver then it is removed beneath or through the Glisson's capsule until the liver surface free of tumor is encountered. The tumor beneath the right hemidiaphragm, the right subhepatic space and the surface of the liver is removed en-bloc forming an envelope. Laterally on the right the dissection includes the peritoneum that covers the right perirenal fat as well as the anterior surface of the right adrenal. Eventually the vena cava, and the right hepatic vein form the base of the specimen (Figures 2, 3).

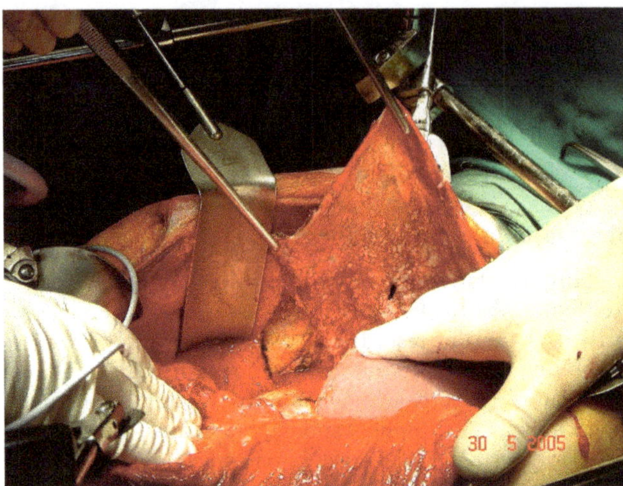

Fig. 2. The peritoneum beneath the right hemidiaphragm with the tumor, and the Glisson's capsule of the right lobe of the liver have been mobilized as an envelope and are ready for resection.

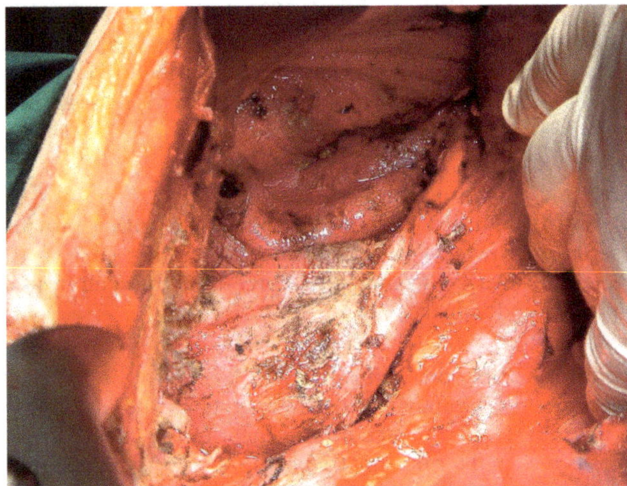

Fig. 3. Specimen of the right subdiaphragmatic peritonectomy procedure. The right lobe of the liver has been turned to the left. The muscular segment of the right hemidiaphragm is exposed free of tumor as well as the anterior surface of the right adrenal and the right kidney. The subhepatic inferior vena cava is visualized.

3.1.4 Left subdiaphragmatic peritonectomy procedure

All the tumor tissue beneath the left hemiaphragm is stripped until the muscular segment of the left hemiaphragm, the anterior surface of the left adrenal, the left kidney, and the tail of the pancreas are visualized free of tumor (Figure 4).

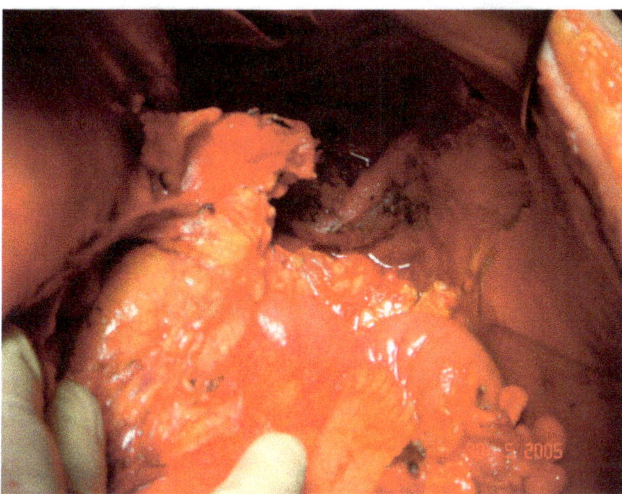

Fig. 4. Specimen of the left subdiaphragmatic peritonectomy procedure. The spleen has been removed. The tail of the pancreas, the undersurface of the left hemidiaphragm, the anterior surface of the left adrenal and the left kidney are exposed.

3.1.5 Greater omentectomy and splenectomy

The greater omentum dissected from the transverse colon and transverse mesocolon permits the exposure of the anterior surface of the body and tail of the pancreas. The branches of the right and left gastroepiploic vessels and the short splenic vessels on the greater curvature of the stomach are clamped and ligated. The splenic artery and vein at the tail of the pancreas are visualized, clamped, divided, and ligated. If the spleen is adherent by tumor of the left hemiaphragm then left subdiaphragmatic peritonectomy procedure must be completed before the spleen and the greater omentum are released (Figure 5, 6).

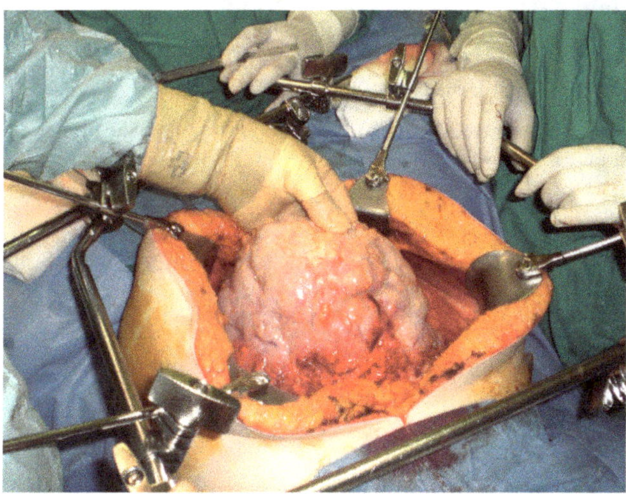

Fig. 5. Omental cake.

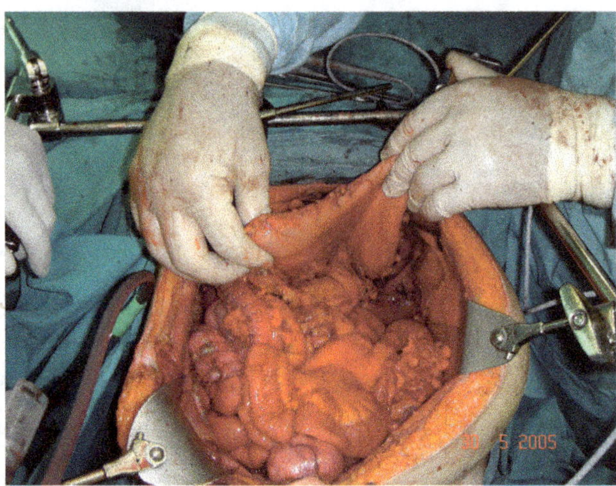

Fig. 6. The base of greater omentectomy and splenectomy (greater curvature of the stomach).

3.1.6 Cholecystectomy and resection of the omental bursa

The gallbladder is removed from its fundus toward the cystic artery and the cystic duct which are ligated, and divided. The anatomical structures of the hepatoduodenal ligament are skeletonized and the covering peritoneum is released. The peritoneum that covers the anterior surface of the inferior vena cava is stripped with the tumor that seeds the foramen of Winslow (Figure 7).

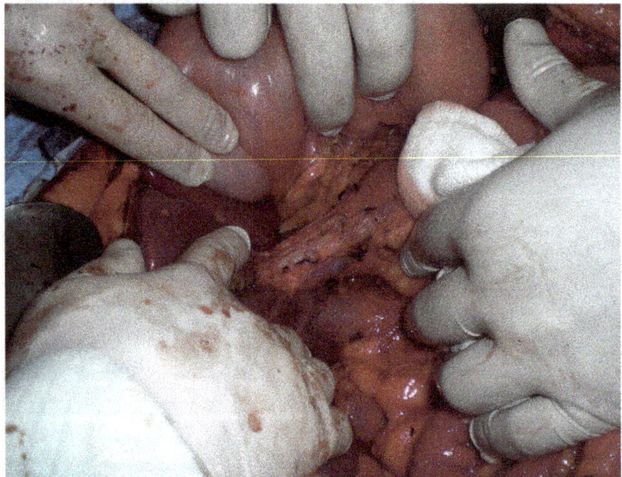

Fig. 7. The skeletonized hepatoduodenal ligament and the anterior surface of the inferior vena cava below the portal vein are exposed free of tumor.

3.1.7 Lesser omentectomy

The lesser omentum is released from the fissure between liver segments 1, 2, and 3, and from the arcade of the right to left gastric artery along the lesser curvature of the stomach.

The fat of the lesser omentum with the tumor are separated and released from the vascular arcade. The anterior vagus must be preserved as much as possible. An accessory left hepatic artery originating from the left gastric artery must also be preserved. After the release of the lesser omentum the complete resection of the omental bursa is possible by division of the peritoneal reflection of the liver to the left of the subhepatic vena cava which is stripped from the superior recess of the omental bursa, from the crus of the right hemidiaphragm, and from beneath the portal vein (Figure 8).

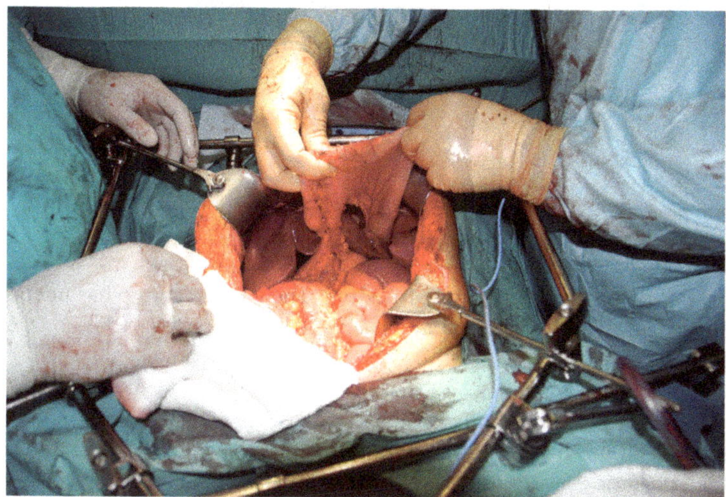

Fig. 8. The base of lesser omentectomy. The arcade of the right gastric and left gastric artery has been preserved.

3.1.8 Pelvic peritonectomy procedure

The peritoneum stripped from the posterior surface of the lower abdominal incision allows the exposure of the posterior muscular wall of the bladder. The urachus is identified, divided, and used for traction of the bladder. In female patients the round ligaments are divided at the point they enter the internal inguinal canal bilaterally. Superiorly the peritoneum is stripped to the duodenum and the ligament of Treitz. The ureters are identified and preserved. In females the ovarian veins are identified and ligated at the lower pole of the kidneys while in males the spermatic veins are preserved. The inferior mesenteric vein is identified and ligated. The inferior mesenteric artery is also identified and ligated just above its origin from the aorta. The colon is divided at the junction of the descending to sigmoid colon and this allows the complete separation of the upper and the lower abdomen. The mesorectum can be easily dissected with the use of a ball-tip electrocautery. The surgeon working in a centripetal fashion may free-up the entire pelvis. The uterine vessels are ligated and divided above the ureters and close to the base of the bladder. The bladder is freed from the cervix and the vagina is encountered. The vagina is divided, the perirectal fat is divided beneath the peritoneal reflection and the tumor occupying the cyl-de-sac of Doudlas is removed en-bloc with the specimen. The mid-rectum is skeletonized and divided (Figure 9).

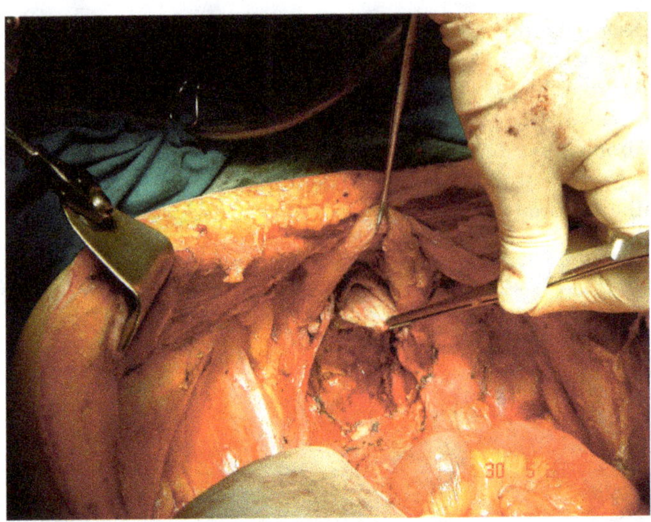

Fig. 9. The base of pelvic peritonectomy procedure. The vaginal stump has not been sutured and is visualized. The bladder is raised by a clamp. The ureters, the sacral bone, and the rectal stump are also visualized.

3.1.9 Bilateral lateral peritonectomy procedure

The peritoneum behind the rectus abdominal muscle is stripped and the base of the specimen is the posterior sheath of the rectus abdominal muscle and the posterior surface of the lateral abdominal muscles.

3.1.10 Resection of other organs

Antrectomy in addition to other peritonectomy procedures is required if the gastric antrum is seeded by tumor. Total gastrectomy is infrequently required in an attempt to achieve complete cytoreduction. Segmental intestinal resection or subtotal colectomy with end-ileostomy may also be performed in order to achieve complete or near complete cytoreduction (Stamou et al, 2003).

3.2 Perioperative intraperitoneal chemotherapy

Even if the macroscopically visible tumor has been completely removed after maximal cytoreductive surgery the microscopic residual tumor will possibly be present at the peritoneal surfaces. The disseminated cancer cells adhere to the peritoneal surfaces and are covered by fibrin, platelets, polymorphonuclear cells, and monocytes that infiltrate fibrin during the healing process. Growth factors released in large amounts stimulate fibroplast proliferation and local collagen production, eventually modulating wound healing promote cancer proliferation and give rise to secondary tumors within 2-3 years after initial surgery (Roberts & Sporn, 1989). In recurrent ovarian cancer it has been demonstrated that in 90% of the patients tumor is found in the vaginal cuff and in 60% tumor is found in the lower part of the abdominal incision (Sugarbaker TA et al, 1996).

The concept about the use of intraperitoneal chemotherapy is based upon the properties of the peritoneal-plasma barrier. Peritoneal plasma barrier is an anatomical and functional

structure. It is consisted by the fluid in the abdominal cavity, the mesothelium, the intervening interstitium, and the blood vessel wall (Jacquet et al, 1994; Sugarbaker, 1991). Most of the cytostatic drugs are large molecular weight substances that are confined for long at the peritoneal surfaces and exert intensively their pharmacologic properties before their absorption into the systemic circulation.
The penetration of intraperitoneal chemotherapy is limited to approximately 1-2 mm into tissues and may result in the eradication of the microscopic residual tumor.

3.2.1 Hyperthermic Intraperitoneal Intraoperative Chemotherapy (HIPEC)

Hyperthermic intraperitoneal intraoperative chemotherapy (HIPEC) enhances cytotoxicity and improves drug penetration. The heat itself has antitumor properties. If HIPEC is performed with the open abdominal technique (Coliseum technique) the surgeon may distribute uniformly the heat and the cytotoxic drugs to the entire peritoneal cavity manually (Figure 10). Renal toxicity of intraperitoneal chemotherapy is avoided by careful monitoring of urine output during perfusion. Side-effects of systemic chemotherapy (nausea, vomiting) are avoided because the patient is under general anesthesia. The time that elapses during hyperthermic perfusion normalizes a number of parameters (hemodynamics, hemostasis, temperature etc) (Sugarbaker, 2005).

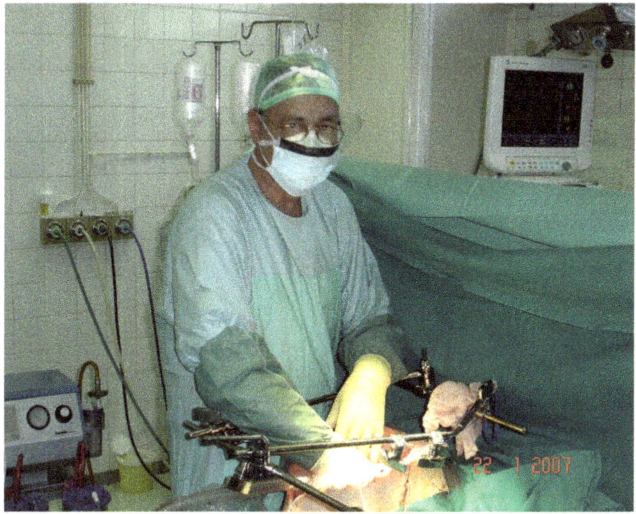

Fig. 10. The surgeon distributes heat and cytotoxic drugs manually to all the peritoneal surfaces.

3.2.2 Early Postoperative Intraperitoneal Chemotherapy (EPIC)

Early postoperative intraperitoneal chemotherapy under normothermia (EPIC) is used with the same intent as HIPEC before intra-abdominal adhesions are formed. The method is used during the first five postoperative days (Sugarbaker, 2005), because the formation of adhesions after days 7-8 do not permit uniform distribution of the cytostatic drugs. The distribution of cytostatic drugs is imperfect with EPIC because the undersurface of the right hemidiaphragm, the corresponding surface of the right lobe of the liver, the anterior surface of the stomach, the folds of small bowel mesentery, and adherent bowel surfaces, the male pelvis, and the abdominal wall are not adequately exposed to cytostatic drugs (Averbach & Sugarbaker, 1996).

The effectiveness of the peritoneal-plasma barrier persists despite extensive stripping of the peritoneal surfaces and the pharmacokinetics of intraperitoneal drug delivery is not changed (Jacquet.& Sugarbaker, 1996a). These results have been reproduced and confirmed by studies on peritoneal transport in experimental animals (Rubin et al, 1988).

3.2.3 Drugs used in HIPEC

The combination of cis-platin (50 mg/m^2) and doxorubicin (15 mg/m^2) is the ideal treatment for both primary and recurrent ovarian cancer. For platinum resistant patients gemcitabine (1000 mg/m^2) or mitomycin-C (10-20 mg/m^2) or oxaliplatin (130 mg/m^2) or melphalan (50-70 mg/m^2) may alternatively be used. The doses are 33% reduced if aggressive chemotherapy has been previously used or the renal function is marginal or the patient is above 60 years of age or there has been extensive intraoperative trauma to the small bowel surfaces or if irradiation has been previously used (Sugarbaker, 2005).

3.2.4 Drugs used in EPIC

5-FU (600 mg/m^2) (maximum dose=1400 mg) with 50 meq sodium bicarbonate or alternatively paclitaxel (20-40 mg/m^2) (maximum dose=80 mg) or docetaxel (20 mg/m^2) (maximum dose=100 mg) are currently in use during EPIC (Sugarbaker, 2005).

4. Patient selection for cytoreductive surgery and perioperative intraperitoneal chemotherapy

The combined treatment with the use of cytoreductive surgery and perioperative intraperitoneal chemotherapy does not offer benefit to all patients. Therefore proper patient selection is required.

4.1 Inclusion criteria

Patients are included for cytoreductive surgery and perioperative intraperitoneal chemotherapy if they meet the following criteria: 1) performance status > 50% according to Karnofsky performance scale, 2) no recent cardiovascular accident, 3) normal hematologic profile, 4) normal hepatic and renal function, 5) absence of a second malignancy at risk for recurrence (except for skin basal-cell carcinoma or in-situ cancer of the cervix adequately treated), 6) absence of chronic or recent acute pulmonary disease, 7) absence of multiple and unresectable extra-abdominal metastases.

4.2 Exclusion criteria

Patients with: 1) performance status < 50%, 2) severe cardiovascular or pulmonary disease, 3) white blood cell count < 4000, 4) platelets < 150.000, 5) urea > 50 mg/dl, 6) creatinine level > 1.5 mg/dl, 7) abnormal hepatic function, 8) presence of a second malignancy at risk for recurrence, 9) pregnancy, 10) drug addiction, 11) presence of tumor at the ligament of Treitz, 12) multiple segmental intestinal obstruction, 13) presence of multiple and unresectable distant metastases, 14) extensive disease at the peritoneal surfaces of the small bowel

making impossible a complete or near-complete cytoredution are excluded from treatment for cytoreductive surgery and perioperative intraperitoneal chemotherapy.
Complete hematological and biochemical profile is preoperatively required as well as whole body bone scanning for the exclusion of osseous metastases.
The presence of resectable distant metastases is not an absolute contraindication for cytoreductive surgery combined with perioperative intraperitoneal chemotherapy. It has been demonstrated that patients with colorectal cancer, peritoneal carcinomatosis, and hepatic metastases who may undergo complete cytoreduction, and R_0 resection of the metastatic lesions are offered significant survival benefit although their long-term survival is not equivalent to survival of patients without distant metastases (Elias et al, 2001).

4.3 Imaging modalities used to detect the extent and distribution of peritoneal malignancy

All imaging modalities have been used in the past to detect peritoneal malignancy. Plain films, ultrasound, magnetic resonance imaging, and CT-scan have been used in excess. CT-scan of the abdomen and pelvis with oral and intrarectal contrast plus intravenous contrast has been the state-of-the-art modality for detecting the extent of the implants of peritoneal malignancy (Archer et al, 1996).

4.3.1 Abdominopelvic Ultrasonography (US)

The first imaging evaluation of women with ovarian cancer and suspected peritoneal carcinomatosis was performed with US (Raptopoulos & Gourtsigiannis, 2001). There is a lack of radiation, the examination is easily accepted from the patient and the availability of the modality is wide. The accuracy of the method is high in detecting ascites and/or peritoneal implants especially at the pelvic walls (Raptopoulos & Gourtsigiannis, 2001; Gonzalez-Moreno et al, 2009). The detailed mapping of cancerous implants in entire peritoneal cavity is time consuming with low specificity. The results of the examination are operator - depended and consequently not always reproducible (Gonzalez-Moreno et al, 2009).

4.3.2 Computed Tomography (CT), Computed Tomography-Enteroclysis (CTE)

CT is the established and worldwide most used imaging method in staging and follow-up of patients with peritoneal carcinomatosis because of high image quality, fast throughput of examinations and lower cost, than other imaging modalities (i.e. MRI, PET, PET/CT) (Raptopoulos & Gourtsigiannis, 2001; Gonzalez-Moreno et al, 2009; Woodward et al, 2004; Coakley et al, 2002; Marin et al, 2010). The last few years the development of technology with the multi-detectors CT (MDCT) has improved significantly the ability to obtain in short-image acquisition very thin slices with high spatial resolution including multiplanar or tridimensional reconstructions (Forstner 2007). The ability of CT to detect peritoneal dissemination depends on the size and morphology of the peritoneal implants. The diagnostic accuracy of CT even MDCT for detecting peritoneal implants is decreased dramatically for lesions smaller than 0.5 cm or for those with a "layered - type" form covering the gastrointestinal tube and especially the small bowel (Gonzalez-Moreno et al, 2009; Coakley et al, 2002).

The assessment of the extent and distribution of the peritoneal carcinomatosis is possible with CT which provides sufficient sensitivity and specificity. However, the sensitivity and specificity at the peritoneal surfaces of the small bowel and its mesentery are not sufficient (Raptopoulos & Gourtsigiannis, 2001; Gonzalez-Moreno et al, 2009; de Bree et al, 2004). Disease at the small bowel constitutes a sentinel, limiting criterion in the decision making process involved cytoreduction because sufficient length of small bowel must remain in place to allow for adequate oral nutrition in the future. Once the extent of peritoneal malignancy at the small bowel is the limit of cytoreductive surgery, the evaluation of the small bowel is a crucial component in the preoperative imaging assessment. Experience tells us that even the most sophisticated CT technology usually underestimates actual small bowel involvement revealed at surgical exploration (Gonzalez-Moreno et al, 2009; de Bree et al, 2004).

Implants of less than 1 cm in size are detected with sensitivity 25-50% when helical-CT is used (Gonzalez-Moreno et al, 2009; de Bree et al, 2004). Multi-detectors CT yield a mean sensitivity of 89% for implants larger than 0.5 cm. The sensitivity decreases to 43% for lesions less than 0.5 cm (Marin et al, 2010).

CTE has been defined as "small bowel distention" by administration of high volume of contrast medium via a naso-gastro-jejunal catheter followed by axial CT acquisition (Maglinte et al, 2007). Thus, CTE is a hybrid technique combining the advantages of conventional enteroclysis and those of CT. The cancerous implants attached to the partially distended intestinal loops, sometimes with insufficient quantity of enteral contrast on conventional CT are very difficult to be depicted. Severe involvement of the entire segments of the small bowel manifested as remarkable wall thickness cannot be revealed, if the intestinal loops are not well-distended. Thus, the study of the small bowel and its mesentery could be more accurate, in detail and facilitated having simultaneously information for both the extent and the distribution of cancerous implants within the peritoneal cavity. At the surface of the stretched loops, the tiny or small in size implants may be depicted. Even, the "layered-type" of small bowel involvement may be demonstrated as remarkable thickness of the strongly enhancing intestinal wall. Small bowel loops dilatation allows mesentery unfolding and consequently the easier demonstration of implanted cancerous lesions.

CTE in patients with peritoneal malignancy is currently under extensive investigation. In a prospective study, forty-five consecutive patients (34 women, 11 males, mean age=57.02 years) with peritoneal malignancy of different primaries who were candidates for cytoreductive surgery and HIPEC underwent CTE before surgery. A modified CTE-Peritoneal Carcinomatosis Index (CTE-PCI) was applied to score the lesion size of the nodules at the small bowel surfaces. CTE-PCI was correlated with surgical–PCI. High sensitivities and specificities were estimated for each part of the small bowel. The sensitivity was 87.5%, 91.3%, 92.3%, 90%, and the specificity was 95.2%, 95.4%, 94.7%, 100% for proximal jejunum, distal jejunum, proximal ileum, and distal ileum respectively. The average sensitivity was 90.3±2.1%, and the average specificity was 96.3±2.5% for the entire small bowel. The kappa coefficient of agreement was found to be statistically significant ($p<0.0001$) in all four parts ranging from 0.597 for proximal jejunum, 0.663 for distal jejunum, 0.470 for proximal ileum, to 0.752 for distal ileum (mean kappa=0.621 ± 0.119) (Courcoutsakis et al, 2010a; Courcoutsakis et al, 2010b) (Figures 11, 12).

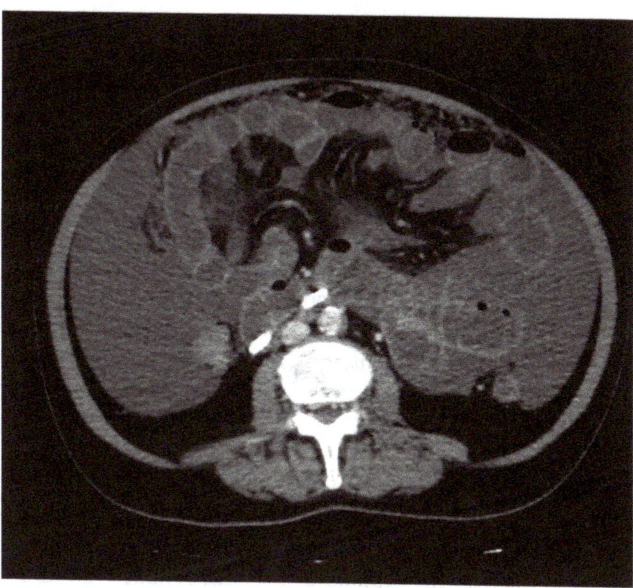

Fig. 11. CT enteroclysis in a patient with ovarian cancer.

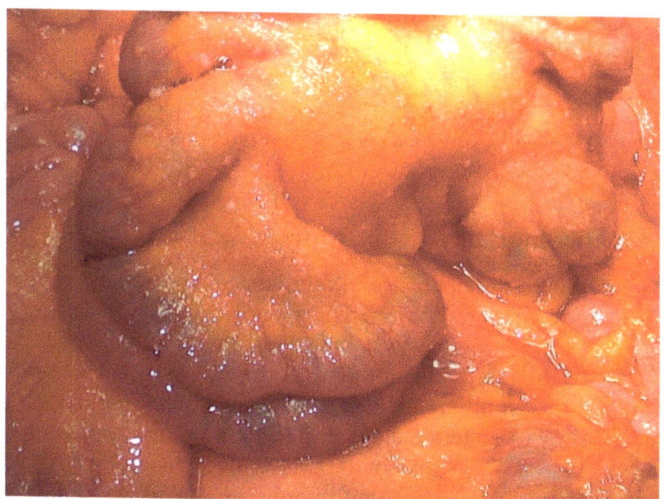

Fig. 12. The corresponding to CT-enteroclysis surgical specimen.

4.3.3 Magnetic Resonance Imaging (MRI)

There are few studies comparing CT to MRI in the peritoneal carcinomatosis evaluation. It has been shown that MRI has significantly improved sensitivity for depicting tumor involving the peritoneum even the subtle peritoneal implants (Forstner, 2007; Low, 2000). In patients with ascites the evaluation of visceral and parietal peritoneum is allowed (Gonzalez-Moreno et al, 2009; Forstner, 2007; Low, 2000). Compared with CT scan, MRI has lower spatial resolution, the acquisition time is longer and influenced by respiratory movement artifacts. On MRI may be obtained multiplanar and tridimensional reconstructions. The clinicians find it harder to interpret, the availability is limited, and the cost is higher. For the evaluation of cancerous implants within the peritoneal cavity specific sequences are needed (i.e. fat-suppression techniques, spoiled-gradient-echo sequence) and the i.v. infusion of gadolinium for tissue enhancement (Gonzalez-Moreno et al, 2009).

The recently introduced MR technique "diffusion-weighted imaging" (DWI) provides quantitative information about tissue cellularity and exploits the restricted water mobility within hypercellular tumors to increase the contrast between these lesions and surrounding tissue. DWI of the peritoneum in patients with ovarian cancer may be helpful for mapping the disease sites, their extent and differentiating tumors from treatment - induced changes (Kyriazi et al, 2010). Larger cohorts are needed to establish the role of the MRI-DWI in peritoneal carcinomatosis.

4.3.4 ^{18} Fluoro Deoxyglucose Positron Emission Tomography (PET), PET/CT

PET has been introduced in the clinical praxis the last decade provoking an innovation in diagnostic oncology. PET uses nuclear medicine in measuring the metabolic assessment of the tumors by counting the selective uptake of the intravenously administrated ^{18} Fluoro-Deoxyglucose. The disadvantages of the method are the poor anatomic resolution, and the non infrequent false positive results. The deficit of the poor spatial resolution is overcome by PET/CT. It has been reported that this hybrid technique is more accurate than PET or CT alone (Gonzale-Moreno et al, 2009, Satoh et al, 2011). This hybrid technique PET/CT may not be commonly used because of disadvantages such as the large size and the high cost of the system, the high cost of the examination, and time expended by the patient (Satoh et al, 2011). There have been only few reports of comparisons of DWI and PET, and the conclusions are controversial (Satoh et al, 2011).

5. Hospital morbidity-mortality

Cytoreductive surgery with perioperative intraperitoneal chemotherapy is associated with high morbidity rate and low mortality rate. The majority of postoperative complications are due to surgery itself. The last decade systemic chemotherapy integrated in this combined treatment has increased the rate of chemotherapy complications which are frequently easily reversed. A large multi-institutional study in patients with peritoneal malignancy of colorectal cancer origin revealed that major complications occurred in approximately 23% of the patients (Glehen et al, 2004). The extent of peritoneal carcinomatosis, and the use of EPIC significantly increase the risk of major complications, as well as the combination of HIPEC and EPIC (Glehen et al 2003; Stephens et al, 1999; Glehen et al, 2003). The most frequent complications are anastomotic leaks or bowel perforation (Glehen et al 2004; Stephens et al, 1999; Glehen et al, 2003; Younan et al, 2005; Kusamura et al, 2006). Other important variables related to postoperative morbidity are the duration of surgery and the number of the performed anastomoses (Stephens et al, 1999). Hematological toxicity is low and does not usually exceed 4% (Stephens et al, 1999).

The rate of postoperative complications in cytoreductive surgery combined with HIPEC does not usually exceed 30-35% although a morbidity rate of 54% has been referred in one

study (Elias et al, 2001). The same high rate of morbidity has been recorded in patients with ovarian cancer treated with cytoreduction and perioperative intraperitoneal chemotherapy (Tentes et al, 2003; Tentes et al, 2006; Raspagliesi et al, 2006; Di Giorgio et al, 2008; Tentes et al, 2010).
In properly selected patients the mortality rate is not high and does not exceed 5% (Piso et al, 2004; Raspagliesi et al, 2006; Tentes et al, 2010). However, if the patients are not properly selected the mortality rate increases dramatically (Tentes et al, 2006). In non-properly selected patients the age > 65 years and the performance status were found to be related to mortality, in addition to extensive peritoneal carcinomatosis that was not completely cytoreduced (Table 1).

1st author	No of patients	Hemato-logical toxicity	Bowel perforation-leak	fistula	bleeding	sepsis	mor-tality
Ryu	57	-	7%	-	-	5%	3%
Rufian	33	-	3%	-	3%	-	0%
Di Giorgio	47	NR	-	7%	4%	NR	4.2%
Ras-pagliesi	40	7.5%	2.5%	-	-	-	8%
Piso	19	-	10%	-	5%	5%	5%
Zanon	30	6%	6%	-	5%	-	3.3%
de Bree	19	0%	-	-			10%
Bae	67	13%	NR	NR	NR	NR	0%
Tentes	29	.9%	10.3%	0%	0%	0%	3.4%
Ceelen	42	NR	NR	NR	NR	NR	0%

NR=not reported

Table 1. Major morbidity and mortality rates in cytoreductive surgery combined with HIPEC in patients with primary or recurrent ovarian cancer.

6. Survival

Several clinical variables have been identified to be related to long-term survival. The completeness of cytoreduction, and the extent of peritoneal dissemination are consistently found to be significant prognostic indicators of survival (Tentes et al, 2003; Piso et al, 2004; Gilly et al, 2006; Di Giorgio et al, 2008; Tentes et al, 2010; Zanon et al, 2004; Rufian et al, 2006). Prior surgical score has been identified as a prognostic indicator of survival in one study (Look et al, 2004).
Median and 5-year survival rate varies from 18-54 months and 12-66% respectively (Piso et al, 2004; Raspagliesi et al, 2006; Di Giorgio et al, 2008; Tentes et al 2010, Ryu et al, 2004; Zanon et al, 2004; Rufian et al, 2006; de Bree et al, 2003; Bae et al, 2007; Ceelen et al, 2009) (Table 2). All these studies are prospective but not randomized (evidence level 4) and demonstrate that the method is feasible, well tolerated by the patients, and the results are equivalent or even improved if compared to historical data.

1st author	year	Patients No	Median FU	Median survival	5-year survival
Ryu	2004	57	47	NR	54
Rufian	2006	33	NR	48	37
Di Giorgio	2008	47	NR	24	16.7
Raspagliesi	2006	40	26	32	12
Piso	2004	19	24	18	15
Zanon	2004	30	19	28	12
de Bree	2003	19	30	54	42
Bae	2007	67	NR	NR	66
Tentes	2010	29	34	34	30
Ceelen	2009	42	NR	37	41.3%

NR=not reported

Table 2. Median follow-up, median and 5-year survival rate in cytoreductive surgery combined with HIPEC for ovarian cancer.

7. Recurrence

The incidence of recurrence is high in ovarian cancer and varies from 42-48% (Di Giorgio et al, 2008; Tentes et al, 2010). The majority of recurrences are loco-regional. The extent of peritoneal carcinomatosis is a prognostic indicator of recurrence (Tentes et al, 2010), and less than 30% of patients with low PCI (<13) develop recurrence.

8. Conclusions

Maximal cytoreductive surgery using standard peritonectomy procedures combined with perioperative intraperitoneal chemotherapy is an effective and promising treatment strategy in women with locally advanced epithelial ovarian cancer. The extent of peritoneal carcinomatosis and the completeness of cytoreduction are the most significant prognostic variables of survival. Proper patient selection is required for women with primary or recurrent ovarian cancer because only those women with limited peritoneal carcinomatosis may undergo complete cytoreduction and may be offered significant survival benefit. A useful tool in patient selection is CT-enteroclysis that shows to have higher sensitivity and specificity in the detection of peritoneal malignancy at the peritoneal surfaces of the small bowel compared to CT-scan.

9. References

Archer A, Sugarbaker PH, & Jelinek J.(1996). Radiology of peritoneal carcinomatosis, In: *Peritoneal Carcinomatosis: Principles of Management,* PH Sugarbaker (ed), p. p. 263-288, Kluwer Academic Publishers, 0-7923-3727-1, Boston

Averbach AM, & Sugarbaker PH. (1996). Methodologic considerations in treatment using intraperitoneal chemotherapy, In: *Peritoneal Carcinomatosis: Principles of Management,* PH Sugarbaker (ed), p. p. 289-309, Kluwer Academic Publishers, 0-7923-3727-1, Boston

Bae JH, Lee JM, Ryu KS, Park YG, Hur SY, Ahn WS, & Namkoong SE. (2007). Treatment of ovarian cancer with paclitaxel- or carboplatin-based intraperitoneal hyperthermic chemotherapy during secondary surgery. *Gynecol Oncol*, Jul 106 (1), 193-200, 0090-8258

Baratti D, Kusamura S, Nonaka D, Langer M, Andreola S, Favaro M, Gavazzi C, Laterza B, & Deraco M. (2007). Pseudomyxoma peritonei: clinical pathological and biological prognostic factors in patients treated with cytoreductive surgery and hyperthermic intraperitoneal chemotherapy (HIPEC). *Ann Surg Oncol*, Feb 15 (2): 526-534

Bergman F. Carcinoma of the ovary (1966). A clinicopathological study of 86 autopsied cases with special reference to the mode of spread. *Acta Obstet Gynecol Scand*, 45 (2): 211-231

Berthet B, Sugarbaker TA, Chang D, & Sugarbaker PH. (1999). Quantitative methodologies for selection of patients with recurrent abdominopelvic sarcoma for treatment. *Eur J Cancer*, Mar 35 (3): 413-419

Brigand C, Monneuse O, Mohamed F, Sayag-Beaujard AC, Isaac S, Gilly FN, & Glehen O (2006). Peritoneal mesothelioma treated by cytoreductive surgery and intraperitoneal hyperthermic chemotherapy: results of a prospective study. *Ann Surg Oncol*, Mar 13 (3): 405-412

Bristow RE, Tomacruz RS, Armstrong DK, Trimble EL, & Montz FJ. (2002). Survival effect of maximal cytoreductive surgery for advanced ovarian carcinoma during the platinum era: a meta-analysis. *J Clin Oncol*, Mar 1, 20(5): 1248-1259

Cannistra SA. (1993). Cancer of the ovary. *N Engl J Med*, Nov 18, 329 (21): 1550-1559

Ceelen WP, Van Nieuwenhoven Y, Van Belle S, Denys H, & Pattyn P.(2009). Cytoreduction and hyperthermic intraperitoneal chemoperfusion in women with heavily pretreated recurrent ovarian cancer. *Ann Surg Oncol*, Dec 29 (Epub ahead of print)

Chi DS, Franklin CC, Levine DA, Akselrod F, Sabbatini P, Jarnagin WR, DeMatteo R, Poynor EA, Abu-Rustum NR, & Barakat RR. (2004) Improved optimal cytoreduction rates for stages IIIC and IV epithelial ovarian, fallopian tube, and primary peritoneal cancer: a change in surgical approach. *Gynecol Oncol*, Sep 94 (3): 650-654

Coakley F, Choi P, Gougoutas A, Pothuri B, Venkatraman E, Chi D, Bergman A, & Hricak H. (2002) Peritoneal metastases: Detection with spiral CT in patients with ovarian cancer. *Radiology*, May 223 (2): 495-499

Courcoutsakis N, Tentes A, Zezos P, Astrinakis E, Korakianitis O, Prasopoulos PK. (2010a). CT-enteroclysis in the preoperative staging of small bowel and mesenteric involvement in patients with peritoneal carcinomatosis candidates for cytoreductive surgery: correlation with surgical findings (initial results) *ESGAR Dresden Germany*, June 2-5th, Book of Abstracts, suppl 1, S13

Courcoutsakis N, Tentes A, Zezos P, Astrinakis E, Korakianitis O, Prasopoulos P. (2010b). CT-Enteroclysis in the preoperative staging of small bowel and mesenteric involvement in patients with peritoneal carcinomatosis candidates for cytoreductive surgery: correlation with surgical findings. A prospective study. *7th International Workshop on Peritoneal Surface Malignancy*, Uppsala, Sweden, September 8 - 10th, Book of Abstracts

de Bree E, Romanos J, Michelakis J, Retakis K, Georgoulias V, Melissas J, & Tsiftsis DD. (2003). Intraoperative hyperthermic intraperitoneal chemotherapy with docetaxel as second-line treatment for peritoneal carcinomatosis of gynaecologic origin. *Anticancer Res*, May-June 23 (3C): 3019-3027

de Bree E, Koops W, Kroger R, van Ruth S, Witkamp AJ, & Zoetmulder FAN. (2004) Peritoneal carcinomatosis from colorectal or appendiceal origin: correlation of preoperative CT with intraoperative findings and evaluation of interobserver agreement. *J Surg Oncol*, May1, 86 (2): 64-73

Deraco M, Nonaka D, Baratti D, Casali D, Rosai J, Younan R, Slvatore A, Cabraa Ad AD, & Kusamura S. (2006). Prognostic analysis of clinicopathologic factors in 49 patients with diffuse malignant peritoneal mesothelioma treated with cytoreductive surgery and intraperitoneal hyperthermic perfusion. *Ann Surg Oncol*, Feb 13(2): 229-237

Di Giorgio A, Naticchioni E, Biacchi D, Sibio S, Accarpio F, Rocco M, Tarquini S, Di Seri M, Ciardi A, Montrucolli D, & Samartino P. (2008). Cytoreductive surgery (peritonectomy procedures) combined with hyperthermic intraperitoneal chemotherapy (HIPEC) in the treatment of diffuse peritoneal carcinomatosis from ovarian cancer. *Cancer*, Jul 15, 113 (2): 315-325

Eisenkop SM, Spirtos NM, Friedman RL, Lin W-CM, Pisani AL, & Perticucci S. (2003). Relative influences of tumor volume before surgery and the cytoreductive outcome on survival for patients with advanced ovarian cancer: a prospective study. *Gynecol Oncol*, Aug 90 (2): 390-396

Elias D, Blot F, El Omany A, Antoun S, Lasser P, Boige V, Rougier P, & Ducreux M. (2001). Curative treatment of peritoneal carcinomatosis arising from colorectal cancer by complete resection and intraperitoneal chemotherapy. *Cance*, Jul 1, 92 (1): 71-76

Elias D, Lefevre JH, Chevalier J, Brouquet A, Marchal F, Classe JM, Ferron G, Guilloit JM, Meeus P, Goere D, & Bonastre J. (2009). Complete cytoreductive surgery plus intraperitoneal chemohyperthermia with oxaliplatin for peritoneal carcinomatosis of colorectal origin. *J Clin Oncol*, Feb 10, 27 (5): 681-685

Forstner R. (2007) Radiological staging of ovarian cancer: imaging findings and contribution of CT and MRI. *Eur Radiol*, Dec 17 (12): 3223-3246

Esquivel J, Farinetti A, & Sugarbaker PH. (1999). Elective surgery in recurrent colon cancer with peritoneal seeding: When to and when not to proceed. *G Chir, Mar 20 (3)*: 81-86

Gilly FN, Cotte E, Brigand C, Monneuse O, Beaujard AC, Freyer G, & Glehen O. (2006). Quantitative prognostic indices in peritoneal carcinomatosis. *EJSO*, Aug 32 (6): 597-601

Glehen O, Osinsky D, Cotte E, Kwiatkowski F, Freyer G, Isaac S, Trillet-Lenoir V, Sayag-Beaujard AC, François Y, Vignal J, & Gilly FN. (2003). Intraperitoneal chemohyperthermia using a Closed abdominal procedure and cytoreductive surgery for the treatment of peritoneal carcinomatosis: morbidity and mortality analysis of 216 consecutive procedures. *Ann Surg Oncol*, Oct 10 (8): 863-869

Glehen O, Kwiatkowski W, Sugarbaker PH, Elias D, Levine EA, De Simone M, Barone R, Yonemura Y, Cavaliere F, Quenet F, Gutman M, Tentes AA, Lorimier G, Bernard JL, Bereder JM, Porcheron J, Gomez-Portilla A, Shen P, Deraco M, & Rat P. (2004). Cytoreductive surgery with perioperative intraperitoneal chemotherapy for the management of peritoneal carcinomatosis from colorectal cancer. A multi-institutional study of 506 patients. *J Clin Oncol*, Aug 15, 22 (16): 3284-3292

Gomez-Portilla A, Sugarbaker PH, & Chang D. (1999). Second look surgery after cytoreductive surgery and intraperitoneal chemotherapy for peritoneal carcinomatosis from colorectal cancer: analysis of prognostic features. *World J Surg,* Jan 23 (1): 23-29

Gonzalez-Moreno S, Gonzalez-Bayon L, Ortega-Perez G, & Gonzalez-Hernando C. (2009) Imaging of peritoneal carcinomatosis. *Cancer J,* May-Jun 15 (13): 184-189

Hacker NF, Berek JS, Lagasse LD, Nieberg RK, & Elashoff RM. (1983). Primary cytoreductive surgery for epithelial ovarian cancer. *Obstet Gynecol,* Apr 61 (4): 413-420

Hoskins WJ, Bundy BN, Thigpen JT, & Omura GA. (1992). The influence of cytoreductive surgery on recurrence-free interval and survival in small-volume stage III epithelial ovarian cancer: a Gynecologic Oncology Group study. *Gynecol Oncol,* Nov 47 (2): 159-166

Hoskins WJ, Mc Guire WP, Brady MF, Homesley HD, Creasman WT, Berman M, Ball H, & Berek JS. (1994). The effect of diameter of largest residual disease on survival after primary cytoreductive surgery in patients with suboptimal residual epithelial ovarian carcinoma. *Am J Obstet Gynecol,* Apr 170 (4): 974-979

Hunter RW, Alexander ND, & Soutter WP. (1992). Meta-analysis of surgery in advanced ovarian carcinoma: is maximum cytoreductive surgery an independent determinant of prognosis? *Am J Obstet Gynecol,* Feb 166 (2): 504-511

Jacquet P, Vidal-Jove J, Zhu B. & Sugarbaker PH. (1994). Peritoneal carcinomatosis from gastrointestinal malignancy: natural history and new peospects for management. *Acta Chir Belg,* Jul-Aug 94 (4): 191-197

Jacquet P, & Sugarbaker PH. Peritoneal-plasma barrier. (1996a), In: *Peritoneal Carcinomatosis: Principles of management,* PH Sugarbaker (ed), p. p. 53-63, Kluwer Academic Publishers, 0-7923-3727-1, Boston

Jaquet P, & Sugarbaker PH. (1996). Clinical research methodologies in diagnosis and staging of patients with peritoneal carcinomatosis, In: *Peritoneal Carcinomatosis: Principles of Management,* P. H. Sugarbaker (ed). p. p. 359-374, Kluwer Academic Publishers, 0-7923-3727-1, Boston

Kusamura S, Younan R, Baratti D, Constanzo P, Favaro M, Gavazzi C, & Deraco M. (2006). Cytoreductive surgery followed by intraperitoneal hyperthermic chemotherapy perfusion: analysis of morbidity and mortality in 209 peritonela surface malignancies treated with closed abdominal technique. *Cancer,* Mar 1, 106 (5): 1144-1153

Kyriazi S, Collins D, Morgan V, Giles S, & de Sousa N. (2010) Diffusion-weighted imaging of peritoneal disease for noninvasive staging of advanced ovarian cancer. *RadioGraphics,* Sep 30 (5): 1269-1285

Look M, Chang D, & Sugarbaker PH. (2004). Long-term results of cytoreductive surgery for advanced and recurrent epithelial ovarian cancers and papillary serous carcinoma of the peritoneum. *Int J Gynecol Cancer,* Jan-Feb, 14 (1): 35-41

Low R. (2000) Extrahepatic abdominal imaging and helical CT in 164 patients. *J Magn Reson Imaging,* Aug 12 (2): 269-277

Maglinte DD, Sandrasegaran K, Lappas JC, & Chioren M. (2007) Enteroclysis. *Radiology,* Dec 245 (3): 661-671

Mahteme H, Hansson J, Berglund A, Pahlman L, Glimelius B, Nygren P, & Graf W. (2004). Improved survival in patients with peritoneal metastases from colorectal cancer: a preliminary study. *Br J Cancer*, Jan 26, 90 (2): 403-407

Marin D, Catalano M, Baski M, Di Martino M, Geiger D, Di Giorgio A, Sibio S, & Passariello R. (2010) 64-section multi-detector row CT in the preoperative diagnosis of peritoneal carcinomatosis: correlation with histopathological findings. *Abdom Imaging*, Dec 35 (6): 694-700

McGuire WP, & Ozols RF. (1998). Chemotherapy of advanced ovarian cancer. *Sem Oncol*, Jun 25 (3): 340-348

Miner T, Shia J, Jaques DP, Klimstra DS, Brennan MF, & Coit DG. (2005). Long-term survival following treatment of pseudomyxoma peritonei: an analysis of surgical therapy. *Ann Surg*, Feb 241 (2): 300-308

Neijt JP, ten Bokkel Huinink WW, van der Burg MEL, van Oosterom AT, Vermorken JB, van Lindert ACM, Heintz APM, Aartsen E, van Lent M, Trimbos JP, & de Meijer AJ. (1991). Long-term survival in ovarian cancer: mature data from the Nederlands Joint Study Group for Ovarian Cancer. *Eur J Cancer*, 27 (11): 1367-1372

Odicino F, Favalli G, Zigliani L, & Pecorelli S. (2001). Staging of gynecologic malignancies. *Surg Clin N Am*, Aug 81 (4): 753-770

Piccart MJ, Bertelsen K, James K, Cassidy J, Mangioni C, Simonsen E, Stuart G, Kaye S, Vergote I, Blom R, Grimshaw R, Atkinson RJ, Swenerton KD, Trope C, Nardi M, Kaern J, Tumolo S, Timmers P, Roy JA, Lhoas F, Lindvall B, Bakon M, Birt A, Andersen JE,Zee B, Paul J, Baron B, & Pecorelli S. (2000). Randomized intergroup trial of cisplatin-paclitaxel versus cisplatin-cyclophosphamide in women with advanced epithelial ovarian cancer: three year results. *J Natl Cancer Inst*, May 3, 92 (9): 699-708

Piso P, Dahlke MH, Loss M, & Schlitt HJ. (2004). Cytoreductive surgery and hyperthermic intraperitoneal chemotherapy in peritoneal carcinomatosis from ovarian cancer. *World J Surg Oncol*, Jun 28, 2: 21

Raptopoulos V, & Gourtsogiannis N. (2001) Peritoneal carcinomatosis. *Eur Radiol*, 11 (11): 2195-2206

Raspagliesi F, Kusamura S, Campos Torres JC, de Souza GA, Ditto A, Zanaboni F, Younan R, Baratti D, Mariani L, Laterza B, & Deraco M. (2006). Cytoreduction combined with intraperitoneal hyperthermic perfusion chemotherapy in advanced/recurrent ovarian cancer patients: the experience of National Cancer Institute of Milan. *EJSO*, Aug 32 (6): 671-675

Reuter NP, Mac Gregor JM, Woodall CE, Sticca RP, William C, Helm MB, Scoggins CR, McMasters KM, & Martin RC. (2008). Preoperative performance status predicts outcome following heated intraperitoneal chemotherapy. *Am J Surg*, Dec 196 (6): 909-913

Roberts AB, & Sporn MB. (1989). Principles of molecular cell biology of cancer: Growth factors related to transformation, In: *Cancer Principles and Practice of Oncology*, De Vita VT, Hellman S, Rosenberg SA (eds)., p. p. 67-80, JB Lippincott, 1989, Philadelphia

Roberts WS. (1996). Cytoreductive surgery in ovarian cancer: why, when, and how? *Cancer Control*, Mar 3 (2): 130-136

Rossi CR, Deraco M, De Simone M, Mocellin S, Pilati P, Foletto M, Cavaliere F, Kusamura S, Gronchi A, & Lise M. (2004). Hyperthermic intraperitoneal intraoperative chemotherapy after cytoreductive surgery for the treatment of abdominal sarcomatosis. Clinical outcome and prognostic factors in 60 consecutive patients. *Cance*, May 1, 100 (9): 1943-1950

Rubin J, Jones Q, Planch A, & Bower JD. (1988). The minimal importance of the hollow viscera to peritoneal transport during peritoneal dialysis in the rat. *Am Soc Artif Intern Organs Transact*, Oct-Dec, 34 (4): 912-915

Rufian S, Munoz-Casares FC, Briceno J, Diaz CJ, Rubio MJ, Ortega R, Ciria R, Morillo M, Aranda E, Muntane J, & Pera C. (2006). Radical surgery-peritonectomy and intraoperative intraperitoneal chemotherapy for the treatment of peritoneal carcinomatosis in recurrent or primary ovarian cancer. *J Surg Oncol*, Sep 15, 94 (4): 316-324

Ryu KS, Kim JH, Ko HS, Kim JW, Ahn WS, Park YG, Kim SJ, & Lee JM. (2004). Effects of intraperitoneal hyperthermic chemotherapy in ovarian cancer. *Gynecol Oncol*, Aug 94 (2): 325-332

Satoh Y, Ichikawa T, Motosugi U, Kimura K, Sou H, Sano K, & Araki T. (2011) Diagnosis of peritoneal dissemination: comparison of 18 F-FDG PET/CT, Diffusion-weighted MRI, and Contrast-Enhanced MDCT. *AJR*, Feb 196 (2): 447-453

Sebbag G, Yan H, Shmookler BM, Chang D, & Sugarbaker PH. (2000). Results of treatment of 33 patients with peritoneal mesothelioma. *Br J Surg*, Nov 87 (11): 1587-1593

Smith JP, & Day TG. (1979). Review of ovarian cancer at the University of Texas Systems Cancer Center, M. D. Anderson Hospital and Tumor Institute. *Am J Obstet Gynecol*, Dec 1, 135 (7): 984-993

Stamou KM, Karakozis S, & Sugarbaker PH. (2003). Total abdominal colectomy, pelvic peritonectomy, and end-ileostomy for the surgical palliation of mucinous peritoneal carcinomatosis from non-gynecologic cancer. *J Surg Oncol*, Aug 83 (4): 197-203

Stephens A, Alderman R, Chang D, Edwards G, Esquivel J, Seggab G, Steves M, & Sugarbaker PH. (1999). Morbidity and mortality analysis of 200 treatments with cytoreductive surgery and hyperthermic intraoperative intraperitoneal chemotherapy using the Coliseum technique. *Ann Surg Oncol*, Dec 6 (8): 790-796

Sugarbaker PH. (1991). Cytoreductive approach to peritoneal carcinomatosis: peritonectomy and intraperitoneal chemotherapy. In: *Postgraduate Advances in Colorectal Surgery*. Forum Medicum, II-X

Sugarbaker PH. (1995). Peritonectomy procedures. *Ann Surg*, Jan 221 (1): 29-42

Sugarbaker PH. (1999). Management of peritoneal surface malignancy: the surgeon's role. *Langenbeck's Arch Surg*, Dec 384 (6): 576-587

Sugarbaker PH. (1999). Successful management of microscopic residual disease in large bowel cancer. *Cancer Chemother Pharmacol*, 43 suppl: S15-25

Sugarbaker PH. (2005). In: *Technical Handbook for the Integration of Cytoreductive Surgery and Perioperative Intraperitoneal Chemotherapy into the Surgical Management of Gastrointestinal and Gynecologic Malignancies*. 4th edition. PH Sugarbaker (ed), p. p. 7-8, Ludann Co, Grand Rapids, Michigan.

Sugarbaker PH. (2006). New standard of care for appendiceal epithelial neoplasms and pseudomyxoma peritonei syndrome? *Lancet Oncol*, Jan 7 (1): 69-76

Tentes AAK, Tripsiannis G, Markakidis SK, Karanikiotis CN, Tzegas G, Georgiadis G, & Avgidou K. (2003). Peritoneal cancer index: a prognostic indicator of survival in advanced ovarian cancer. *EJSO*, Feb 29 (1): 69-73

Tentes AAK, Mirelis CG, Markakidis SK, Bekiaridou KA, Bougioukas IG, Xanthoulis AI, Tsalkidou EG, Zafiropoulos GH, & Nikas IH. (2006). Long-term survival in advanced ovarian carcinoma following cytoreductive surgery with standard peritonectomy procedures. *Int J Gynecol Cancer*, Mar-Apr, 16 (2): 490-495

Tentes AAK, Korakianitis O, Kakolyris S, Kyziridis D, Veliovits D, Karagiozoglou C, Sgouridou E, & Moustakas K. (2010). Cytoreductive surgery and periopeartive intraperitoneal chemotherapy in recurrent ovarian cancer. *Tumori*, May-Jun 96 (3): 411-416

Verwaal VJ, Bruin S, Boot H, van Slooten G, & van Tinteren H. (2008). 8-year follow-up of randomized trial: cytoreduction and hyperthermic intraperitoneal chemotherapy versus systemic chemotherapy in patients with peritoneal carcinomatosis of colorectal cancer. *Ann Surg Oncol*, Sep 15 (9): 2426-2432

Woodward P, Hosseinzadeh K, & Saenger J. (2004) Radiologic staging of ovarian carcinoma with pathologic correlation. *Radiographics*, Jan-Feb 24 (1): 225-246

Yan TD, Brun EA, Cerruto CA, Haverik N, Chand D, & Sugarbaker PH. (2007). Prognostic indicators for patients undergoing cytoreductive surgery and perioperative intraperitoneal chemotherapy for diffuse malignant peritoneal mesothelioma. *Ann Surg Oncol*, Jan 14 (1): 41-49

Yancik R. (1993). Ovarian cancer: age contrasts in incidence, histology, disease stage at diagnosis, and mortality. *Cancer*, Jan 15, 71 (2suppl): 517-523

Yonemura Y, Fujimura T, Nishimura G, Falla R, Sawa T, Katayama K, Tsugawa K, Fushida S, Miyazaki I, Tanaka M, Endou Y, & Sasaki T. (1996). Effects of intraoperative chemohyperthermia in patients with gastric cancer with peritoneal dissemination. *Surgery*, Apr 119 (4): 437–444

Yonemura Y, Bandou E, Kinoshita K, Kawamura T, Takahashi S, Endou Y, & Sasaki T. (2003). Effective therapy for peritoneal dissemination in gastric cancer. *Surg Oncol Clin N Am*, Jul 12 (3): 635-648

Yu W, Whang I, Sih I, Averbach A, Chang D, & Sugarbaker PH. (1998). Prospective randomized trial of early postoperative intraperitoneal chemotherapy as an adjuvant to resectable gastric cancer. *Ann Surg*, Sep 228 (3): 347-354

Younan R, Kusamura S, Baratti D, Oliva GD, Costanzo P, Favaro M, Gavazzi C, & Deraco M. (2005). Bowel complications in 203 cases of peritoneal surface malignancies treated with peritonectomy and closed-technique intraperitoneal hyperthermic perfusion. *Ann Surg Oncol*, Nov 12 (11): 910-918

Zanon C, Clara R, Chiappino I, Bortolini M, Cornaglia S, Simone P, Bruno F, De Riu L, Airoldi M, & Pedani F. (2004). Cytoreductive surgery and intraperitoneal chemohyperthermia for recurrent peritoneal carcinomatosis from ovarian cancer. *World J Surg*, Oct 28 (10): 1040-1045

9

Management of Recurrent or Persistent Ovarian Cancer

Constantine Gennatas
Areteion Hospital, University of Athens
Greece

1. Introduction

Approximately 70-80% of patients with epithelial ovarian cancer will relapse after first-line chemotherapy with a platinum and taxane-based combination. These patients require further treatment and they may benefit from local and/or systemic therapy. The prognosis is poor and the management of relapsed ovarian cancer remains a difficult problem open to research [National Cancer Institute (NCI), 2010].

Most patients with epithelial ovarian carcinoma receive postoperative chemotherapy, either as adjuvant treatment after complete removal of all visible disease or because of residual tumor. Evaluation after chemotherapy completion includes CA 125 and imaging with chest-X-Ray or CT scanning of the chest and CT scanning or MRI of the abdomen. The limitations of this evaluation are well known. In the past several institutions practiced a "second-look laparotomy", which several times revealed widespread intra-abdominal disease in patients with a negative metastatic work-up. Early detection of persistent disease by second-look laparotomies after completing first-line treatment is no longer practiced, as it had no effect on patients' outcome. The time to first relapse varies from a few months to several years (NCI, 2010). The median interval to first recurrence is 18 to 24 months. Half of the recurrences occur more than 12 months from the end of the first-line therapy, and one quarter of all recurrences occur at less than 6 months. Regarding recurrent sites at first relapse, the primary disease site is involved in fifty-five percent of the patients. Recurrence can also been noted in retroperitoneal or distant nodes, liver, spleen, brain, and bones. In order to clarify prognostic factors and to determine the best treatment approach grouping of recurrent patients has been applied. The results are not clear yet and more publications are needed. (Martin 2009; NCI 2011; Ushijima, 2010).

2. The management of patients with persistent or recurrent disease

Patients with persistent detectable disease after surgery and first-line chemotherapy with a platinum derivative and taxane combination are candidates for further treatment. They have a partial response of residual disease or they have developed progressive disease during first-line chemotherapy. Another group includes patients in complete remission after surgery and first-line chemotherapy who eventually relapse. The management of patients with persistent or recurrent disease is very difficult. In the case of persistent disease the question is what is the proper next step including surgery, chemotherapy and research protocols. In the case of relapse after a complete response to upfront therapy the first question related to these patients is the best follow-up, the second the time to start treatment and the third the choice of treatment. The goal of treatment today is not the cure but the maintaining or improving the quality of life and prolonging patients' survival. (NCI, 2010; Ushijima, 2010).

As the results of the recurrent disease management remain disappointing the question of maintenance therapy after initial therapy has been raised. After the completion of the initial therapy, surgery and chemotherapy, the majority of patients are in complete remission. This remission in most cases does not last and patients develop recurrent disease. Instead of terminating therapy at this point, the question is if a maintenance, low toxicity therapy, can improve disease free progression and the overall survival. (Gardner & Jewell 2011). Two studies examined the use of paclitaxel in maintenance or consolidation treatment without significant results. There are two ongoing studies with paclitaxel or CT-2103, a polyglutamated taxane and the second with the addition of bevacizumab. Finally vaccines are being studied and they represent a hope to improve today's results (Gardner & Jewell 2011).

2.1 The follow-up of patients completing postoperative chemotherapy

History, physical examination and serial CA 125 determinations at intervals of 1 to 3 months have been accepted as a reasonable follow-up program for patients who are in clinical complete remission. Increases in CA 125 represent a common method to detect disease relapse but as its limitations are well known imaging procedures are also included in many Institutions. (NCI, 2010).

2.2 Detection of disease recurrence and the proper time to start treatment

A well-known analysis of a trial by the Medical Research Council and European Organization for Research and Treatment of Cancer examined the consequences of early institution of treatment for recurrence versus treatment delayed until clinical symptoms appeared. The median survival of all patients registered was 70.8 months. The study concluded that there was no benefit in the detection of early presence of disease by CA 125 (NCI, 2010; Ozols et al., 2003). This is also consistent with the failure of currently tested therapeutic modalities to alter outcome by routine second-look laparotomies and early detection of persistent disease after initial treatment. However it is difficult in everyday practice to follow-up patients with evidence of recurrent disease without treatment and most Oncologists treat their patients without waiting for the symptoms of their disease.

2.3 Therapeutic options

Therapeutic options include local modalities, surgery and radiation therapy, and systemic therapy.

2.3.1 Local modalities: Surgery

Primary cytoreductive surgery and combination chemotherapy are the cornerstones of the initial treatment for epithelial ovarian cancer. Despite advances in the use of chemotherapeutic and biologic agents, surgery remains an important modality in the treatment of recurrent disease as well. (Ramirez et al., 2011). Surgery for clinical recurrence is defined as secondary cytoreductive surgery and it is similar to surgery for persistent disease at the completion of chemotherapy. The role of secondary cytoreductive surgery for persistent and/or recurrent disease remains unclear. Complete response to chemotherapy for recurrent ovarian cancer is rare, and shrinkage of the tumor does not always prolongs survival while a surgical approach may offer a clear clinical benefit to properly selected patients. So while the results of chemotherapy remain unsatisfactory, especially in platinum resistant patients, several authors have published encouraging results with surgery and the question remains what are the selection criteria for secondary debulking. Are the theoretical and clinical benefits of primary cytoreduction the same in patients with recurrent disease? Do they apply to platinum sensitive and platinum resistant patients as well? What is the definition of limited recurrent disease? How much we can trust the preoperative work-up? What are the results of the cytoreductive surgery in terms of complete resection, optimal resection (residual ≤ 1 cm) or suboptimal resection (residual ≥1 cm) and what is the relation of these results to the post recurrence survival? Several authors have reported a significant median survival benefit in patients with no or minimal residual disease that ranges from 38 to 61 months compared to 4.5 months to 27 months for suboptimal cytoreduction. In a retrospective study fifty five patients were included who met the following inclusion criteria: A complete clinical response to primary therapy, ≥ 12 months between initial diagnosis and recurrence, and ≤ 5 recurrence sites on preoperative imaging studies. The conclusions of this study were the definition of localized recurrent ovarian cancer as patients with 1 or 2 radiographic recurrence sites and that in a select population with a diagnosis-to-recurrence interval ≥ 18 months and complete secondary cytoreduction the associated median post recurrence survival was approximately 50 months. (Salani et al., 2007).

Due to a lack of large randomized trials, conclusive and universally accepted data are limited regarding the benefits of secondary cytoreductive surgery. A patient with a rapid, multifocal recurrence is unlikely to obtain any clinical benefit from surgery. Secondary cytoreduction should be considered for the subgroup of patients with progressive -free interval of ≥12 to 18 months from completion of adjuvant chemotherapy, localized recurrence amenable to complete cytoreduction, potential chemosensitive disease, and good performance status. As with primary debulking, resection to no gross residual disease is the most important prognostic factor. Patients with optimal secondary cytoreduction survived for 16 to 60 months, compared to 8 to 27 months for those patients with residual diseases >1 cm. However the benefit of surgery, compared to chemotherapy alone, is unclear because of a lack of data. The biology of the cancer is certainly another significant cofounding factor (Bae et al., Hoskins et al., 1989; Markman et al, 2004; Frederick et al.; Harter et al; Munkarah & Coleman, 2004).

A subgroup of patients may be candidates for tertiary debulking, based on similar selection criteria used for secondary debulking. (Fotopoulou et al., 2010; Frederick et al 2011). At secondary reduction, bowel or other organ resections are often also performed. More than 30% of surgeries included bowel resection and some of them accompanied considerable morbidity, such as colostomy or pelvic exenteration (Ushijima, 2010).

2.3.2 The management of complications

Small and/or large bowel obstruction is a rather common complication in patients with advanced disease. Surgery in these cases remains controversial and requires careful patient selection. Patients are usually end-stage and malnourished after a period of nausea, vomiting and constipation. The causes of obstruction are often multifactorial and include mechanical blockage, dense mesenteric infiltration, peritoneal carcinomatosis and adhesions from previous surgery (Ramirez et al., 2011). Surgical procedures include bowel resection, colostomy and intestinal bypass. Even with palliative surgery to remove obstruction, the re-obstruction rate ranges between 10 and 50% (Ramirez et al., 2011). Several patients will definitely benefit from palliative surgery and the absence of the following factors have been associated with successful palliation: 1) More than 3 liters of ascites, 2) Multifocal obstruction, 3) palpable bulky tumors, and 4) preoperative weight loss more than 9 Kg. There are authors who do not agree with these criteria and it remains very important to individualize the approach to a patient with bowel obstruction. Certain patients are candidates for percutaneous gastrostomy only or intravenous hydration and end-stage care (Pothuri et al., 2003; Ramirez et al, 2011).

2.3.3 Local modalities: Radiation therapy

The role of radiation therapy in patients with recurrent ovarian cancer has not been defined. It can be used in selected cases for symptoms palliation.

2.4.1 Systemic therapy

Chemotherapy options for patients with persistent or recurrent disease are subdivided as follows: 1) Platinum-sensitive recurrence: for patients whose disease recurs more than 6 months after cessation of the induction (usually retreated with a platinum (cisplatin or carboplatin) and referred to as potentially platinum sensitive. 2) Platinum-refractory or platinum-resistant recurrence: for patients who progress prior to cessation of induction therapy (platinum refractory) or within 6 months after cessation (platinum resistant); in these patients, platinum derivatives are generally deemed toxic and not sufficiently useful to be part of the treatment plan (NCI, 2010).

2.4.2 Platinum-sensitive recurrence

It has long been recognized that individuals with malignant disease who respond to chemotherapy and who experience a long treatment-free interval before initiation of a second-line treatment program may respond again to the same drug(s) as used in the initial treatment regimen. Ovarian cancer is no exception to this highly clinically relevant observation. (Markman et al, 2004). A number of studies have revealed that secondary responses to platinum-based chemotherapy occur in this setting in as many as 50% to 80% of patients, based on the duration of the treatment-free interval. (Markman et al, 2004). A retrospective study conducted at the Cleveland Clinic has addressed the following question:" Can the duration of the second response in an individual patient be reasonably accurately predicted based on knowledge of the length of the prior response or treatment-free interval?" This study has confirmed the importance of the duration of prior response in defining the opportunity for secondary responses to platinum-based treatment. It has also demonstrated that the duration of response to the initial or prior platinum-based chemotherapy regimen is highly predictive of the upper limit of the duration of response to a subsequent platinum treatment program, assuming that the same or similar drugs are used as in the previous treatment program. The authors note that the large majority of patients in these series received either single-agent carboplatin in the second-line setting or the same drug regimen (carboplatin-paclitaxel) used in the previous course of chemotherapy. For patients who exhibited an objective response, treatment was frequently discontinued after six courses of therapy. Therefore, it is possible that if platinum had been delivered in combination with an agent not previously administered to that individual or if the drug had been continued in the responding patient population, the duration of response might have been longer. (Markman et al, 2004). They suggest that more data are required. However, they note, although prolonging second-line therapy or adding a new drug may improve the duration of response, either approach also has the potential to increase both the toxicity and the cost of treatment without having any meaningful impact on the patient's quality of life, time to symptomatic disease progression, or overall survival. (Markman et al, 2004). These series have been unable to accurately predict the duration of secondary response to platinum chemotherapy for individual patients based on the length of the initial or immediately preceding remission. Although this may have been because of the limited number of patients in each previous response duration category, it is also possible that inherent substantial heterogeneity associated with the recurrent tumor (e.g. the rate of growth of platinum-resistant cells present within the sensitive tumor cell population) makes it unrealistic that a reliable predictive model for individual patient management can be developed. (Markman et al, 2004). This study has several potential implications for clinical trials design for second-line chemotherapy.

Several studies that have been conducted in patients with recurrent platinum sensitive ovarian carcinoma, have reinforced using carboplatin as the treatment core for patients with platinum-sensitive recurrences (Muggia, 1989). Cisplatin is occasionally used, particularly in combination with other drugs, because of its lesser myelosuppression, but this advantage over carboplatin is counterbalanced by its greater intolerance. Oxaliplatin, initially introduced with the hope that it would overcome platinum resistance, has activity mostly in platinum-sensitive patients (Piccart et al., 2000) but has not been compared with carboplatin alone or in combinations. With all platinums, outcome is in generally better the longer the initial interval without recurrence from the initial platinum-containing regimens (Markman M et al., 2004).

However the clinical benefit based on the progression free survival (PFS) and the overall survival (OS) is in generally limited.

The combination of Carboplatin and pegylated-liposomal doxorubicin have resulted in a median PFS of 9 months and a median OS of 31 months (Ferrero et al, 2007). The combination of Carboplatin and Epirubicin versus Carboplatin produced a very limited difference in OS 17 versus 15 months (Bolis et al, 2001). A triple combination of Cisplatin, doxorubicin and cyclophosphamide (CAP) that has been used in the past as first-line treatment of choice versus paclitaxel revealed a significant difference in both PFS 15.7 versus 9 months and in OS 34.7 versus 25.8 months (Cantù et al., 2002). The addition of Gemcitabine to Carboplatin was compared to Carboplatin alone. The PFS was 8,6 versus 5.8 month and the OS 18 versus 17 months (Pfisterer et al, 2006).

In an international, multicenter trial 802 patients were randomized to receive paclitaxel plus platinum chemotherapy or conventional platinum-based chemotherapy. The paclitaxel plus platinum combination seems superior in terms of PFS and median OS. The PFS was 11 versus 9 months and the OS 24 versus 19 months in the two groups (Parmar et al, 2003). Accordingly, because of this randomized experience, carboplatin plus paclitaxel is considered the standard regimen for platinum-sensitive recurrence in the absence of residual neurotoxicity.

Platinum derivatives remain the most important drugs in the management of recurrent ovarian carcinoma. It is of interest that on occasion, patients with platinum-sensitive recurrences relapsing within 1 year have been included in trials of nonplatinum drugs. In one such trial, comparing the pegylated liposomal doxorubicin (PLD) to topotecan, the subset of patients who were platinum sensitive had better outcomes with either drug (and in particular with PLD) relative to the platinum-resistant cohort (Gordon et al., 2004).

2.4.3 Platinum-refractory or platinum-resistant recurrence

Clinical recurrences that take place during or within 6 months of completion of a platinum-containing regimen are considered platinum-refractory or platinum-resistant recurrences respectively. Patients with originally platinum- sensitive disease eventually also become platinum-resistant. Anthracyclines (particularly when formulated as PLD), taxanes, topotecan, and gemcitabine are used as single agents for these recurrences. These agents in generally convey a marginal benefit. Patients with platinum-resistant disease should be encouraged to enter clinical trials. Treatment with paclitaxel historically provided the first agent with consistent activity in patients with platinum-refractory or platinum-resistant recurrences (Kohn et al., 1994; McGuire et al., 1989, Einzig et al., 1992, Thigpen JT et al., 1994, Trimble EL et al., 1993).

Subsequently, randomized studies have indicated that the use of topotecan achieved results that were comparable to those achieved with paclitaxel. In phase II studies, topotecan administered intravenously 1.5mg/m^2 on days 1 to 5 of a 21-day cycle yielded objective response rates ranging from 13% to 16.3% and other outcomes that were equivalent or superior to paclitaxel (Ten Bokkel Huinink W et al, 1997, Kudelka AP et al.; 1996, Creemers et al.; 1996, Bookman et al., 1998). Substantial myelosuppression follows administration in most cases. Other toxic effects include nausea, vomiting, alopecia, and asthenia. A number of schedules are under evaluation in an effort to decrease hematologic toxicity (NCI, 2010). Topotecan was compared with pegylated liposomal doxorubicin in a randomized trial of 474 patients and demonstrated similar response rates, PFS, and OS at the time of the initial report, contributed primarily by the platinum-resistant subsets (Gordon et al., 2001).

A phase II study of Pegylated liposomal doxorubicin (PLD) given IV 50mg/m^2 once every 21 to 28 days demonstrated one complete response and eight partial responses in 35 patients with platinum-refractory or paclitaxel-refractory disease (response rate = 25.7%). In general, liposomal doxorubicin has few acute side effects other than hypersensitivity. The most frequent toxic effects are usually observed after the first cycle and are more pronounced following dose rates exceeding 10 mg/m^2 per week and include stomatitis and hand-foot syndrome. Neutropenia and nausea are minimal, and alopecia rarely occurs. (Muggia et al., 1997). Liposomal doxorubicin and topotecan have been compared in a randomized trial of 474 patients with recurrent ovarian cancer. Response rates (19.7% versus 17.0%; P = .390), PFS (16.1 weeks vs. 17.0 weeks; P = .095), and OS (60 weeks versus. 56.7 weeks; P = .341) did not differ significantly between the liposomal doxorubicin and topotecan arms, respectively. Survival was longer for the patients with platinum-sensitive disease who received liposomal doxorubicin (Gordon et al., 2001,2004).

Docetaxel has shown activity in paclitaxel-pretreated patients and is a reasonable alternative to weekly paclitaxel in the recurrent setting (Berkenblit et al., 2004).

Several phase II trials of gemcitabine as a single agent administered IV on days 1, 8, and 15 of a 28-day cycle have been reported. The response rate ranges from 13% to 19% in evaluable patients. Responses have been observed in patients whose disease are platinum refractory and/or paclitaxel refractory as well as in patients with bulky disease. Leukopenia, anemia, and thrombocytopenia are the most common toxic effects. Many patients report transient flu-like symptoms and a rash following drug administration. Other toxic effects, including nausea, are usually mild (Friedlander et al., 1998; Lund et al., 1994; Mutch et al., 2007, Shapiro et al., 1996).

Ovarian cancer patients generally receive paclitaxel in front-line induction regimens. Retreatment with paclitaxel, particularly in weekly schedules, indicates an activity comparable to those of the preceding drugs. If there is residual neuropathy upon recurrence, this may shift the choice of treatment towards other agents. In a phase III study, 235 patients who did not respond to initial treatment with a platinum-based regimen but who had not previously received paclitaxel or topotecan, were randomly assigned to receive either topotecan as a 30-minute infusion daily for 5 days every 21 days or paclitaxel as a 3-hour infusion every 21 days. The overall objective response rate was 20.5% for those patients who were randomly assigned to treatment with topotecan and 13.2% for those patients who were randomly assigned to treatment with paclitaxel ($P = .138$). Both groups experienced myelosuppression and gastrointestinal toxic effects. Nausea and vomiting, fatigue, and infection were observed more commonly following treatment with topotecan, whereas alopecia, arthralgia, myalgia, and neuropathy were observed more commonly following paclitaxel (Ten Bokkel Huinink et al., 1997).

2.4.4 Other drugs used to treat platinum-refractory or platinum-resistant recurrence

This group includes drugs that have limited activity in platinum-resistant cases but they are in use in every day practice as there are patients who need successive chemotherapeutic regimens. 1) Etoposide. It can be given intravenously or orally. It has limited activity. 2) Cyclophosphamide. It was used as first-line therapy in combination with platinum derivatives in the before the paclitaxel era. It has uncertain activity in platinum resistant cases. 3) Hexamethylmelamine (Alteramine) is an alkylating prodrug, has also uncertain activity in platinum resistant cases. 4) Irinotecan. It is cross - resistant to topotecan. 5) Oxaliplatin. Partially cross -resistant to the other platinum derivatives. 6) Vinorelbine. 25-30mg/m^2 IV on days 1 and 8 every 21 days. Vinorelbine can also be given orally. It has erratic activity. 7) 5-fluorouracil and capecitabine. May be useful in mucinous tumors. (Vasey et al., 2003). 8) Tamoxifen. Has minimal activity. May be useful in certain cases either after chemotherapy or in older patients who do not tolerate or refuse to receive chemotherapy 9) Trabectedin (*Yondelis*) a new drug for advanced soft-tissue sarcomas in combination with liposomal doxorubicin has shown significant activity in patients with relapsed ovarian carcinoma and has been approved for use in certain countries. It was however rejected by a US Food and Drug Administration (FDA) advisory committee. Further clinical trials are needed. 10) Thalidomide an antiangiogenic agent in combination with Topotecan appears to improve response rate in patients with recurrent ovarian cancer. The results of phase III are needed (Downs Jr LS 2007).

2.4.5 Hyperthermic intraperitoneal chemotherapy

Patients with widespread peritoneal carcinomatosis present a very difficult problem as cytoreductive surgery has limited results. A retrospective study suggests that the combination of cytoreductive surgery and hyperthermic intraperitoneal chemotherapy is feasible and has potential benefits. A randomized trial is needed to establish its role in the management of these difficult cases (Chua, et al 2009). Similar results were reported in a pilot study of Oxaliplatin-based hyperthermic intraperitoneal chemotherapy in recurrent epithelial ovarian cancer. It proved to be feasible, relatively safe and effective in combination with chemotherapy and surgery in cases with peritoneal carcinomatosis (Frenel, et al 2011). Larger studies are needed (Roviello, et al 2010).

2.4.6 New drugs – Targeted therapy

Certain studies evaluating the efficacy of antiangiogenic agents in ovarian cancer have been reported including vascular endothelial growth factor (VEGF) pathway inhibitors, monoclonal antibodies, tyrosine kinase inhibitors and inhibitors of other angiogenic factors and vascular disrupting agents. Angiogenesis is a critical component of tumor development and proliferation. Agents that target the angiogenic process are of considerable interest in the treatment of ovarian cancer. Bevacizumab is a humanized monoclonal antibody against VEGF and possesses minimal single-agent activity in common epithelial cancers such as colorectal, non-small-cell lung cancer and breast cancer. The combination of Bevacizumab with chemotherapy has revealed significant improvement in the outcome in several tumors, leading to registration. Bevacizumab possesses more single-agent activity in epithelial ovarian cancer than in any other epithelial tumor, apart from renal cancer, where the vascular biology is specifically relevant to this therapeutic approach. Clinical trials have confirmed Bevacizumab effectiveness but that also revealed significant toxicity including bowel perforation. (Kaye ., 2007; Teoh et al., 2011; Monk et al., 2006).

Three phase II studies have shown activity for Bevacizumab, an antibody to vascular endothelial growth factor (VEGF). The first study included 62 patients who had received only one or two prior treatments (these last patients had received one additional platinum-based regimen because of an initial interval of 12 months or greater after first-line regimens and also had to have a performance status of 0 or 1)(Burger et al., 2007). Patients received a dose of 15 mg/kg every 21 days; there were two complete responses and 11 partial responses, a median PFS of 4.7 months, and an OS of 17 months. This activity was noted in both platinum-sensitive and platinum-resistant subsets. The second study only included patients with platinum-resistant disease using an identical dose schedule, but the study was stopped because five of 44 patients experienced bowel perforations, one of them fatal; seven partial responses had been observed (Cannistra et al., 2007). This increased risk of bowel perforations was associated with three or more prior treatments (Monk et al., 2006; Kaye 2007). The third study included 70 patients who received 50 mg of oral cyclophosphamide daily, in addition to bevacizumab (10 mg/kg every 2 weeks); 17 partial responses were observed and four patients had intestinal perforations. (Garcia et al., 2008). Studies by the Gynecologic Oncology Group are evaluating the efficacy of the drug added to the initial treatment and at first recurrence in the platinum-resistant setting. Bevacizumab will probably be approved for clinical use in the near future. As neovascularization is a complicated process other antiangiogenic agents have been developed to overcome resistance to VEGF blockade, and several are undergoing clinical trials (Teoh et al., 2011). Future studies must answer to the following questions: The role of bevacizumab in first-line treatment and in the management of recurrent disease, the results of the combination with chemotherapy, risk factors for bowel perforation, the appropriate dose 15mg/Kg every three weeks or less and criteria for patient selection for bevacizumab treatment. (Kaye., 2007; Teoh et al., 2011; Monk et al., 2006).

Several targeted therapeutic agents are under evaluation in ongoing studies. They include the following groups of agents: 1) Antiangiogenic agents, 2) mTOR inhibitors, 3) PARP inhibitors and 4) Histone Deacetylase inhibitors.

1. Antiangiogenic agents include: a) Bevacizumab which has already been presented and will probably be approved for clinical use in the near future. b) VEGF-Trap a potent angiogenesis inhibitor fusion protein is under study. c) Agents that block the VEGF receptor. These agents include sorafenib and sunitinib, small molecules that block tyrosine kinase activity located in the cytoplasmic domain of VEGF receptor (VEGFR). Some of these molecules block VEGFR specifically, whereas others, such as sorafenib and sunitinib, block both VEGFR and the platelet-derived growth factor (PDGFR), thought to be involved in later phases of tumor angiogenesis relating to vessel maturation. (Gardner & Jewell, 2011).
2. mTOR inhibitors. Dysregulation of mTOR signaling occurs in many tumors and has been found to be activated in gynecological cancers. Increased AKT/PI3K activity with constitutive downstream activation of the mTOR pathway has been found in ovarian tumor specimens and ovarian cancer cell lines. Inhibition of mTOR by agents such temsirolimus, everolimus and deforolimus are in clinical trials.(Gardner & Jewell, 2011).
3. PARP inhibitors. Inhibition of poly(adenosine diphosphate [ADP]-ribose) polymerase (PARP), a key enzyme in the DNA repair, may lead to the accumulation of breaks in double-stranded and cell death. Therefore, PARP inhibitors have been developed and are potentially exciting agents in the treatment of ovarian cancer, especially cancers with BRCA1 and BRCA2 mutations. Initial reports have been encouraging A phae II, randomized double-blind, multicenter study is assessing the efficacy of an oral PARP inhibitor olaparib (AZD2281) in the treatment of patients with platinum-sensitive serous ovarian cancer following treatment with two or more platinum-containing regimens. (Gardner & Jewell, 2011).
4. Histone Deacetylase Inhibitors. Aberrant histone modifications such as hypoacetylation have been associated with malignancy through the transcriptional silencing of tumor suppressor genes. Belinostat is a histone deacetylase inhibitor (HDAC) that can alter the acetylation level of histone and nonhistone proteins. Such epigenetic modulation may sensitize drug-resistant tumor cells to other antineoplastic agents, as suggested in preclinical studies. A phase II study is examining the use of belinostat in combination with carboplatin among patients with recurrent or persistent platinim-resistant disease. (Gardner & Jewell, 2011). These new targeted biologic agents, particularly those involved with the vascular endothelial growth factor pathway and those targeting the poly (ADP-ribose) polymerase (PARP) enzyme, hold great promise for improving the outcome of ovarian cancer. (Jelovac & Armstrong 2011).

2.4.7 Microarray – Based gene expression studies in ovarian cancer

Despite recent improvements in treatment, ovarian cancer remains the No. 1 cause of death among gynecologic cancer in the United States. In more than 90% of patients with localized disease, surgery alone is curative. However, in most patients, the tumor has disseminated beyond the ovaries by the time the cancer is diagnosed. For these patients combined modality treatment, surgery and chemotherapy, is necessary and first-line chemotherapy has yielded response rates of greater than 80%. Unfortunately the median progression-free survival has been only 18 months in these patients and, in most with advanced cancer, the disease eventually relapses and the patient dies. Studies evaluating various cytotoxic agents in recurrent ovarian cancer have generally shown responses of 10% to 28% with limited effect on overall survival. This has prompted the search for novel strategies for treatment of ovarian cancer. (Chon & Lancaster, 2011).

Since 1987 microarray technology has been deeply incorporated in research settings and is developing an increasing presence in clinical arenas. Prior to the era of microarrays, the approach to understanding carcinogenesis largely focused on studying one gene at a time. Measuring the expression of thousands of genes at the same time using microarrays has answered many questions that were impossible to resolve previously. Gene expression assays are now used in daily clinical practice in the care of many patients who are newly diagnosed with breast cancer. In ovarian cancer, gene expression profiles have so far been used to examine differential gene expression patterns between histology subtypes. Several studies have sought to identify gene expression signatures that correlate with clinical outcome, to determine which genes affect survival and relapse, and to generate biomarkers that could predict patient response to chemotherapy. Data from these studies have deepened and widened our understanding of the biology of ovarian cancer despite some challenges. Studies on the role of microarray analysis to identify gene expression profiles associated with prognostic values and prognostic and predictive molecular markers will help identify patient groups who could benefit more from individualized treatment rather than the current standard first-line chemotherapy. In addition, identification of biomarkers associated with early detection of disease and molecular subsets will also improve overall survival for patients with ovarian cancer, as the early signs of the disease are often undetectable. (Chon & Lancaster, 2011).

2.4.8 Ovarian cancer: The future

Over the last several decades, clinical trials have led in 2006, for the first time, to a median overall survival of greater than 5 years in advanced - stage patients treated in a randomized controlled trial (Gardner & Jewell, 2011). Clinical trials continue to address important questions including the following issues: 1) The combination of surgery and chemotherapy. 2) The identification of new targeted therapeutics. 3) The route and timing of chemotherapy administration. 4) The quality of life endpoint 5) Tissue acquisition for translational studies. (Gardner & Jewell, 2011).

Quality of life studies. Persistent or recurrent ovarian cancer is not a curable disease today. The first aim of the Oncologist must be the improvement or maintenance of the quality of patients' life and the second the survival increase. There are at least 78 ongoing studies on quality of life today. The burden of disease and the effects of treatment have been increasingly recognized. Clinical trials are increasingly including quality of life components in trial designs in an effort to increase the duration of life and improve its quality at the same time. (Gardner & Jewell, 2011). Health - related quality of life (HRQOL) addresses important aspects of the patient's life including physical, social, psychological, financial, and sexual issues, as well as the side effects of the chemotherapeutic medications that we rely on for treatment. (Grzankowski & Carney, 2011). HRQOL assessment plays an important role in medical care, and this is especially significant in ovarian cancer treatment as 80% of newly diagnosed patients present with advanced disease and require extensive surgical and chemotherapeutic treatment regimens that are associated with significant morbidity. (Grzankowski & Carney, 2011). HRQOL data can be utilized in clinical trials, with an endpoint of improvement of HRQOL. The data can also be used as a tool in standardizing the efficacy and tolerability of treatment. In addition, information from the HRQOL assessments may help identify the need for changes in treatment regimens that may have otherwise been overlooked and can aid in the deciding when to pursue need for further treatment versus palliative care. (Grzankowski & Carney, 2011). Prolongation of life, without regard for the quality of that life, is not a universally desired goal. When considering aggressive, life-prolonging treatments and end-of-life decisions, it is necessary to consider each individual's assessment of what makes life worth living. Overall HRQOL assessment can help patients with ovarian cancer maintain autonomy when faced with the difficult decision between aggressive, life - prolonging treatments versus end-of-life decisions. As medical, pharmaceutical, and surgical techniques continue to prolong life much longer than our predecessors would have imagined, it is now the role of today's physicians to encompass quality of life into their ever-changing role as health care providers and patient advocates. To reach such positive outcomes, the use of an interdisciplinary treatment team approach is vital to each patient's needs. To optimize treatment decisions for patients with ovarian cancer, clinicians need to be familiar with differences between regimens in terms of toxicity, dosage, and administration, and emerging data from HRQOL assessments. (Grzankowski & Carney, 2011).

While decisions surrounding the diagnosis and treatment of cancer are difficult and cost is not usually the most pressing concern of decision makers, the increasing burden of the rising cost of healthcare demands attention. As newer, higher-cost therapies become available, formal evaluation of the costs and benefits of these new treatments in comparison to existing and established strategies should be a high priority. (Sfakianos et al, 2011).

2.5.1 Treatment options for patients with persistent or recurrent disease

There are today three available treatment options, as presented above, for patients with persistent or recurrent disease than can be used alone or in combination:

a. Secondary cytoreduction.
b. Chemotherapy. For patients with platinum-sensitive disease treatment with a cisplatinum or carboplatin combination is indicated. For patients with platinum-refractory or platinum-resistant disease treatment with other effective drugs must be used.
c. Clinical trials.

3. Conclusions

Patients with persistent or recurrent ovarian cancer have a lethal chronic disease. Treating them is challenging, and despite the recent advances many controversies remain. Research findings continue to resolve many of these issues. Secondary cytoreduction, especially complete, combined with further adjuvant therapy at the time of relapse may improve clinical outcome in selected patients. There are several treatment choices from first relapse to terminal state; however these choices cannot be made uniformly. They should be decided on an individual basis depending directly on the patients' condition. Patients with recurrent platinum-sensitive ovarian cancer have significant response rates and longer PFS when treated with combination platinum-based chemotherapy. Most recurrent patients with platinum resistant disease have little chance for a long PFS, but treatment may contribute to extending their overall survival.

Finding the optimal treatment remains a research goal.

4. References

Bae, J.; Lim MC.; Choi, JH.; Song, YJ.; Lee KS.; Kang, S.; Seo, SS & Park SY. (2009). Prognostic factors of secondary cytoreductive surgery for patients with recurrent epithelial ovarian cancer. *J Gynecol Oncol,* Vol. 20,No. 2, (June 2009), pp. 101-106

Berkenblit, A.; Seiden, MV.; Matulonis, UA.; Penson RT, Krasner CN, Roche M, Mezzetti L, Atkinson T & Cannistra SA. (2004). A phase II trial of weekly docetaxel in patients with platinum-resistant epithelial ovarian, primary peritoneal serous cancer, or fallopian tube cancer. *Gynecol Oncol,* Vol. 95, No.3, (December 2004), pp. 624-631

Bolis, G.; Scarfone, G.; Giardina, G.; Villa, A.; Mangili, G.; Melpignano, M.; Presti, M.; Tateo, S.; Franchi, M.; & Parazzini, F.(1998). Carboplatin alone vs carboplatin plus epidoxorubicin as second-line therapy for cisplatin- or carboplatin-sensitive ovarian cancer. *Gynecol Oncol,* Vol 81, No.1, (Apr 2001), pp.3-9.

Bookman, MA .; Malmström, H.; Bolis, G.;, Gordon A.; Lissoni, A.; Krebs, JB & Fields, S Z. (1998). Topotecan for the treatment of advanced epithelial ovarian cancer: an open-label phase II study in patients treated after prior chemotherapy that contained cisplatin or carboplatin and paclitaxel. *J Clin Oncol,* Vol. 16, No. 10, (October 1998), pp. 3345-3352

Burger, RA.; Sill, MW.; Monk, BJ.; Greer, BE & Sorosky, JI.(2007). Phase II trial of bevacizumab in persistent or recurrent epithelial ovarian cancer or primary peritoneal cancer: a Gynecologic Oncology Group Study. *J Clin Oncol,* Vol.25, No.33, (November 2007), pp. 5165-5171

Cannistra, SA.; Matulonis, UA.; Penson, RT.; Hambleton, J.; Dupont, J.; Douglas, J.; Burger, RA.; Armstrong, D.; Wenham R & McGuire W (2007). Phase II study of bevacizumab in patients with platinum-resistant ovarian cancer or peritoneal serous cancer. *J Clin Oncol* Vol. 25, No.33, (November 2007), pp.5180-5186

Cantù, MG.; Buda, A.; Parma, G.; Rossi, R.; Floriani, I.; Bonazzi, C.; Dell'Anna, T.; Torri, V et Colombo N.(2002).Randomized controlled trial of single-agent paclitaxel versus cyclophosphamide, doxorubicin, and cisplatin in patients with recurrent ovarian cancer who responded to first-line platinum-based regimens. *J Clin Oncol* Vol.20, No. 5, (March 2002), pp. 1232-1237

Chua, TC.; Robertson, G.; Liauw, W.; Farrell, R.; Yan, TD & Morris, DL. (2009). Intraoperative hyperthermic intraperitoneal chemotherapy after cytoreductive surgery in ovarian cancer peritoneal carcinomatosis; systematic review of current results. *J Cancer Res Clin Oncol,* Vol. 135, No. 12, (December 2009), pp. 1637-1645

Creemers, GJ.; Bolis, G.; Gore, M.; Scarfone, G.; Lacave, AJ; Guastalla, JP.; Despax, R.; Favalli, G.; Kreinberg, R.; Van Belle, S.; Hudson, I.; Verweij, J.; Ten Bokkel Huinink, WW et al. (1996). Topotecan, an active drug in the second-line treatment of epithelial ovarian cancer: results of a large European phase II study. *J Clin Oncol* Vol.14, No.12, (December 1996), pp. 3056-3061

Downs, L.; Argenta, PA.; Ghebre, R.; Geller, MA.; Bliss, L.; Boente, MP.; Nahhas, WA.; Abu-Ghazeleh, SZ.; Dwight Chen, M & Carson, LF.(2008). A prospective randomized trial of thalidomide with topotecan compared with topotecan alone in women with recurrent epithelial ovarian carcinoma. *Cancer,* Vol. 112, No. 2, (January 2008), pp. 331-339

Einzig, AI.; Wiernik, PH.; Sasloff, J.; Runowicz, CD & Goldberg GL (1992). Phase II study and long-term follow-up of patients treated with taxol for advanced ovarian adenocarcinoma. *J Clin Oncol,* Vol 10, No.11, (November 1992), pp. 1748-1753

Ferrero, JM.; Weber, B.; Geay, J.;, Lepille, D.; Orfeuvre, H.; Combe, M.; Mayer, F.; Leduc, B.; Bourgeois, H.; Paraiso, D & Pujade-Lauraine E.(2007)l. Second-line chemotherapy with pegylated liposomal doxorubicin and carboplatin is highly effective in patients with advanced ovarian cancer in late relapse: a GINECO phase II trial. *Ann Oncol,* Vol. 18, No.2, (November 2007), pp. 263-268

Frederick, PJ.; Ramirez, PT.; McQuinn, L.; Milam, MR.; Weber, DM.; Coleman, RT.; Gershensom, DM & Landen, CN Jr.(2011), Preoperative factors predicting survival after secondary cytoreduction for recurrent ovarian cancer. *Int J Gynecol Cancer,* Vol. 21, No. 5, (July 2011), pp. 831-836

Frenel, JS.; Leux, C.; Pouplin, L.; Ferron, G.; Berton Rigaud, D.; Bourdouloux, E.; Dravet, F.; Jaffre, I & Classe, JM.(2011), oxaliplatin-based hyperthermic intraperitoneal chemotherapy in primary or recurrent epithelial ovarian cancer; A pilot study of 31 patients. *J Surg Oncol,* Vol. 103, No. 1, (January 2011), pp. 10-16

Friedlander, M.; Millward, MJ.; Bell, D.; Bugat, R.; Harnett, P.; Moreno, JA.; Campbell, L.; Varette, C.; Ripoche V & Kayitalire L. (1998) A phase II study of gemcitabine in platinum pre-treated patients with advanced epithelial ovarian cancer..*Ann Oncol.* Vol. 9, No. 12, (December 1998), pp.1343-1345

Fotopoulou C.; Richter R.; Braicu IE.; Schmidt, SC.; Neuhaus P.; Lichtenegger, W & Sehouli J. (2011). *Ann Surg Oncol,* Vol 18, No. 1 (January 2011), pp. 49-57

Garcia, AA.; Hirte, H.; Fleming, G.; Yang, D.; Tsao-Wei, DD.; Roman, L.; Groshen, S.; Swenson, S.; Markland,F.; Gandara, D.; Scudder, S.; Morgan, R.; Chen, H.; Lenz, HJ et Oza, AM.(2008). Phase II clinical trial of bevacizumab and low-dose metronomic oral cyclophosphamide in recurrent ovarian cancer: a trial of the California, Chicago, and Princess Margaret Hospital phase II consortia. *J Clin Oncol* , Vol.26, No.1, (January 2008), pp. 76-82

Gardner, J & Jewell EL.(2011). Current and Future Directions of Clinical Trials for Ovarian Cancer.*Cancer Control,* Vol. 18, No. 1, (January 2011), pp. 44-51

Gordon, AN.; Fleagle, JT.; Guthrie, D.; Parkin, DE.; Gore, ME & Lacave, AJ(2001). Recurrent epithelial ovarian carcinoma: a randomized phase III study of pegylated liposomal doxorubicin versus topotecan. *J Clin Oncol,* Vol. 19, No.14, (July 2001), pp. 3312-3322

Gordon, AN.; Tonda, M.; Sun, S.; Rackoff W & Doxil Study 30-49 Investigators.(2004). Long-term survival advantage for women treated with pegylated liposomal doxorubicin compared with topotecan in a phase 3 randomized study of recurrent and refractory epithelial ovarian cancer. *Gynecol Oncol* , Vol.95, No.1, (October 2004), pp. 1-8

Grzankowski, K. & Carney, M. (2011). Quality of life in Ovarian Cancer. *Cancer Control,* Vol.18, No.1 (January 2011), pp. 52-58.

Harter, P.; du Bois, A.; Hahmann, M.; hasenburg, A.; Burges, A.; Loibl, S.; Gropp, M.; Huober, J.; Fink, D.; Schroder, W.; Muenstedt, K.; Schmalfeldt, B.; Emons, G.; Pfisterer, J.; Wollschlaeger, K.; Meerpohl, HG.; Breitbach, GP.; Tanner, B et Sehouli, J. Arbeitsgemeinschaft Gynaekologische Onkologie Ovarian Committee; AGO

Ovarian Cancer Study Group. (2006). *Ann Surg Oncol*,Vol. 13, No. 12, (December 2006), pp. 1702-1710

Hoskins, WJ.; Rubin, SC.; Dulaney, E.; Chapman, D.; Almadrones, L.; Saigo, P.; Markman, M.; Hakes, T.; Reichman, B & Jones, WB.(1989). Influence of secondary cytoreduction at the time of second-look laparotomy on the survival of patients with epithelial ovarian carcinoma. *Gynecol Onco,* Vol. 34, No.3, (Sep 1989), pp. 365-71

Jelovac, D & Armstrong D.(2011). Recent progress in the diagnosis and treatment of ovarian cancer. *CA: A Cancer Journal for Clinicians*, Vol. 61, No. 3, (May-June 2011), pp. 183–203

Kaye SB. (2007). Bevacizumab for the treatment of epithelial ovarian cancer: will this be its finest hour? *J Clin Oncol,* Vol. 25, No.33, (November 2007) pp. 5150-5152

Kohn, EC.; Sarosy, G.; Bicher, A.; Link, C.; Christian, M.; Steinberg, SM.; Rothenberg, M.; Adamo, DO.; Davis, P. & Ognibene, FP.(1994). Dose-intense taxol: high response rate in patients with platinum-resistant recurrent ovarian cancer. *J Natl Cancer Inst* , Vol.86, No. 1, (January 1994), pp. 18-24

Kudelka, AP.; Tresukosol, D.; Edwards, CL.; Freedman, RS.; Levenback, C.; Chantarawiroj, P.; Gonzalez de Leon, C.; Kim, EE.; Madden, T.; Wallin, B.; Hord, M.; Verschraegen, C.;Raber, M & Kavanagh, JJ. (1996). Phase II study of intravenous topotecan as a 5-day infusion for refractory epithelial ovarian carcinoma. *J Clin Oncol,* Vol. 14, No. 5, (May 1996), pp. 1552-1557

Lund, B.; Hansen, OP.; Theilade, K.; Hansen, M et Neijt, JP (1994). Phase II study of gemcitabine (2',2'-difluorodeoxycytidine) in previously treated ovarian cancer patients. *J Natl Cancer Inst,* Vol.86, No. 20, (October 1994), pp. 1530-1533

Markman, M.; Markman, J.; Webster, K.; Zanotti, K.; Kulp, B.; Peterson, G. & Belinson, J. (2004). Duration of response to second-line, platinum-based chemotherapy for ovarian cancer: implications for patient management and clinical trial design. *J Clin Oncol,* Vol. 22, No. 15, (August 2004), pp. 3120-3125

Martin,LP.; & Schilder RJ. (2009). Management of recurrent ovarian carcinoma: current status and future directions. *Semin Oncol,* Vol. 36, No. 2, (April 2009), pp. 112-125

McGuire, WP.; Rowinsky, EK.; Rosenshein, NB.; Grumbine, FC.; Ettinger, DS.; Armstrong, DK & Donehower,RC.(1989). Taxol: a unique antineoplastic agent with significant activity in advanced ovarian epithelial neoplasms. *Ann Intern Med,* Vol. 111, No. 4, (August 1989), pp. 273-279

Monk, BJ.; Han, E.; Josephs-Cowan, CA.; Pugmire G & Burger, RA. (2006) Salvage bevacizumab (rhuMAB VEGF)-based therapy after multiple prior cytotoxic regimens in advanced refractory epithelial ovarian cancer. *Gynecol Oncol,* Vol.102, No.2, (August 2006), pp. 140-144

Muggia, FM. (1989).Overview of carboplatin: replacing, complementing, and extending the therapeutic horizons of cisplatin. *Semin Oncol,* Vol.16, 2 Suppl 5, (April1989), pp. 7-13

Miller, P.; Groshen, S.; Tan, M.; Roman, L.; Uziely, B.; Muderspach, L.; Garcia, A.; Burnett, A.; Greco, FA.; Morrow, CP.; Paradiso LJ & Liang, LJ.(1997) Phase II study of liposomal doxorubicin in refractory ovarian cancer: antitumor activity and toxicity modification by liposomal encapsulation. *J Clin Oncol,* Vol.15, No.3,(March 1997), pp. 987-993

Munkarah, AR & Coleman, Rt.(2004). Critical evaluation of secondary cytoreduction in recurrent ovarian cancer. *Gynecol Oncol,* Vol. 95, No. 2, (November 2004), pp. 273-280

Mutch, DG.; Orlando, M.; Goss, T.; Teneriello, MG.; Gordon, AN.; McMeekin, SD.; Wang, Y.; Scribner, DR Jr.; Marciniack, M.; Naumann, RW & Secord, AA.(2007) Randomized phase III trial of gemcitabine compared with pegylated liposomal doxorubicin in patients with platinum-resistant ovarian cancer. *J Clin Oncol,* Vol.25, No. 19, (July 2007), pp. 2811-2818

National Cancer Institute (NCI). Recurrent or persistent Epithelial Cancer Treatment. http: cancer.gov/cancertopics/pdq/treatment/ovarianepithelial/HealthProfessional. Accessed July 9, 2011

Ozols, RF.; Bundy, BN.; Greer, BE.; Fowler, JM.; Clarke-Pearson, D.; Burger, RA.; Mannel, RS.; DeGeest, K.; Hartenbach, EM.; Baergen, R.; Gynecologic Oncology Group et al.(2003). Phase III trial of carboplatin and paclitaxel compared with cisplatin and paclitaxel in patients with optimally resected stage III ovarian cancer: a Gynecologic Oncology Group study. *J Clin Oncol,* Vol. 21, No. 17, (September 2003), pp. 3194-3200

Parmar, MK.; Ledermann, JA.; Colombo, N.; du Bois, A.; Delaloye, JF.; Kristensen, GB.; Wheeler, S.; Swart, AM.; Qian, W.; Torri, V.; Floriani, I.; Jayson, G.; Lamont, A.; Tropé, C.; ICON and AGO Collaborators.(2003). Paclitaxel plus platinum-based chemotherapy versus conventional platinum-based chemotherapy in women with relapsed ovarian cancer: the ICON4/AGO-OVAR-2.2 trial. *Lancet.* Vol. 361, No. 9375, (June 2003), pp. 2099-2106

Piccart, MJ.; Green, JA.; Lacave, AJ.; Reed, N.; Vergote, I.; Benedetti-Panici, P.; Bonetti, A.; Kristeller-Tome, V.; Fernandez, CM.; Curran, D.; Van Glabbeke, M.; Lacombe, D.; Pinel, MC. & Pecorelli, S. (2000). Oxaliplatin or paclitaxel in patients with platinum-pretreated advanced ovarian cancer: A randomized phase II study of the European Organization for Research and Treatment of Cancer Gynecology Group. *J Clin Oncol,* Vol. 18 , No.6, (March 2000), pp.1193-1202

Pfisterer, J.; Plante, M.; Vergote, I.; du Bois, A.; Hirte, H.; Lacave, AJ.; Wagner, U.; Stähle, A.; Stuart, G.; Kimmig, R.; Olbricht, S.; Le, T.; Emerich, J.; Kuhn, W.; Bentley, J.; Jackisch, C.; Lück, HJ.; Rochon, J.; Zimmermann, AH.; Eisenhauer, E.; AGO-OVAR; NCIC CTG; EORTC GCG.(2006). Gemcitabine plus carboplatin compared with carboplatin in patients with platinum-sensitive recurrent ovarian cancer: an intergroup trial of the AGO-OVAR, the NCIC CTG, and the EORTC GCG. *J Clin Oncol,* Vol. 24, No. 29, (October 2006), pp. 4699-4707.

Pothuri, B; Vaidya, A.; Aghajanian, C et al. (2003). Palliative surgery for bowel obstruction in recurrent ovarian cancer: an updated series. *Gynecol Oncol,* Vol. 89, No. 2 (2003), pp.306-313.

Ramirez, I.; Chon, HS & Apte, SM.(2011). The Role of Surgery in he Management of Epithelial Ovarian Cancer. *Cancer Control,* Vol. 18, No. 1, (January 2011), pp. 22-30.

Roviello, E.; Pinto, e.; Corso, G.; Pedrazzani, C.; Caruso, S.; Fillippeschi, M.; petrol, R.; Marsill, S.; Mazzei, MA & Marrelli, d.(2010). Safety and potential benefit of hyperthermic intraperitoneal chemotherapy (HIPEC) in peritoneal carcinomatosis from primary or ecurrent ovarian caner. *J Surg Oncol,* Vol. 102, No. 6, (November 2010), pp. 663-670

Salani, R.; Santillan A, ZahuraK ML.; Gluntoli II, RL.; Gardner GJ, Armstrong DK & Bristow RE. (2007). Secondary Cytoreductive Surgery for Localized, Recurrent Epithelial Ovarian Cancer. Analysis of Prognostic Factors and Survival Outcome. *Cancer,* Vol. 109, No. 4, (February 2007), pp. 685-691

Shapiro, JD.; Millward, MJ.; Rischin, D.; Michael, M.; Walcher, V.; Francis, PA. et Toner, GC. (1996). Activity of gemcitabine in patients with advanced ovarian cancer: responses seen following platinum and paclitaxel. *Gynecol Oncol,* Vol. 63, No. 1, (October 1996), pp. 89-93

Sfakianos, GP & Havrilesky LJ.(2011). A Review of Cost-Effectiveness Studies in Ovarian Cancer.*Cancer Control,* Vol. 18, No. 1, (January 2011), pp.59-64.

Ten Bokkel Huinink, W.; Gore, M.; Carmichael, J.; Gordon, A.; Malfetano, J.; Hudson, I.; Broom, C.; Scarabelli, C.; Davidson, N.; Spanczynski, M.; Bolis, G.; Malmström, H.; Coleman, R.; Fields, SC & Heron, JF. (1997). Topotecan versus paclitax,el for the treatment of recurrent epithelial ovarian cancer. *J Clin Oncol,* Vol.15, No.6, (June 1997), pp. 2183-2193

Thigpen, JT.; Blessing, JA.; Ball, H.; Hummel, SJ et Barrett, RJ. (1994). Phase II trial of paclitaxel in patients with progressive ovarian carcinoma after platinum-based chemotherapy: a Gynecologic Oncology Group study. *J Clin Oncol,* Vol. 12, No.9, (September 1994), pp.1748-1753

Trimble, EL.; Adams, JD.; Vena, D.; Hawkins, MJ.; Friedman, MA.; Fisherman, JS.; Christian, MC.; Canetta, R.; Onetto, N. & Hayn, R.(1993). Paclitaxel for platinum-refractory ovarian cancer: results from the first 1,000 patients registered to National Cancer Institute Treatment Referral Center 9103. *J Clin Oncol,* Vol.11, No. 12, (December 1993) pp. 2405-2410

Ushijima K. (2009). Treatment for Recurrent Ovarian Cancer—At First Relapse. *Journal of Oncology,* Volume 2010 (Article IDJ Oncol. 2010; 2010:497429. Epub 2009 Dec 24.497429, 7 pages doi:10.1155/2010/497429

Vasey, PA.; McMahon, L.; Paul, J.; Reed, N & Kaye, SB.(2003). A phase II trial of capecitabine (Xeloda) in recurrent ovarian cancer. *Br J Cancer,* Vol. 89, No. 10, (November 2003), pp. 1843-1848

10

Minimally Invasive Surgical Procedures for Patients with Advanced and Recurrent Ovarian Cancer

Samir A. Farghaly
The Joan and Sanford I. Weill/ The Graduate School of Medical Sciences and The New York Presbyterian Hospital - Weill Cornell Medical Center, Cornell University, New York, NY USA

1. Introduction

Estimated, 225,000 new cases of ovarian cancer in the world in 2011, with approximately 140,000 deaths. In the United States of America, ovarian cancer is the second most gynecological cancer. It is the most common cause of gynecological cancer related death primarily because most patients present with advanced disease. 65-70% of patients are diagnosed at an advanced stage, conferring a 5-year survival rate of 30-55%. Epithelial ovarian cancer (EOC) remains the most lethal gynecologic cancer in the United States. In 2010, approximately 21,880 new cases and 13,850 deaths occurred. There is no proven screening test for this disease. Many women present with vague symptoms, including abdominal bloating, change in bowel or bladder habits, early satiety, or abdominal pain. It is diagnosed at advanced stage for about 75% of patients [1]. It spreads along the peritoneal surfaces to the upper abdomen by direct extension or by peritoneal implantation [2]. Metastases to the diaphragm, especially to the right hemi-diaphragm, are common in patients with advanced ovarian cancer. About 40% of patients with advanced ovarian cancer present with bulky metastatic diaphragmatic disease. About 19% of patients are diagnosed with International Federation of Obstetrics and Gynecology (FIGO) [Table 1.] stage I disease, in which the tumor is confined to one or both ovaries. (1). Stage I disease is usually diagnosed incidentally during laparoscopic or laparotomy surgery for benign-looking ovarian tumors, but, following complete staging, it is upstaged in 30% of patients due to microscopic metastatic disease.(2,3). FIGO guidelines have stated that the standard management for apparent early-stage disease is complete surgical staging, including total abdominal hysterectomy, bilateral salpingo-oophorectomy, pelvic and para-aortic lymph node dissection, infracolic omentectomy, multiple peritoneal washing, and multiple peritoneal biopsies (4). Initial evaluation includes a thorough history and physical examination, imaging studies such as MRI and computerized tomography scanning, assessment of tumor markers such as CA-125, biopsies, cystoscopy and colonoscopy. The standard treatment for primary ovarian cancer consists of maximum cytoreductive effort to reduce residual tumor (RT), followed by platinum-based chemotherapy (3, 4). It has been shown that cytoreduction has a more significant influence on survival than the extent of a metastatic disease observed before surgery (5). This target has value in the primary cytoreduction (3), and in interval debulking surgery after neoadjuvant chemotherapy (6), in addition to in secondary cytoreduction in platinum-sensitive recurrent ovarian cancer patients (7). Extensive upper abdominal debulking surgery increases the rate of optimal cytoreduction and it is related with improved survival rates in advanced ovarian cancer undergoing primary cytoreduction and interval debulking surgery (8). Hepatic resection (9), splenectomy (10) and (11), video-assisted thoracic surgery (12), and diaphragmatic resection (13), (14), (15), (16), (17), (18) and (19) have been considered as components of primary cytoreduction when necessary.

Stage I: Growth limited to the ovaries
IA Growth limited to one ovary: no ascites present containing malignant cells. No tumor on the external surface; capsule intact. IB Growth limited to both ovaries: no ascites present containing malignant cells. No tumor on the external surfaces; capsules intact. IC* Tumor either stage IA or IB, but with tumor on surface of one or both ovaries, or with capsule ruptured, or with ascites present containing malignant cells, or with positive peritoneal washings.
Stage II: Growth involving one or both ovaries with pelvic extension.
IIA Extension and/or metastases to the uterus and/or tubes. IIB Extension to other pelvic tissues. IIC* Tumor either stage IIA or IIB, but with tumor on surface of one or both ovaries, or with capsule(s) ruptured, or with ascites present containing malignant cells, or with positive peritoneal washings.
Stage III: Tumor involving one or both ovaries with histologically confirmed peritoneal implants outside the pelvis and/or positive retroperitoneal or inguinal nodes. Superficial liver metastases equals stage III. Tumor is limited to the true pelvis but with histologically proven malignant extension to small bowel or omentum.
IIIA Tumor grossly limited to the true pelvis, with negative nodes, but with histologically confirmed microscopic seeding of abdominal peritoneal surfaces, or histologic proven extension to small bowel or mesentery. IIIB Tumor of one or both ovaries with histologically confirmed implants, peritoneal metastasis of abdominal peritoneal surfaces, none exceeding 2 cm in diameter; nodes are negative. IIIC Peritoneal metastasis beyond the pelvis > 2 cm in diameter and/or positive retroperitoneal or inguinal nodes.
Stage IV: Growth involving one or both ovaries with distant metastases. If pleural effusion is present, there must be positive cytology to allot a case to stage IV. Parenchymal liver metastasis equals stage IV.
* In order to evaluate the impact on prognosis of the different criteria for allotting cases to stage IC or IIC, it would be of value to know if rupture of the capsule was spontaneous, or caused by the surgeon; and if the source of malignant cells detected peritoneal washings, or ascites.

Table 1. Carcinoma of the ovary: figo classification (rio de janerio 1988)

2. Minimally invasive surgery in advanced ovarian cancer

Laparoscopic assisted surgery can be utilized in the surgical management of apparent early-stage ovarian cancer, in assessing resectability of advanced disease prior to laparotomy, and also in second-look procedures.

Several studies showed that laparoscopy is safe and feasible in the surgical management of apparent early-stage ovarian cancer. (20-23) In a Study comparing laparoscopic treatment of gynecologic malignancies with traditional laparotomy for early-stage ovarian cancer, it was observed (24) that the acceptable survival rates with decreased morbidity and shorter hospitalization: 91.6% with disease-free survival and overall survival of 100% at 46 months. The advantages of laparoscopy are faster recovery with early return of bowel function and a shorter hospital stay. Laparoscopy can be useful, when deciding whether to proceed with primary cytoreductive surgery or neoadjuvant chemotherapy in advanced epithelial ovarian cancer. In a study of 87 patients who underwent diagnostic laparoscopy, 53 were considered resectable.(25). Of these 53 patients, 96% were optimally cytoreduced. Laparoscopy seems to be an acceptable method for assessing disease resectability. Operative time of 120 to 240 minutes has been reported with laparoscopic staging of ovarian cancer (26). Surgical complications could include vascular and gastrointestinal injuries, and possibly port site metastases (27). There is a concerqn that ovarian cancer mass my rupture while trying to remove it. Ovarian cyst rupture has been reported in 12% to 25% of patients undergoing laparoscopy(,28,29) and rupture may cause intra-abdominal dissemination. Several studies have suggested that cyst rupture increase recurrence rate and decrease survival (30,31). To avoid any spillage, the ovarian mass should be placed in a laparoscopic bag and retrieved through the umbilical port or through a colpotomy. Minimally invasive robot- assisted laparoscopic surgery, utilizing da Vinci surgical system (Figures 1 and 2), has been employed to duplicate traditional open procedures via small incisions in the skin with surgical outcomes equivalent or superior to a traditional surgical approach. Robotic surgery enables the operator to control the robotic system alone and to perform more precise and complex operations. The da Vinci Surgical System provides surgeons with 1) intuitive translation of the instrument handle to the tip movement, thus eliminating the mirror-image effect, 2) visualization with high quality 3-dimensional images and stable camera platform, 3) scaling, 4) tremor filtering, 5) coaxial alignment of eyes, hand, and tooltip images, 6) EndoWrist with a 360-degree range of motion, 7) comfortable, ergonomically ideal operating position.

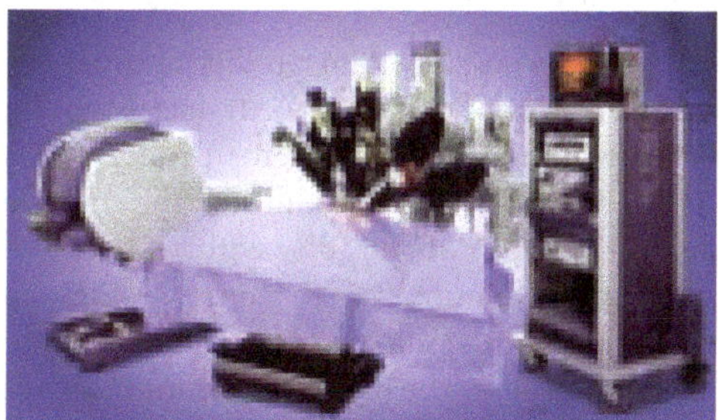

Fig. 1. Da Vinci Surgical System

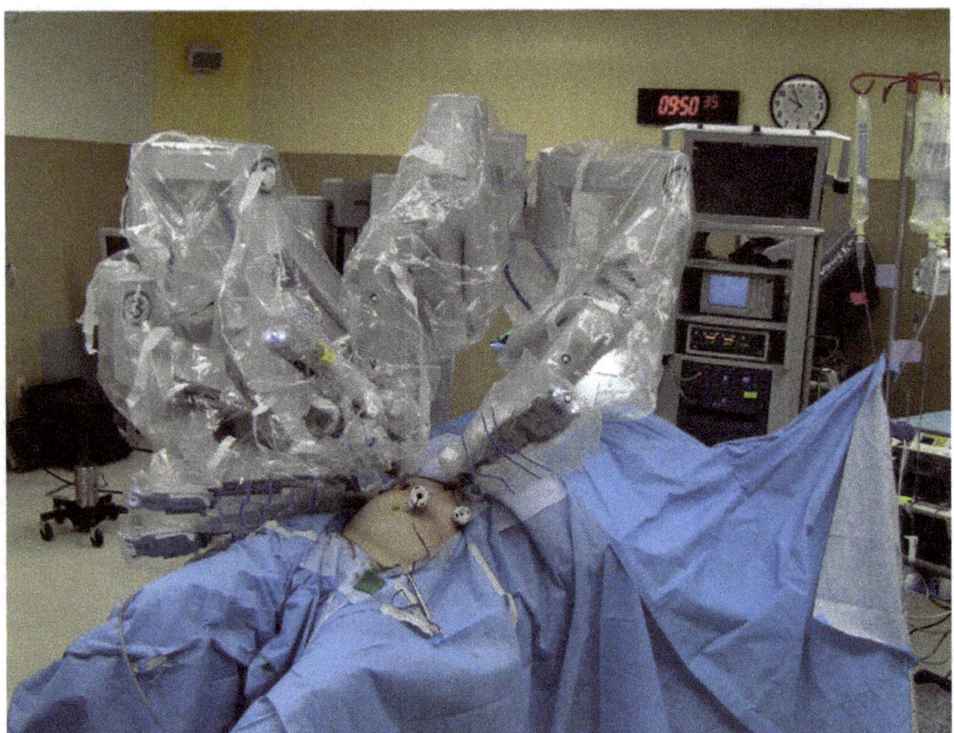

Fig. 2. Robotic platform docked off patient's right shoulder in 10 degree reverse Trendelenburg position, and 10 degree rotation to left.

It has been demonstrated that minimally invasive surgery is associated with less blood loss , shorter hospital stay, less post operative pain , improved cosmesis, and faster recovery compared to traditional approaches (32), (33). 10 cases were reported with an operative time of 207 minutes, blood loss of 355 cc and nodal yield of 27 (34). It was observed that the operative time in robotic radical hysterectomy was 241 minutes and blood loss of 71 cc, and no conversion to laparotomy reported (35).

3. Laparoscopic assesment of disease extent and potential for resectability

Staging laparoscopy (S-LPS) has been shown to predict optimal cytoreduction in primary and recurrent ovarian cancer (36), (37), (38), (39). It has been shown that an objective evaluation of the complete debulking is available for primary advanced cases utilizing a laparoscopic predictive index score (40- 41). In addition, the inclusion of S-LPS can reduce the risk of explorative laparotomies to about 10%, with respect to 20% and 30% obtained with the classical criteria of evaluation of response. S-LPS could increase optimal cytoreduction in 20% of patients with stable disease. The explanation to this, could be the presence of radiological artifacts due to the effects of chemotherapy, such as adherences or fibrosis secondary to tumor shrinkage, which would probably alter the diagnostic performances of conventional images. The laparoscopic predictive score of surgical outcome has been shown to be reliable in selected group of patients (41-42). The laparoscopic parameters meeting the inclusion criteria have been mesenteral retraction, bowel and stomach infiltration, and superficial liver metastases. Excluding bowel infiltration, these results confirmed others (43-44). It is clear that, S-LPS has an important role in the prediction of optimal cytoreduction in advanced ovarian cancer patients at primary diagnosis.

4. Laparoscopic re-assesment and 2nd look surgery

Second-look surgical reassessments in patients with advanced ovarian cancer have been performed to identify patients who had a complete pathologic response to chemotherapy, as demonstrated by numerous biopsies that were negative for persistent cancer. . The surgical method involved a laparotomy with extensive exploration of the abdomen, including multiple peritoneal washings, multiple biopsies, and, more than often, additional retroperitoneal lymph node sampling (45). With the current chemotherapy regimens, 75 - 80% of patients with optimally cytoreduced disease have a complete clinical response to primary chemotherapy, but only 50% of these patients are found to have a negative second look (46),(47). About one-half of all patients, who achieve a negative second look develop recurrent disease. It has been shown that, there is no survival benefit to the second-look procedure (48-51). Laparoscopy had been used to perform second-look evaluations in patients with ovarian cancer. Initial studies of second look by laparoscopy reported inadequate visualization; a high false-negative rate of between 11 and 55%; a high rate of complications, primarily bowel injuries, of 2 to 9%; and a higher recurrence rate following negative second-look laparoscopy (52 -55). More recent studies, however, have shown that laparoscopic second-look evaluations are equivalent to those performed by laparotomy, but are associated with significantly lower blood loss, decreased operating time, short hospital stay, and decreased hospital charges (56), (57). The current purpose of laparoscopic second-look surgery is to identify 3 patients categories: (1) those with microscopic diseases, (2) those with resectable disease that can successfully be rendered microscopic, and (3) those with gross, unresectable disease. In general, laparoscopy is an efficient and accurate technique for surgical reassessment following primary therapy in advanced ovarian cancer patients. Despite initial good response rates with primary chemotherapy, the majority of patients with advanced ovarian cancer will die of their disease. As approximately 50% of patients with a pathologically negative second look will eventually suffer from recurrent disease, as these patients all have microscopic disease. Studies have found, that patients with microscopic disease at second-look surgical reassessment have a good prognosis and a 5-year survival rate of 50 to 70% with continued therapy. Furthermore, patients who are successfully cytoreduced to microscopic disease at the time of second look have a prognosis equivalent to those found to have microscopic disease (58-61). Therefore, this group represents a subset of patients who have an overall better prognosis and may potentially be curable with effective therapy. Studies have suggested a potential benefit to consolidation/salvage therapy in this group of patients (62,63). It appears that microscopic disease may be missed by laparoscopy compared with laparotomy, but as all patients in this group (both negative-second-look and microscopically positive second-look patients) may benefit from consolidation therapy, the small advantage of a more accurate diagnosis of microscopic disease does not warrant laparotomy. It has been shown that, the rate of positive retroperitoneal nodes as the only evidence of disease at second look was only 3.8% (64). Several studies have shown that second-look laparoscopy was considered a promising candidate to replace second-look laparotomy which has been considered as standard treatment (65-67). In most initial studies which were conducted involving a small number of patients, second look laparoscopy did not produce satisfactory results and inappropriate operative field was reported to reach up to 12% and resulted in a false negative rate between 29.1% and 55% (65,68,69). It has been shown that patients in complete remission after chemotherapy underwent laparotomy and histological examination right after suspicious lesions were detected by second-look laparoscopy. As a result, the positive and negative predictive values of laparoscopy were 100% (six of six cases) and 86% (two false-negative out of 14 cases), respectively. Thorough observation of intraperitoneal lesions was available in 95% of patients in the LT group and only in 41% of patients in the LPS group due to intraperitoneal adhesions after previous surgeries. Though this study has some limitations in which postoperative survival rates were not compared with the results of the operation, it suggested that second look laparoscopy was less reliable than second-look laparotomy (67). Russo reported similar results (70). In a retrospective study by Husain on 150 cases of second look laparoscopy (71), the procedure was reported to be safe and accurate as a second-look operation. Also, the authors observed that the complication rates were reportedly low when laparoscopy was performed on patients who had received a primary debulking operation, and the recurrence rates of laparoscopic second-look in patients with histologically negative findings and a negative predictive value were also reported to be equivalent to those in patients who underwent laparotomic second-look (71). Second-look laparoscopy is thought to have disadvantages including limited access to lesions due to adhesions formed after previous surgeries, inappropriate operative fields and difficulty in manual examination of lesions. However, it has several advantages to offset these disadvantages. These are:

1. When using second-look laparoscopy not for removal of lesions but for diagnosis, the preoperative imaging procedure enables the extent and duration of operation to be predicted equivalently to those in non-invasive surgery,
2. Enlarged laparoscopic images enable the detection of minute lesions,
3. A certain degree of adhesion due to previous surgeries does not affect the performance of experienced laparoscopists (76), (77).

Currently, advanced laparoscopic procedures are increasingly being utilized as an alternative to laparotomy in gynecological surgery.(72-74). A meta-analysis of 27 prospective randomized trials has proven the benefits of laparoscopic compared with abdominal gynecologic surgery: decreased pain, decreased surgical-site infections (decreased relative risk 80%), decreased hospital stay (2 days less), quicker return to activity (2 weeks sooner), and fewer postoperative adhesions (decreased 60%).(75)

5. Minimally invasive thoracic surgery for patients with advanced ovariian cancer

In advanced and recurrent ovarian cancer, the presence of macroscopic intrathoracic disease may alter patient management, particularly if less than 1–2 cm intrathoracic tumor deposits. That would leave the patient with suboptimal residual disease at the conclusion of maximum intra-abdominal cytoreduction. It has been reported that rate of optimal primary debulking ranges from 27% to 51% (78), (79) and (80). The benefits of debulking in patients with malignant pleural effusions compared with other stage IV disease criteria have been evaluated. In a study of 84 patients with stage IV disease, including 38% of those patients with malignant pleural effusions, in a study it was reported a median survival of 38.4 months in optimally debulked patients (≤ 1 cm) and 10.3 months for patients with suboptimal residual disease (P = 0.0004) (79). On univariate analysis, there was no difference in median survival comparing patients with pleural effusion and other stage IV criteria. Although several retrospective reviews have demonstrated a survival benefit to optimal intra-abdominal debulking in patients with malignant pleural effusions, these patients still have decreased survival when compared with patients who have disease confined to the abdomen. Evaluating optimally cytoreduced stage IIIC and stage IV patients, it has been reported (82) reported a median survival of 58 months for patients who had stage IIIC disease and 30 months for patients with stage IV disease (p = 0.016). In patients with symptomatic malignant pleural effusions, video-assisted thoracic surgery (VATS) provides therapeutic benefits, as thoracoscopic pleurodesis is an effective technique for performing pleurodesis, particularly when using talc as the sclerosant. It was observed that the use of more extensive ablative techniques and radical upper abdominal procedures is required to achieve optimal cytoreduction (83). The involvement of the diaphragm in patients with ovarian cancer is the limiting factor preventing optimal cytoreduction (84). Diaphragmatic superficial tumor studding can be ablated or resected using diaphragmatic peritonectomy. Several authors have described the use of extensive diaphragmatic resections for full thickness or deeply invasive diaphragmatic disease (85, (86). VATS may be helpful in evaluating the extent of superficial and full thickness diaphragmatic disease and can then be used to plan appropriate intra-abdominal surgical approaches. In patients with isolated pleural-based disease, VATS can also facilitate intrathoracic cytoreduction. The outcomes of 30 patients who underwent thoracoscopy either by a transdiaphragmatic approach at laparotomy was observed, or through the chest wall prior to a planned abdominal procedure (81). In this series, 33% (10/30) underwent pleural implant ablation and/or tumor excision, which influenced the final cytoreductive outcome (87). VATS should be considered for incorporation into the standard management algorithm for patients with advanced ovarian cancer and pleural effusion. The rate of pleural involvement is underestimated in patients with advanced ovarian cancer. Preoperative computed tomography (CT) identified only one third of patients who had macroscopic pleural nodules by video-assisted thoracoscopy (VAT) (88). Occult pleural involvement may be present in up to 84% of patients with abdominal diaphragmatic involvement. (89). Without routine pleural exploration, failure to remove thoracic lesions occurs in up to one third of patients (89). It has been reported that VAT is feasible and safe in patients with advanced ovarian cancer (87).

Pleural metastases are common in patients with ovarian malignancies and pleural effusions. Previously reported rates range from 42% to 65%, Video-assisted thoracoscopy is better than CT for evaluating pleural involvement. In a retrospective study of 12 patients with large pleural effusions, chest CT detected pleural lesions in only 2 of 6 patients who had pleural disease by VAT.(87).

Routine examination of the pleural cavity may improve staging accuracy, even in patients with limited abdominal involvement. In another study, the result of VAT influenced treatment decisions in 33% of patients, (87).

Pleural involvement has been shown to influence patient outcomes (90). In a retrospective study, median survival after optimal cytoreductive surgery was 58 months in patients with stage IIIC disease and 30 months in those with stage IV disease (P = 0.016). This survival difference may be attributed to residual intrathoracic disease responsible for decreased efficacy of complete abdominal cytoreduction or to tumor aggressiveness in patients with stage IV disease. Extensive thoracic cytoreductive surgery has been suggested in combination with abdominal surgery. It has been reported (91) that performing VAT may translate into therapeutic benefits in 30% of cases. Other studies found better survival in patients who underwent complete cytoreductive surgery (91), (92).

Ovarian cancer usually spreads along different routes: lymphatic, haematogenous and transcaelomic. One of its features is the possible peritoneal and pleural dissemination. Mediastinal lymph node metastasis predicts poor prognosis (93). CPLN colonization is frequently associated with intrathoracic disease, which presents as right-sided pleural effusion. This is explained by the anatomic arrangement of abdominal lymphatic drainage, which follows a clockwise route, involving first the thoracic lymphatic stations on the right side. Metastatic calcification of supradiaphragmatic nodes from ovarian primary, is an interesting phenomenon, and is reported with an incidence up to 35%. Calcified intrathoracic nodes in patients with previous ovarian serous adenocarcinoma cannot be ruled out as granulomatous disease, but metastatic deposits must be excluded. Progressive growth of the involved station will point out to the latter. FDG-PET scan proves to be unreliable because granulomatous lymphadenitis which show an increased FDG-uptake.

Surgery for patients with ovarian cancer is carried to achieve histologic diagnosis, disease staging, and prolonged survival, and Videothoracoscopy is a reliable procedure for that. The minimally invasive approach enables thorough exploration of the entire pleural cavity, easy resection of any small nodes sited within the pericardial fat, and removal of bilateral CPLN growths. Resection of isolated node metastases could improve outlook for slow growing tumors. It has been shown that ovarian tumor growth rate seems a sound parameter (93).

6. Laparooscopic assisted diaphragmatic and hepatic surgery in patients with advanced ovarian cancer

Advanced ovarian cancer spreads along the peritoneal surfaces to the abdomen, and often it involves the upper abdomen by direct extension or by peritoneal implantation. Metastases to the diaphragm, especially to the right hemi-diaphragm, are common in patients with advanced ovarian cancer, and up 40% of patients with advanced ovarian cancer present with bulky metastatic diaphragmatic disease. The current standard treatment for primary ovarian cancer consists of maximum cytoreductive effort to reduce residual tumor (RT), followed by platinum-based chemotherapy (94), (95). It has been observed that cytoreduction has a more significant influence on survival than the extent of a metastatic disease observed before surgery(96); this target has value not only in the primary cytoreduction (94), but also in interval debulking surgery after neoadjuvant chemotherapy (97), and in secondary cytoreduction in platinum-sensitive recurrent ovarian cancer patients (98). It is accepted that upper-abdominal spread of disease represents a major limit to achieve an optimal residual disease after primary cytoreduction (99). Extensive upper abdominal debulking surgery increases the rate of optimal cytoreduction and it is related with improved survival rates in advanced ovarian cancer undergoing primary cytoreduction and interval debulking surgery (100). Thus, hepatic resection(99), splenectomy [102] and [103], video-assisted thoracic surgery [104], and diaphragmatic resection [105], [106], [107], [108], [109], [110] and [111] have been advocated as components of radical primary cytoreduction . The aim of surgery in advanced or recurrent ovarian cancer patients should be the removal of any macroscopic intra-abdominal disease. It has been shown (94) that each decrease of 10% in residual tumor volume is followed by an increase of 5.5% in median survival in advanced ovarian cancer patients. The diaphragmatic implants can be resected with various surgical techniques, as ABC, peritonectomy or muscle resection. As previously suggested [112], [115]. The complete understanding of the upper abdominal anatomy and of the liver mobilization maneuvers are essential to allow exploration and radical debulking of the diaphragm, and minimizing the risk of major vessels injuries (retro-hepatic caval vein, supra-hepatic veins, diaphragmatic vessels) with severe haemorrhage. It has been reported that the most frequent complication is pleural effusion (42.5%) (114). It was observed, using multivariate analysis, that pleural effusion was statistically well predicted only by hepatic mobilization. Data from 2 reports [107], [113] showed that pulmonary complications represented the main morbidity of diaphragmatic surgery and suggest that the respiratory status of patients with diaphragmatic perforation should be carefully observed postoperatively. The insertion of intra-operative chest tube should be considered in patients undergoing complete liver mobilization and large diaphragmatic peritoneal or full thickness resection. Moreover, a strict early post-operative pulmonary follow-up should reduce the rate of chest complications. In metastatic ovarian carcinoma, involving the dome of the right hepatic lobe are encountered, and this requires radical full-thickness resection of a portion of the muscular diaphragm. Secondary cytoreductive surgery is an acceptable treatment paradigm for patients with platinum sensitive [progression-free survival (PFI) at least 6 to 12 months], recurrent ovarian cancer, who have a good performance status and can subsequently undergo platinum-based salvage chemotherapy [116]. Optimally resected patients have an 18 to 25 months survival advantage over those left with bulky disease ([117), (118] and completely resected patients have overall median survival in excess of 44 months [119], (120). Hepatic resection of recurrent ovarian and fallopian tube cancers has been reported by Yoon et al [119} with a series of 24 patients collected over 14-years in a single institution. Most (88%) were completely resected and the median survival was 62 months (range, 6 to 94). Fifty percent of patients also required diaphragm resection in this series [121]. Robotic-assisted major and minor hepatic resections have been described for management of benign and malignant liver lesions. It has been reported that conversion to laparotomy was low (5.7%), mean estimated blood loss 262 ml, mortality 0%, and morbidity 21.4% [122]. The majority of the malignant lesions were hepatobiliary primary or metastatic cancers, and only two cases required a partial diaphragm resection.

Port placement for this procedure requires careful preoperative planning based on the anatomic location of the hepatic lesion. The camera should be triangulated 11 cm from the operative table. The laparoscopic Habib 4X® can be useful for cauterization of surrounding parenchyma, especially for lesions deeper in the liver. Diaphragm resection performed by laparotomy results in a pneumothorax that can be evacuated using a red rubber tube and suction from a syringe applied just prior to tying the running suture, while the lung is temporarily hyperinflated. A study [121] reported on management and outcomes from 9 laparoscopic diaphragm injuries or resections accumulated over a 10-year experience. In all cases, a 14 Fr rubber catheter was introduced through a port and placed to water seal while the anesthesiologist hyperinflated the lungs, expelling excess $CO2$ from the chest cavity prior to tying the final diaphragm suture. Only one patient had a pneumothorax on postextubation chest X-ray and it resolved spontaneously. Based on their experience and, they recommended reserving chest tubes only for patients symptomatic with greater than 30% pneumothorax. In general, performance of hepatic and diaphragm resections for recurrent ovarian cancer can be associated with considerably extended patient survival when followed by platinum-based chemotherapy. This procedure is successfully performed with robotic-assisted laparoscopy. The technique involves, general anesthesia, the patient is placed in a supine position, and 5 trocars are used. Pneumoperitoneum to 12 mmHg is established. A 12-mm trocar for the robotic camera is placed above or below the umbilicus by the Hassen method. Three additional 8-mm trocars are placed at the left upper quadrant (LUQ) epigastric, and right upper quadrant (RUQ) areas under the laparoscopic guidance, respectively. A 12-mm trocar for an assistant was also placed at the LUQ area. Insertion sites of trocars are slightly different for each case because of additional procedures. The 4-arm da Vinci surgical robot system is brought into position and docked following port placement. The operator moved to the console to control the robotic arms. The assistant remained at the patient's left side to change robotic instruments and perform clipping, stapling, intraoperative ultrasonography, and choledochoscope through the 12-mm LUQ trocar site. 30° robotic camera was used. After exploration of the abdominal cavity, intraoperative ultrasonography is used to examine the remaining liver to search for undetectable lesions and obtain adequate surgical resection margins, and hepatic resection is performed.

A closed suction drain catheter is placed in the subhepatic space. The specimen was placed in an endoscopic retrieval bag and removed through a left subcostal mini-laparotomy incision extending from the port site.

Robotic surgery enables the operator to control the robotic system alone and to perform more precise and complex operations, and possibility of remote site surgery (123- 124). Robotic liver surgery provides access to fine structures of the liver and allows visualization of blood vessels and ducts. Three-dimensional vision offers the advantage of improved depth-perception and accuracy. Robotic surgery has several limitations: 1) high cost, 2) inadequate coverage by medical insurance, 3) lack of tactile sense, that can impair surgeons' capacity to make intuitive decisions, 4) lack of training systems, 5) heavy robotic arms and equipments, 6) time-consuming set up, and 7) difficulty in converting to open surgery. (125-126).

In addition, resected hepatic parenchymal metastasis in patients with primary epithelial ovarian carcinoma have favorable outlook with an actuarial 3 year cancer survival of 78% after resection. From surgical standpoint, the use of parenchymal -sparing segmental resections and decrease in the number of hepatic segments resected have substantial influence on decline in blood loss, the use of blood products and, hospital stay (3). Moreover, laparoscopic surgery or robotic assisted laparoscopic surgery is ideal for these cases. The same oncologic rules would apply, including "non -touch technique, RO radical resection and, the achievement of tumor-free surgical margin. Moreover, it was observe that overall morbidity, biliary leakage, transfusion rates, and mortality revealed no difference between the clamp crushing and other alternative transaction techniques (127), (128).

7. Minimally invasive Splenectomy in advanced ovarian cancer

To achieve optimal cytoreductive results in patients with advanced-stage ovarian cancer, splenectomy may be required when disease involves the hilum, capsule, or parenchyma of the spleen. In patients with extensive omental involvement extending into the splenic hilum, complete removal of the omentum can be safer, with less blood loss, if the spleen is removed en bloc with the omentum.

With the focus on attempting radical cytoreduction to less than 5 mm residual tumor, The frequency with which splenectomy is conducted has increased. The major associated complications of splenectomy include pleural effusions, pneumonia, thrombocytosis with thromboembolism, pancreatic injury, and postoperative sepsis.

The benefit of ultra- radical surgical cytoreduction in the management of ovarian cancer, with the goal of microscopic or minimal residual disease, has been established.

- The minimally invasive robotic surgical technique for splenectomy, involves placing the patient in an incomplete lateral right decubitus position with an anti-Trendelenbourg inclination of about 30°. A patient-side cart with robotic arms is positioned on the left side of the operating table. A 12 mm Hg pneumoperitoneum is created using an open technique and by inserting a Verses needle in the same point and the needle is then replaced with a 15 mm trocar. A 30° laparoscope is used in all cases. Three additional trocars are used. A lateral approach is used. At the start of the procedure the abdominal cavity is examined to detect any accessory spleens, which are identified and removed. The first step consists of the dissection of the inferior splenic pole and ligature of the lower polar vessels, followed by the dissection and ligature of the short gastric vessels. The second step is to approach the splenic pedicle next to the hilum; the ligature of hilar vessels is performed as far as possible from the pancreatic tail.
- This part of the procedure is more precise. The splenorenal ligaments are divided up to the splenodiaphragmal attachments. The splenic ligament dissection is performed using an ultrasonic device , and the hilar and short gastric vessels are dissected using an endovascular stapler. The surgical specimens are removed, laparoscopically, through an enlarged median supra or subumbilical incision using an endobag, and the drain is removed within 48 hours, to avoid the risk of postoperative infections.

  For optimal laparoscopic splenectomy, first, a gentle dissection to avoid incidental hemorrhages or parenchymal rupture due to traction on the spleen and cellular dissemination; second, accurate hemostasis and transection of the hilar vessels, and the identification and removal of accessory spleens that can cause the failure of the surgical procedure. For successful laparoscopic splenectomy, the semi lateral right decubitus position associated with a lateral approach to the splenic hilum reduces the risks of intraoperative bleeding, which is an important reason for conversion to laparotomy. Vaccination in the splenectomized is an important topic. *Streptococcus pneumonia* is the major pathogen in postsplenectomy sepsis, accounting for 50% to 90% of all infections (129). It has been observed that 31% of patients who had an overwhelming postsplenectomy infection (OPSI) had previously received the appropriate pneumococcal vaccine. OPSIs are rare but well-described, life-threatening events that can occur after splenectomy (131), (132). The incidence of postoperative infection has been estimated to be 3.2%, with a mortality rate of 1.3% (131). When an OPSI occurs, the mortality rate increases to 50% or higher (130). Aggressive early management of postoperative infection is critical to patient survival (129). The interval from the time of a splenectomy to an episode of OPSI varies, from 24 days to 65 years (130). The classic manifestation of OPSI is a brief episode of fever with mild nonspecific symptoms that rapidly evolve into overwhelming septic shock. It is important to initiate empiric broad-spectrum antibiotic therapy against *Serratia pneumonia, Haemophilus influenzae,* and

Neisseria meningitides, and await blood culture results. Preoperatively, patients should receive the pneumococcal vaccine (Pneumovax), *H influenzae* vaccine (if available), and meningococcal vaccinations approximately 10 to 14 days before surgery to maximize immunity (131). Patients who do not receive the vaccine preoperatively should receive the appropriate vaccinations in the immediate postoperative period.

Minor lacerations to the tail of the pancreas that do not involve the major ducts are managed with closed suction drainage. The splenic capsule should not be closed as there is no evidence that will decrease morbidity (132).

8. Minimally invasive colorectal surgery in patients with advanced ovarian cancer

Several studies have compared laparoscopic versus open rectal excision for rectal cancer (133). There were no difference in morbidity, rate of pelvic sepsis and mortality in both groups (134), (135). Histopathologic assessment of the rectal reflects the quality of resection in rectal cancer surgery. Both distal and circumferential resection margins are risk factors of recurrence after rectal excision. (136), (137). It has been shown that laparoscopic approach for rectal cancer is an oncologic safe procedure (138). The surgical technique for rectal metastatic involvement , secondary to advanced ovarian cancer is as follows: patients have a mechanic bowel preparation the day before the operation and prophylactic antibiotics are given at the time of surgery. High ligation of the inferior mesenteric artery and mobilization of the splenic flexure are performed. For upper third rectal tumors, a 5-cm mesorectal excision with end-to-end colorectal anastomosis is performed, for mid and low rectal tumors, TME with pouch supra-anal or anal anastomosis is performed, and abdominoperineal excision is performed when the levator muscle is invaded. Mesorectal excision includes complete removal of the mesorectum circumferentially with preservation of the hypogastric and pelvic plexuses. Extra facial anatomic dissection of the mesorectum is performed. The rectum is transected with a linear stapler, or transanally according to the level of the tumor. For very low tumors, intersphincteric resection is performed to achieve sphincter preservation with clear distal margin. The anastomosis is fashioned using a mechanical circular stapler. A colonic pouch is performed when feasible. A loop ileostomy is performed when the anastomosis is below 5 cm from the anal verge. Pelvic suction drain is inserted. In addition, the distal part of rectal dissection is performed by the perineal approach and a manual coloanal anastomosis is done. The goal of this minimally invasive procedure is to optimize obtaining distal and circumferential safe margins, and to decrease pitfalls due to a difficult laparoscopic low stapling.

Postoperative analgesia is ensured by intravenous morphine chloridrate (patient-controlled administration) at a maximum of 4 mg per hour with a single dose of 1 mg and free interval of 10 minutes for 1 to 2 days. Nasogastric tube is removed at the end of the surgical procedure, fluids intake on postoperative day 1, oral solid food at postoperative day 2 or 3, and bladder catheter removal on postoperative day 3.

The rectal specimen is examined in the operative room to assess distal resection margin, then addressed freshly to the pathologic department pinned on a cork board with moderate tension. The surface of the mesorectum is inked before slicing to assess the circumferential resection margin. Microscopic assessment included tumor infiltration through the bowel wall (pT), presence of positive lymph nodes, and distal and circumferential resection margins. The resection margin is considered as negative if >1 mm (R0) and positive if <=1 mm (R1).

9. Minimally invasive lower urinary tract surgery in invasive ovarian cancer

In patients with advanced or recurrent ovarian cancer, who have metastatic lower urinary tract involvement, robotic assisted laparoscopic surgery is beneficial. The advantage of using the robotic system is that it enables the surgeon to dissect deeply in the narrow pelvic floor. Also, it offers a better visualization with the binocular optics generating 3-D stereoscopic vision. The utilization of harmonic scalpel allows for control of the pelvic sidewall vessels and transaction of the ligaments attachments around the pelvic structures. The articulating wristed robotic instrument allows for fine sewing. Robotic surgery for advanced ovarian cancer can be achieved by rotating the operating table and relocking the robot at the patient's head. This position will allow dissection and removal of the paraaortic lymph nodes, resection of the upper abdominal metastases, and debulking of diaphragm and live involvement (139). It has been shown that robotic radical prostatectomy; provide a significant advantage in terms of its learning curve especially to surgeons with little or no advanced laparoscopic experience (140). It required only 12 cases to achieve proficiency in performing robotic assisted radical prostatectomy. Total cystectomy with urinary diversion remains the treatment of choice for organ -confined muscle invasive cancer of the urinary bladder. Gil et al. (141) reported laparoscopic radical cystectomy, bilateral lymphadenectomy, and ileal conduit diversion, with the entire procedure carried out by intracorporeal laparoscopic technique. There have been few case reports of laparoscopic anterior pelvic exenteration (142), (143). It has been shown that the procedure is feasible and if combined with intracorporal urinary diversion. The overall morbidity and hospitalization considerably decreased. It is worth noting that, the goal of extensive surgery; anterior pelvic exenteration should always be resection of the tumor with tumor free margin. Farghaly (144) described the following Technique for urinary bladder invasion in advanced and recurrent ovarian cancer: Once the patient is anesthetized, she is placed in the low lithotomy position in yellowfin stirrups and her arms tucked at her side. After prepping and draping the patient, a standard V-care ® Uterine Manipulator (Conmed Endosurgery, Utica, NY) is placed and a foley catheter is inserted into the urinary bladder. A 3-cm incision is made at the umbilicus, a Gelport ® is inserted into the incision and trocars are introduced through the port with robotic instruments. The patient is then placed in the steep trendelenberg position and the da Vinci ® surgical system (Intitutive Surgical, Sunnyvale, CA) is docked between her legs. A 10-mm robotic 30 degree scope is used through the 10-mm port and robotic monopolar Hook and bipolar Maryland instruments are used through the triangulated robotic ports to perform the procedure. The assistant intermittently places an endoscopic suction device directly through the port. Ovarian cancer tumor and local metastases are debulked to less than 1cm in diameter. The round ligaments are ligated bilaterally, and retroperitoneal spaces are developed. The infundibulopelvic ligaments are skeletonized and transected. A bladder flap is developed, and the uterine arteries and their tributaries are skeletonized and ligated. Pelvic and para-aortic lymph nodes are dissected. The anatomical margins for the lymph node dissection were: medially the ureter, laterally the body of the psoas muscle and genitofemoral nerve, posteriorly, the obturator nerve, inferiorly, the deep circumflex iliac vein, and cephalic of the midportion of the common iliac artery. The superior limit of the para-aortic dissection is the inferior mesenteric artery. The bladder is dissected with its covering. Peritoneum in the cave of Retzius and ureters are clipped and cut. The vagina is cut with harmonic shears and this cut is extended anteriorly into the urethera and the entire specimen is disconnected. The paracolpos is cut with Ligasure till the levator ani muscle with endopelvic fascia is seen. The entire specimen; uterus, ovarian tumor tissues, fallopian tubes and all lymph nodes removed through the vagina by placing it in endocatch bag, and the vagina is packed to prevent carbon dioxide gas leak. The urinary resvoir is formed by dissecting the terminal ileum about 12 cm from the ileocecal valve and the large colon is dissected 15-20 cm distal to the hepatic flexure. The transection site of the large colon is performed before the middle colonic artery. The distal portion of the ileum is used for continent mechanism of the resvoir. The isolated bowel tract is washed using normal saline solution, ringer lactate and antiseptic proidone-iodine solution. The isolated bowel tract is then filled with 200 ml. of normal saline, and 6 teniamyotomies are performed. The tenia is sectioned across the whole width to the subumblical layer with, 6 cm between each teniamyotomy. The teniamyotomies are left open in order to increase the resvoir capacity of the pouch. The spatulated ureters are sutured together at the medial side of spatulation to create a trapezoidal plane which is anastomosed to the resvoir as the distal ileum is used as efferent segment of the pouch. The distal ileum is cannulated with 14 Fr catheter. The ileocecal valve is reinforced with 2/0 prolene suture. The tapered ileum is then brought to the anterior abdominal wall.

Pelvic drain is introduced through the 10mm port and ports were removed under vision. The vagina is closed by intracorporeal suturing with 2-0 vicryl and by taking continuous interlocking sutures. The fascia is closed using 0 vicryl suture and the skin is closed with running 4-0 monocryl subcuticular stitch. Estimated operative time 4.6 hours, and average blood loss 210 ml. The pelvic drain is kept for 24-48 hours depending on the drainage. Hospital stay is about 5 days.

This technique offers benefits such as improved surgeon dexterity, enhanced ergonomics and 3-D optics. The utilization of ileal conduit formation for urinary diversion is technically feasible with good result. Also, it is safe, cost effective, with acceptable operative, pathological and short and long term clinical outcome. It retains the advantage of minimally invasive surgery

10. Minimally invasive Surgery for small bowel involvement in patients with ovarian cancer

Cytoreductive surgery and hyperthermic intraperitoneal chemotherapy have an important role in the management of patients with peritoneal surface and small bowel involvement in patients with advanced stage ovarian cancer. The patterns of intraceolomic dissemination, combined with loco-regional cancer therapies directed at small microscopic residual disease constitute the basis of this therapy. Heat and intraperitoneal chemotherapy given at the time of surgery after a cytoreduction of the peritoneal tumors has resulted in a significant improvement of quality and a prolongation of life in selected patients. The robot -assisted laparoscopic or laparoscopic technique involves greater omentectomy. The greater omentum is mobilized off the transverse colon and its hepatic and splenic flexures are excised using the Harmonic scalpel (Ethicon Inc, Guaynabo, Puerto Rico). The gastrosplenic ligament is transected close to the splenic hilum. Bowel resections are performed with an Endo GIA 3.5/60 mm cartridge (US Surgical, Norwalk, Connecticut). The bowel mesentery is transected with the Harmonic scalpel (Ethicon Inc, Guaynabo, Puerto Rico). At the end of the laparoscopic stage of the procedure, a 5 cm periumbilical midline laparotomy is performed and the specimens are extracted. Two inflow and 2 outflow perfusion catheters are placed and the skin at the laparotomy and port sites is closed with a running Nylon stitch. Hyperthermic intraperitoneal chemotherapy with cisplatin and adriamycin or mitomycin C for 90 minutes at 43°C is administered using Thermasolutions (Thermasolutions Inc, Pittsburgh, Pennsylvania) perfusion system. At the completion of the heated perfusion, gastrointestinal anastomosis is performed.

11. References

[1] S.M. Eisenkop and N.M. Spirtos, What are the current surgical objectives, strategies, and technical capabilities of gynecologic oncologists treating advanced epithelial ovarian cancer. Gynecol. Oncol. 82 (2001), pp. 489–497.

[2] O. Zivanovic, E.L. Eisenhauer, Q. Zhou, A. Iasonos, P. Sabbatini and Y. Sonoda et al., The impact of bulky upper abdominal disease cephalad to the greater omentum on surgical outcome for stage IIIC epithelial ovarian, fallopian tube, and primary peritoneal cancer, Gynecol. Oncol. 108 (2008), pp. 287–292.

[3] Jemal A, Siegel R, Ward E, et al. Cancer statistics, 2006. CA Cancer J Clin 2006; 56:106–30.

[4] Young RC, Decker DG, Wharton JT, et al. Staging laparotomy in early ovarian cancer. JAMA 1983; 250:3072–6.

[5] Stier EA, Barakat RR, Curtin JP, et al. Laparotomy to complete staging of presumed early ovarian cancer. Obstet Gynecol 1996; 87:737–40.

[6] Staging announcement. FIGO cancer committee. Gyencol Oncol 1986; 50:383–5.

[7] R.E. Bristow, R.S. Tomacruz, D.K. Armstrong, E.L. Trimble and F.J. Monts, Survival effect of maximal cytoreductive surgery for advanced ovarian carcinoma during the platinum era: a meta-analysis, J. Clin. Oncol. 20 (2002), pp. 1248–1259.

[8] G.D. Aletti, 8. S.C. Dowdy, B.S. Gostout, M.B. Jones, C.R. Stanhope and T.O. Wilson et al., Aggressive surgical effort and improved survival in advanced-stage ovarian cancer, Obstet. Gynecol. 107 (2006), pp. 77–85.

[9] S.M. Eisenkop and N.M. Spirtos, Procedures required to accomplish complete cytoreduction of ovarian cancer: is there a correlation with "biological aggressiveness" and survival, Gynecol. Oncol. 82 (2001), pp. 435–441

[10] F. Fanfani, G. Ferrandina, G. Corrado, A. Fagotti, H.V. Zakut and S. Mancuso et al., Impact of interval debulking surgery on clinical outcome in primary unresectable FIGO stage IIIc ovarian cancer patients, Oncology 65 (2003), pp. 316–322.

[11] R. Salani, A. Santillan, M.L. Zahurak, R.L. Giuntoli II, G.J. Gardner and D.K. Armstrong et al., Secondary cytoreductive surgery for localized, recurrent epithelial ovarian cancer: analysis of prognostic factors and survival outcome, Cancer 109 (2007), pp. 685–691.

[12] G.D. Aletti, S.C. Dowdy, K.C. Podratz and W.A. Cliby, Surgical treatment of diaphragm disease correlates with improved survival in optimally debulked advanced stage ovarian cancer, Gynecol. Oncol. 100 (2006), pp. 283–287.

[13] M.A. Merideth, W.A. Cliby, G.L. Keeney, T.G. Lesnick, D.M. Nagorney and K.C. Podratz, Hepatic resection for metachronous metastases from ovarian carcinoma, Gynecol. Oncol. 89 (2003), pp. 16–21

[14] S.M. Eisenkop, N.M. Spirtos and W.C. Lin, Splenectomy in the context of primary cytoreductive operations for advanced epithelial ovarian cancer, Gynecol. Oncol. 100 (2006), pp. 344–348

[15] P.M. Magtibay, P.B. Adams, M.B. Silverman, S.S. Cha and K.C. Podratz, Splenectomy as part of cytoreductive surgery in ovarian cancer, Gynecol. Oncol. 102 (2006), pp. 369–374

[16] M.M. Juretzka, N.R. Abu-Rustum, Y. Sonoda, R.J. Downey, R.M. Flores and B.J. Park et al., The impact of video-assisted thoracic surgery (VATS) in patients with suspected advanced ovarian malignancies and pleural effusion, Gynecol. Oncol. 104 (2007), pp. 670–674.

[17] F.J. Montz, J.B. Schlaerth and J.S. Berek, Resection of diaphragmatic peritoneum and muscle: role in cytoreductive surgery for ovarian cancer, Gynecol. Oncol. 35 (1989), pp. 338–340

[18] S.J. Kapnick, C.T. Griffiths and N.J. Finkler, Occult pleural involvement in stage III ovarian carcinoma: role of diaphragmatic resection, Gynecol. Oncol. 39 (1990), pp. 135–138

[19] W. Cliby, S. Dowdy, S.S. Feitoza, B.S. Gostout and K.C. Podratz, Diaphragm resection for ovarian cancer: technique and short-term complications, Gynecol. Oncol. 94 (2004), pp. 655–660

[20] Ghezzi F, Cromi A, Uccella S, et al. Laparoscopy versus laparotomy for the surgical management of apparent early stage ovarian cancer. Gynecol Oncol. 2007; 105(2):409-413.

[21] Chi DS, Abu-Rustum NR, Sonoda Y, et al. The safety and efficacy of laparoscopic surgical staging of apparent stage I ovarian and fallopian tube cancers. Am J Obstet Gynecol. 2005;192(5):1614-1619.

[22] Park JY, Kim DY, Suh DS, et al. Comparison of laparoscopy and laparotomy in surgical staging of early-stage ovarian and fallopian tubal cancer. Ann Surg Oncol. 2008;15(7):2012-2019.

[23] Nezhat FR, Ezzati M, Chuang L, et al. Laparoscopic management of early ovarian and fallopian tube cancers: surgical and survival outcome. Am J Obstet Gynecol. 2009;200(1):83.e1-6.

[24] Tozzi R, Köhler C, Ferrara A, et al. Laparoscopic treatment of early ovarian cancer: surgical and survival outcomes. Gynecol Oncol. 2004;93(1): 199-203.

[25] Angioli R, Palaia I, Zullo MA, et al. Diagnostic open laparoscopy in the management of advanced ovarian cancer. Gynecol Oncol. 2006;100(3): 455-461.

[26] Childers JM, Lang J, Surwit EA, et al. Laparoscopic surgical staging of ovarian cancer. Gynecol Oncol. 1995;59(1):25-33.

[27] Ramirez PT, Wolf JK, Levenback C. Laparoscopic port-site metastases: etiology and prevention. Gynecol Oncol. 2003;91(1):179-189.

[28] Havrilesky LJ, Peterson BL, Dryden DK, et al. Predictors of clinical outcomes in the laparoscopic management of adnexal masses. Obstet Gynecol. 2003; 102(2):243-251.

[29] Canis M, Botchorishvili R, Manhes H, et al. Management of adnexal masses: role and risk of laparoscopy. Semin Surg Oncol. 2000; 19(1):28-35.

[30] Bakkum-Gamez JN, Richardson DL, Seamon LG, et al. Influence of intraoperative capsule rupture on outcomes in stage I epithelial ovarian cancer. Obstet Gynecol. 2009;113(1):11-17.

[31] Vergote I, De Brabanter J, Fyles A, et al. Prognostic importance of degree of differentiation and cyst rupture in stage I invasive epithelial ovarian carcinoma. Lancet. 2001;357(9251):176-182.

[32] Abu-Rustum N; Gemigani M, Moore K et al. Total laparoscopic radical hysterectomy with lymphadenectomy using the argon-beam coagulator: pilot data and comparison to laparotomy. Gynecol Oncol 2003; 91; P. 402-9
[33] Magrina J, Mutone N, Weaver A et al. Laparoscopic lymphadenectomy and vaginal or laparoscopic hysterectomy with bilateral salpingo-ophrectomy for endometrial cancer: morbidity and survival. Am J Obstet Gynecol 1999; 181; P. 376-81
[34] Kim YT, Kim SW, Hyung WJ et al. Robotic radical hysterectomy with Pelvic lymphadenectomy for cervical carcinoma: a pilot study. Gynecolo Oncol 2008; 108 (2):312-16
[35] Sert B, and Abeler V. Robotic radical hysterectomy in early -stage cervical carcinoma patients, comparing results with total laparoscopic radical hysterectomy cases; the future is now. Int J Med Robot 2007; 3; P.224-28
[36] Fanning J, Fenton B, Purohit M. Robotic radical hysterectomy . Am J Obstet Gynec ;2008; 198; P.1-4
[37] R. Angioli, I. Palaia, M.A. Zullo, L. Muzii, N. Manci and M. Calcagno et al., Diagnostic open laparoscopy in the management of advanced ovarian cancer, Gynecol. Oncol. 100 (2006), pp. 455–461.
[38] X. Deffieux, D. castaigne and C. Pomel, Role of laparoscopy to evaluate candidates for complete cytoreduction in advanced stages of epithelial ovarian cancer, Int. J. Gynecol. Cancer 16 (suppl. 1) (2006), pp. 35–40.
[39] A. Fagotti, F. Fanfani, M. Ludovisi, R. Lo Voi, G. Bifulco and A.C. Testa et al., Role of laparoscopy to assess the chance of optimal cytoreductive surgery in advanced ovarian cancer patients: a pilot study, Gynecol. Oncol. 96 (2005), pp. 729–735.
[40] Vazzielli and V. Carone et al., Prospective validation of a laparoscopic predictive model for optimal cytoreduction in advanced ovarian carcinoma, Am. J. Obstet. Gynecol. 199 (6) (2008), pp. 642.e1–642.e6.
[41] A. Fagotti, F. Fanfani, C. Rossitto, D. Lorusso, A.M. De Gaetano and A. Giordano et al., A treatment selection protocol for recurrent ovarian cancer patients: the role of FDG-PET/CT and staging laparoscopy, Oncology 75 (3-4) (2008), pp. 152–158.
[42] A. Fagotti, G. Ferrandina, F. 42. Fanfani, A. Ercoli, D. Lorusso and M. Rossi et al., A laparoscopy-based score to predict surgical outcome in patients with advanced ovarian carcinoma: a pilot study, Ann. Surg. Oncol. 13 (2006), pp. 1156–1161.
[43] Brun, R. Rouzier, S. Uzan and E. Darai, External validation of a laparoscopic-based score to evaluate respectability of advanced ovarian cancers: clues for a simplified score, Gynecol. Oncol. 110 (2008), pp. 354–359.
[44] Ozols RF, Rubin SC, Thomas G, Robboy S: Epithelial Ovarian Cancer. In Hoskins WJ, Perez CA, Young RC (eds): Principles and Practice of Gynecologic Oncology, 2nd ed. Philadelphia, Lippincott–Raven, 1997, pp 919–986
[45] Cain JM, Saigo PE, Pierce VK, Clark DG, Jones WB, Smith DH, Hakes TB, Ochoa M, Lewis JL Jr: A review of second-look laparotomy for ovarian cancer. Gynecol Oncol 23:14 -25, 1986
[46] Ozols RF, Bundy BN, Fowler J, et al.: Randomized phase III study of cisplatin (CIS)/paclitaxel (PAC) versus carboplatin (CARBO/PAC) in optimal stage III epithelial ovarian cancer (OC): a Gynecologic Oncology Group trial (GOG 158). Proc Am Soc Clin Oncol 18:356a, 1999 (Abstract 1373)

[47] Rubin SC, Hoskins WJ, Hakes TB, Markman M, Cain JM, Lewis JL Jr: Recurrence after negative second-look laparotomy for ovarian cancer: analysis of risk factors. Am J Obstet Gynecol 159:1094 -1098, 1988

[48] Rubin SC, Hoskins WJ, Saigo PE, Chapman D, Hakes TB, Markman M, Reichman B, Almadrones L, Lewis JL Jr: Prognostic factors for recurrence following negative second-look laparotomy in ovarian cancer patients

[49] Rubin SC, Randall TC, Armstrong KA, Chi DS, Hoskins WJ: Ten year follow-up of ovarian cancer patients after second-look laparotomy with negative findings. Obstet Gynecol 93:21–24, 1999

[50] Nicoletto MO, Tumolo S, Talamini R, Salvagno L, Franceschi S, Visona E, Marin G, Angelini F, Brigato G, Scarabelli C, Carbone A, Cecchetto A, Prosperi A, Rosabian A, Giusto M, Cima GP, Morassut S, Nascimben O, Vinante O, Fiorentino MV: Surgical second look in ovarian cancer: arandomized study in patients with laparoscopic complete remission—a Northeastern Oncology Cooperative Group–Ovarian Cancer Cooperative Group Study. J Clin Oncol 15(3):994 -999, 1997

[51] Quinn MA, Bishop GJ, Campbell JJ, Rodgerson J, Pepperell RJ: Laparoscopic follow-up of patients with ovarian cancer. Br J Obstet Gynaecol 87:1132–1139, 1980

[52] Ozols RF, Fisher RI, Anderson T, Makuch R, Young RC: Peritoneoscopy in the management of ovarian cancer. Am J Obstet Gynecol 140:611- 619, 1981

[53] Berek JS, Griffiths CT, Leventhal JM: Laparoscopy for second-look evaluation in ovarian cancer. Obstet Gynecol 58:192–198, 1981

[54] Gadducci A, Sartori E, Maggino T, Zola P, Landoni F, Fanucchi A, Palai N, Alessi C, Ferrero AM, Cosio S, Cristofani R: Analysis of failures after negative second look in patients with advanced ovarian cancer: an Italian multicenter study. Gynecol Oncol 68:150 -155, 1998

[55] Casey AC, Farias-Eisner R, Pisani AL, Cirisano FD, Kim YB, Muderspach L, Futoran R, Leuchter RS, Lagasse LD, Karlan BY: What is the role of reassessment laparoscopy of gynecologic cancers in 1995? Gynecol Oncol 60:454–461, 1996

[56] Abu-Rustum NR, Barakat RR, Siegel PL, Venkatraman E, Curtin JP, Hoskins WJ: Second-look operation for epithelial ovarian cancer: Laparoscopy or laparotomy? Obstet Gynecol 88:549 -553, 1996

[57] Copeland LJ, Gershenson DM, Wharton JT, Atkinson EN, Sneige N, Edwards CL, Rutledge FN: Microscopic disease at second-look laparotomy in advanced ovarian cancer. Cancer 55:472- 478, 1985

[58] Hoskins WJ, Rubin SC, Dulaney E, Chapman D, Almadrones L, Saigo P, Markman M, Hakes T, Reichman B, Jones WB, et al.: Influence of cytoreductive surgery at the time of second-look laparotomy on the survival of patients with epithelial ovarian cancer. Gynecol Oncol 34:365–371, 1989

[59] Lippman SM, Alberts DS, Slymen DJ, Weiner S, Aristizabal SA, Luditch A, Davis JR, Surwit EA: Second-look laparotomy in epithelial ovarian carcinoma. Prognostic factors associated with survival duration. Cancer 61(12):2571–2577, 1988.

[60] Williams L, Brunetto VL, Yordan E, DiSaia PJ, Creasman WT: Secondary cytoreductive surgery at second-look laparotomy in advanced ovarian cancer: a Gynecologic Oncology Group Study. Gynecol Oncol 66(2):171–178, 1997

[61] Barakat RR, Almadrones L, Venkatraman ES, Aghajanian C, Brown C, Shapiro F, Curtin JP, Spriggs D: A phase II trial of intraperitoneal cisplatin and etoposide as

consolidation therapy in patients with Stage II-IV epithelial ovarian cancer following negative surgical assessment. Gynecol Oncol 69:17-22, 1988

[62] Markman M, Reichman B, Hakes T, Lewis JL Jr, Jones W, Rubin S, Barakat R, Curtin J, Almadrones L, Hoskins W: Impact on survival of surgically defined favorable responses to salvage intraperitoneal chemotherapy in small-volume residual ovarian cancer. J Clin Oncol 10:1479-1484, 1992

[63] Barter J, Barnes WA: Second Look Laparotomy, in Rubin SC, Sutton SP (eds.): Ovarian Cancer, New York, McGraw-Hill, 1993

[64] Abu-Rustum NR, Barakat RR, Siegel PL, Venkatraman E, Curtin JP, Hoskins WJ. Second-look operation for epithelial ovarian cancer: laparoscopy or laparotomy? Obstet Gynecol. 1996;884:549-53.

[65] Husain A, Chi DS, Prasad M, Abu-Rustumz N, Barakat RR, Brown CL, et al. The role of laparoscopy in second-look evaluations for ovarian cancer. Gynecol Oncol. 2001;80:44-7.

[66] Clough K, Ladonne JM, Nos C, Renolleau C, Validire P, Durand JC. Second look for ovarian cancer: laparoscopy or laparotomy? A prospective comparative study. Gynecol Oncol. 1999;72:411-17.

[67] Berek JS, Griffith CT, Leventhal JM. Laparoscopy for second-look evaluation in ovarian cancer. Obstet Gynecol. 1981; 58:192-8.

[68] Lele S, Piver MS. Interval laparoscopy prior to second-look laparotomy in ovarian cancer. Obstet Gynecol. 1986;68: 345-9.

[69] Fanning J, Fenton B, Purohit M. Robotic radical hysterectomy. Am J Obstet Gynecol. 2008;198:649-650.

[70] Russo A, Cirelli G, Cassese E, Delli Ponti D, Sgambata R, Cecere F, et al. Second-look in ovarian cancer: laparoscopy or laparotomy? Minerva Ginecol. 2001;53: 146-54.

[71] Husain A, Chi DS, Prasad M, Abu-Rustum N, Barakat RR, Brown CL, et al. The role of laparoscopy in second-look evaluations for ovarian cancer. Gynecol Oncol. 2001;80: 44-7.

[72] Fanning J, Fenton B, Switzer M, Johnson J, Clemons J. Laparoscopically assisted vaginal hysterectomy for uteri weighing 1,000g or more. JSLS. 2008;12:376-379. [

[73] Fanning J, Trinh H. Feasibility of laparoscopic ovarian debulking at recurrence in patients with prior laparotomy debulking. Am J Obstet Gynecol. 2004;190:1394-1397. [PubMed]

[74] Johnson N, Barlow D, Lethaby A, Tavender E, Curr E, Garry R. Surgical approach to hysterectomy for benign gynaecological disease. Cochrane Database Syst Rev. 2005;1:DC003677.

[75] Curtin, R. Malik, E.S. Venkatraman, R.R. Barakat and W.J. Hoskins, Stage IV ovarian cancer: impact of surgical debulking, Gynecol. Oncol. 64 (1) (1997), pp. 9-12.

[76] g, Z.Y. Zhang and S.M. Cai et al., Cytoreductive surgery for stage IV epithelial ovarian cancer, J. Exp. Clin. Cancer Res. 18 (4) (1999), pp. 449-454.

[77] P.C. Liu, I. Benjamin and M.A. Morgan et al., Effect of surgical debulking on survival in stage IV ovarian cancer, Gynecol. Oncol. 64 (1) (1997), pp. 4-8.

[78] R.E. Bristow, F.J. Montz, L.D. Lagasse, R.S. Leuchter and B.Y. Karlan, Survival impact of surgical cytoreduction in stage IV epithelial ovarian cancer, Gynecol. Oncol. 72 (3) (1999), pp. 278-287

[79] R. Eitan, D.A Levine and N. Abu-Rustum et al., The clinical significance of malignant pleural effusions in patients with optimally debulked ovarian carcinoma, Cancer 103 (7) (2005), pp. 1397–1401

[80] D.S. Chi, C.C. Franklin and D.A. Levine et al., Improved optimal cytoreduction rates for stages IIIC and IV epithelial ovarian, fallopian tube, and primary peritoneal cancer: a change in surgical approach, Gynecol. Oncol. 94 (3) (2004), pp. 650–654.

[81] S.M. Eisenkop, R.L. Friedman and H.J. Wang, Complete cytoreductive surgery is feasible and maximizes survival in patients with advanced epithelial ovarian cancer: a prospective study, Gynecol. Oncol. 69 (2) (1998), pp. 103–108.

[82] G.D. Aletti, S.C. Dowdy, K.C. Podratz and W.A. Cliby, Surgical treatment of diaphragm disease correlates with improved survival in optimally debulked advanced stage ovarian cancer, Gynecol. Oncol. 100 (2) (2006), pp. 283–287.

[83] D.F. Silver, Full-thickness diaphragmatic resection with simple and secure closure to accomplish complete cytoreductive surgery for patients with ovarian cancer, Gynecol. Oncol. 95 (2) (2004), pp. 384–387

[84] Chi DS, Abu-Rustum NR, Sonoda Yet al. The benefit of video-assisted thoracoscopic surgery before planned abdominal exploration in patients with suspected advanced ovarian cancer and moderate to large pleural effusions. Gynecol Oncol. 2004;94:307-311

[85] S.M. Eisenkop, Thoracoscopy for the management of advanced epithelial ovarian cancer–a preliminary report, Gynecol. Oncol. 84 (2) (2002), pp. 315–320

[86] Kapnick SJ, Griffiths CT, Finkler NJ. Occult pleural involvement in stage III ovarian carcinoma: role of diaphragm resection. Gynecol Oncol. 1990;39:135-138.

[87] Eitan R, Levine DA, Abu-Rustum Net al. The clinical significance of malignant pleural effusions in patients with optimally debulked ovarian carcinoma. Cancer. 2005;103:1397-1401.

[88] Bristow RE, Tomacruz RS, Armstrong DKet al. Survival effect of maximal cytoreductive surgery for advanced ovarian carcinoma during the platinum era: a meta-analysis. J Clin Oncol. 2002;20:1248-1259.

[89] Munkarah AR, Hallum AV 3rd, Morris Met al. Prognostic significance of residual disease in patients with stage IV epithelial ovarian cancer. Gynecol Oncol. 1997;64:13-17.

[90] Blanchard P, Plantade A, Pagés C, Afchain P, Louvet C, Tournigand C, de Gramont A. Isolated lymph node relapse of epithelial ovarian carcinoma: Outcomes and prognostic factors. Gynecol Oncol. 2007;104:41–5.

[91] Lim MC, Lee HS, Jung DC, Choi JY, Seo SS, Park SY. Pathological diagnosis and cytoreduction of cardiophrenic lymph node and pleural metastasis in ovarian cancer patients using video-assisted thoracic surgery. Ann Surg Oncol. 2009;16:1990–6.

[92] Uzan C, Morice P, Rey A, Pautier P, Camatte S, Lhommè C, Haie-Meder C, Duvillard P, Castaigne D. Outcomes after combined therapy including surgical resection in patients with epithelial ovarian cancer recurrence(s) exclusively in lymph nodes. Ann Surg Oncol. 2004;11(7):658–64

[93] O. Zivanovic, E.L. Eisenhauer, Q. Zhou, A. Iasonos, P. Sabbatini and Y. Sonoda et al., The impact of bulky upper abdominal disease cephalad to the greater omentum on

surgical out come for stage IIIC epithelial ovarian, fallopian tube, and primary peritoneal cancer, Gynecol. Oncol. 108 (2008), pp. 287-292

[94] R.E. Bristow, R.S. Tomacruz, D.K. Armstrong, E.L. Trimble and F.J. Monts, Survival effect of maximal cytoreductive surgery for advanced ovarian carcinoma during the platinum era: a meta-analysis, J. Clin. Oncol. 20 (2002), pp. 1248-1259

[95] G.D. Aletti, S.C. Dowdy, B.S. Gostout, M.B. Jones, C.R. Stanhope and T.O. Wilson et al., Aggressive surgical effort and improved survival in advanced-stage ovarian cancer, Obstet. Gynecol. 107 (2006), pp. 77-85.

[96] S.M. Eisenkop and N.M. Spirtos, Procedures required to accomplish complete cytoreduction of ovarian cancer: is there a correlation with "biological aggressiveness" and survival, Gynecol. Oncol. 82 (2001), pp. 435-441

[97] F. Fanfani, G. Ferrandina, G. Corrado, A. Fagotti, H.V. Zakut and S. Mancuso et al., Impact of interval debulking surgery on clinical outcome in primary unresectable FIGO stage IIIc ovarian cancer patients, Oncology 65 (2003), pp. 316-322.

[98] R. Salani, A. Santillan, M.L. Zahurak, R.L. Giuntoli II, G.J. Gardner and D.K. Armstrong et al., Secondary cytoreductive surgery for localized, recurrent epithelial ovarian cancer: analysis of prognostic factors and survival outcome, Cancer 109 (2007), pp. 685-691

[99] S.M. Eisenkop and N.M. Spirtos, What are the current surgical objectives, strategies, and technical capabilities of gynecologic oncologists treating advanced epithelial ovarian cancer?, Gynecol. Oncol. 82 (2001), pp. 489-497.

[100] G.D. Aletti, S.C. Dowdy, K.C. Podratz and W.A. Cliby, Surgical treatment of diaphragm disease correlates with improved survival in optimally debulked advanced stage ovarian cancer, Gynecol. Oncol. 100 (2006), pp. 283-287.

[101] M.A. Merideth, W.A. Cliby, G.L. Keeney, T.G. Lesnick, D.M. Nagorney and K.C. Podratz, Hepatic resection for metachronous metastases from ovarian carcinoma, Gynecol. Oncol. 89 (2003), pp. 16-21[105] S.M.

[102] Eisenkop, N.M. Spirtos and W.C. Lin, Splenectomy in the context of primary cytoreductive operations for advanced epithelial ovarian cancer, Gynecol. Oncol. 100 (2006), pp. 344-348.

[103] P.M. Magtibay, P.B. Adams, M.B. Silverman, S.S. Cha and K.C. Podratz, Splenectomy as part of cytoreductive surgery in ovarian cancer, Gynecol. Oncol. 102 (2006), pp. 369-374

[104] M.M. Juretzka, N.R. Abu-Rustum, Y. Sonoda, R.J. Downey, R.M. Flores and B.J. Park et al., The impact of video-assisted thoracic surgery (VATS) in patients with suspected advanced ovarian malignancies and pleural effusion, Gynecol. Oncol. 104 (2007), pp. 670-674

[105] F.J. Montz, J.B. Schlaerth and J.S. Berek, Resection of diaphragmatic peritoneum and muscle: role in cytoreductive surgery for ovarian cancer, Gynecol. Oncol. 35 (1989), pp. 338-340

[106] S.J. Kapnick, C.T. Griffiths and N.J. Finkler, Occult pleural involvement in stage III ovarian carcinoma: role of diaphragmatic resection, Gynecol. Oncol. 39 (1990), pp. 135-138.

[107] S. Dowdy, S.S. Feitoza, B.S. Gostout and K.C. Podratz, Diaphragm resection for ovarian cancer: technique and short-term complications, Gynecol. Oncol. 94 (2004), pp. 655-660.

[108] E.L. Eisenhauer, M.I. D'Angelica, N.R. Abu-Rustum, Y. Sonoda, W.R. Jarnagin and R.R. Barakat et al., Incidence and management of pleural effusion after diaphragm peritonectomy or resection for advancer Mullerian cancer, Gynecol. Oncol. 103 (2006), pp. 871–877.
[109] G.D. Aletti, S.C. Dowdy, K.C. Podratz and W.A. Cliby, Surgical treatment of diaphragm disease correlates with improved survival in optimally debulked advanced stage ovarian cancer, Gynecol. Oncol. 100 (2006), pp. 283–287.
[110] K. Devolder, F. Amant, P. Neven, T. van Gorp, K. Leunen and I. Vergote, Role of diaphragmatic surgery in 69 patients with ovarian cancer, Int. J. Gynecol. Cancer. 18 (2008), pp. 363–368.
[111] P.E. Colombo, A. Mourregot, M. Fabbro, M. Gutowski, B. Saint-Aubert and F. Quenet et al., Aggressive surgical strategies in advanced ovarian cancer: a monocentric study of 203 stage IIIC and IV patients, Eur. J. Surg. Oncol. 35 (2009), pp. 135–143.
[112] G. Deppe, V.K. Malviya, G. Boike and A. Hampton, Surgical approach to diaphragmatic metastases from ovarian cancer, Gynecol. Oncol. 24 (1986), pp. 258–260
[113] S.M. Kehoe, E.L. Eisenhauer and D.S. Chi, Upper abdominal surgical procedures: liver mobilization and diaphragm peritonectomy/resection, splenectomy, and distal pancreatectomy, Gynecol. Oncol. 111 (2008), pp. S51–S55.
[114] S.C. Dowdy, R.T. Loewen, G. Aletti, S.S. Feitoza and W. Cliby, Assessment of outcomes and morbidity following diaphragmatic peritonectomy for women with ovarian carcinoma, Gynecol. Oncol. 109 (2008), pp. 303–307
[115] E. Chereau, M. Ballester, F. Selle, A. Cortez, C. Pomel and E. Darai et al., Pulmonary morbidity of diaphragmatic surgery for stage III/IV ovarian cancer, BJOG 116 (2009), pp. 1062–1068.
[116] Janicke F, Holscher M, Kuhn W, von Hugo R, Pache L, Siewert JR, Graeff H. Radical surgical procedure improves survival time in patients with recurrent ovarian cancer. Cancer 1992;70:2129–36.
[117] Gadducci A, Iacconi P, Cosio S, Fanucci A, Cristofani R, Genazzani AR. Complete salvage surgical cytoreduction improves further survival of patients with late recurrent ovarian cancer. Gynecol Oncol 2000;79:344–9.
[118] Eisenkop SM, Friedman RL, Spirtos NM. The role of secondary cytoreductive surgery in the treatment of patients with recurrent epithelial ovarian carcinoma. Cancer 2000;88:144–53.
[119] Yoon SS, Jarnagin WR, Fong Y, DeMatteo RP, Barakat RR, Blumgart LH, Chi DS. Resection of recurrent ovarian or fallopian tube carcinoma involving the liver. Gynecol Oncol 2003;91:383–8.
[120] Giulianotti PC, Coratti A, Sbrana F, Addeo P, Bianco FM, Busch NC, Annechiarico M, Benedetti E. Robotic liver surgery: Results for 70 resections. Surgery 2011;149: 29–39.
[121] Idrees K, Bartlett DL. Robotic liver Surgery. Surg Clin N Am 2010;90:761–74.
[122] Aron M, Colombo Jr JR, Turna B, Stein RJ, Haber G-P, Gill IS. Diaphragmatic repair and/or reconstruction during upper abdominal urologic laparoscopy. J Urol 2007;178:2444–50.
[123] Vidovszky TJ, Smith W, Ghosh J, Ali MR. Robotic cholecystectomy: learning curve, advantages, and limitations. J Surg Res. 2006;136:172–178.

[124] Hashizume M, Tsugawa K. Robotic surgery and cancer: the present state, problems and future vision. Jpn J Clin Oncol. 2004;34:227–237
[125] D'Annibale A, Morpurgo E, Fiscon V, Trevisan P, Sovernigo G, Orsini C, et al. Robotic and laparoscopic surgery for treatment of colorectal disease. Dis Colon Rectum. 2004;47:2162–2168.
[126] Nguyen MM, Das S. The evolution of robotic urologic surgery. Urol Clin North Am. 2004;31:653–658. vii
[127] Jarngin WR, Gonenm, Fong Y et al. Improvement in perioperative outcome after hepatic resection: Analysis of 1803 consecutive cases over the past decade. Ann Surg 2002, 236 (4), P. 397-407
[128] Rahbari NN, Koch M, Schmidt T et al. Meta-analysis of the clamp-crushing technique for transaction of the parenchyma in elective hepatic resection: back to where we started. Ann Surg Oncol 2009, 16 (3), 630-9
[129] Farghaly SA. Observation on the surgical aspect of resection of Noncolorectal Vonneuroendocrine Hepatic Parenchymal Metastasis in Patients with Primary Epithelial Ovarian Carcinoma. Gynecol Oncol 2009,;115 (2): 319
[130] G.D. Aletti, S.C. Dowdy, B.S. Gostout, M.B. Jones, C.R. Stanhope and T.O. Wilson et al., Aggressive surgical effort and improved survival in advanced-stage ovarian cancer, Obstet Gynecol 107 (2006), pp. 77–85.
[131] A.M. Lynch and R. Kapila, Overwhelming postsplenectomy infection, Infect Dis Clin North Am 10 (1996), pp. 693–707141..
[132] Gelmini R, Romano F, Quaranta N, Caprotti R, Tazzioli G, Colombo G, Saviano M, Uggeri F. Suturless and stapless laparoscopic splenectomy using radiofrequency: Ligasure device. Surg Endosc 2006;20:991–994.–986.
[133] W. Krivit, Overwhelming postsplenectomy infection, Am J Hematol 2 (1977), pp. 193–201.
[134] E.C. Ellison and P.J. Fabri, Complications of splenectomy. Etiology, prevention, and management, Surg Clin North Am 63 (1983), pp. 1313–1330.
[135] Birbeck KF, Macklin CP, Tiffin NJ, et al. Rates of circumferential resection margin involvement vary between surgeons and predict outcomes in rectal cancer surgery. Ann Surg. 2002;235:449–457
[136] Nagtegaal ID, Quirke P. What is the role for the circumferential margin in the modern treatment of rectal cancer? J Clin Oncol. 2008;26:303–312
[137] Braga M, Frasson M, Vignali A, et al. Laparoscopic resection in rectal cancer patients: outcome and cost-benefit analysis. Dis Colon Rectum. 2007;50:464–471.
[138] Bandera CA and Magrina F. Robotic surgery in Gynecologic Oncology. Obstet Gynecol 2009;1: 25-30
[139] Ahlering TE, Skarecky D, Lee D, Llayman RV. Successful transfer of open surgical skills to a laparoscopic environment using a robotic interface: initial experience with laparoscopic radical prostatectomy. J Urol 2003; 5: 1738-1741
[140] Gill I, Fergany A, Klein E et al. Laparoscopic radical cystectomy with ileal conduit performed completely intracorporeally; the initial 2 cases. Urology 2000; 56:26-29
[141] Lin MY, Fan EW, Chiuaw et al. Laparoscopy –assisted transvaginal total exenteration for locally advanced cervical cancer with bladder invasion after radiotherapy. J Endourol 2004; 9: 867-870

[142] Pomel C, Rouzier M, Pocard A et al. Laproscopic total pelvic exenteration for cervical cancer . Gynecol Oncol. 2003;91(3):616-8

[143] Farghaly SA. Robotic-assisted laparoscopic anterior pelvic exenteration in patients with advanced ovarian cancer: Farghaly's Technique. Eur J Gynecol Oncol 2010; 31(4): 361-3

[144] Verwaal VJ, Bruin S, Boot H, et al. 8-year follow-up of randomized trial: cytoreduction and hyperthermic intraperitoneal chemotherapy versus systemic chemotherapy in patients with peritoneal carcinomatosis of colorectal cancer Ann Surg Oncol. 2008;15(9):2426–2432

11

Antiprogestins in Ovarian Cancer

Carlos M. Telleria and Alicia A. Goyeneche
Division of Basic Biomedical Sciences,
Sanford School of Medicine,
The University of South Dakota, Vermillion, South Dakota
USA

1. Introduction

The overall goal of this chapter is to provide evidence for the feasibility of repositioning antiprogestin compounds originally utilized for reproductive medicine toward ovarian cancer therapy. This disease is the most deadly of the female reproductive track; at the time of diagnosis, in the majority of cases abnormal growths have progressed outside the ovaries and into the nearby fallopian tubes, uterus, and peritoneal cavity. Thus, the majority of diagnosed patients require cytoreductive surgery followed by platinum-based chemotherapy (Bukowski et al.,2007; DiSaia&Bloss,2003; Martin,2007; Naora&Montell,2005; Ozols,2006a). The efficacy of this therapy, however, is limited by the elevated toxicity of the platinum derivatives (Cepeda et al.,2007), the development of mechanisms to escape drug toxicity (Cepeda et al.,2007; Kelland,2007), and the repopulation or regrowth of cells between treatment intervals (Kim&Tannock,2005), all of which lead to the recurrence of the disease. The majority of relapsing patients are platinum-resistant, with very limited chemotherapeutic options, and a median survival time of about only two years (Gordon et al.,2004; Modesitt&Jazaeri,2007; Ozols,2006b; Pectasides et al.,2006; Wilailak&Linasmita,2004). The five-year survival for ovarian cancer patients is extremely disappointing, ranging from 37% to 45% (Jemal et al.,2006). Hence, new therapeutic interventions to overcome the limitations of platinum-based therapy for ovarian cancer patients are greatly needed.

2. Mifepristone: A prototypical antiprogestin

The synthetic steroid RU-38486 or simply RU-486, now named mifepristone, was first synthesized in the mid-1980s when investigators were in the pursuit of synthesizing an antiglucocorticoid agent to treat Cushing's syndrome (Spitz,2006); however, because in preclinical studies with pregnant animals the compound had a remarkable capacity to interrupt pregnancy, its ability to oppose progesterone action in the uterus was inferred. As a result, mifepristone was rapidly repositioned for reproductive medicine, to exploit largely its antiprogesterone and, consequently, contraceptive properties. Mifepristone became the first prototypical antiprogestin clinically approved for early termination of pregnancy in the United States in 2000. In this context, mifepristone blocks progesterone receptors in the uterus (Philibert et al.,1985), thus increasing the sensitivity to myometrial contractions induced by prostaglandin analogues, leading to early interruption of pregnancy (Benagiano et al.,2008a).

Mifepristone has also been used for other reproductive indications, such as oral contraception, menstrual regulation, and emergency contraception (Benagiano et al.,2008b; Ho et al.,2002). More recently, mifepristone emerged as a treatment of endocrine-related diseases such as endometriosis and uterine leiomyoma (Moller et al.,2008); it diminishes the pain associated with pelvic endometriosis (Fedele&Berlanda,2004; Kettel et al.,1994) and reduces the size of uterine fibroids, improving quality of life without evidence of endometrial hyperplasia (Eisinger et al.,2009; Murphy et al.,1995; Steinauer et al.,2004).

3. Mifepristone is a valuable therapeutic alternative in oncology

The antiprogestin activity of mifepristone has been extensively studied; however, it is evident that the contraceptive effect of the compound jeopardized its investigation for other medical uses, in particular, its application in oncology, which is now emerging. In non-reproductive tissues, it was reported that mifepristone inhibited the growth of gastric cancer cells (Li et al.,2004), meningioma cells *in vitro* and *in vivo* (Grunberg et al.,2006; Grunberg et al.,1991; Matsuda et al.,1994; Tieszen et al.,2011), glioblastoma and osteosarcoma cells (Tieszen et al.,2011), and non-small lung cell carcinoma cell lines (Weidner, Hapon & Telleria, unpublished observations).

In reproductive tissues, mifepristone blocked the growth of cervical adenocarcinoma cells *in vitro* and *in vivo* (Jurado et al.,2009), and inhibited cell proliferation killing benign and malignant endometrial cancer cells (Han&Sidell,2003; Murphy et al.,2000; Narvekar et al.,2004; Schneider et al.,1998). In prostate cancer, the antiprogestin blocked growth of androgen-sensitive and androgen-insensitive LNCaP and PC-3 cells (El Etreby et al.,2000a; El Etreby et al.,2000b; Liang et al.,2002; Tieszen et al.,2011). In breast cancer, mifepristone inhibited the growth of T-47D (Musgrove et al.,1997), MCF-7, and MDA-MB-231 cells (Tieszen et al.,2011); particularly in MCF-7 cells, mifepristone had an additive lethal effect when associated with the antiestrogen tamoxifen (El Etreby et al.,1998), as well as a synergistic lethal interaction with the Chk-1 inhibitor 7-hydroxystaurosporine (UCN-01) (Yokoyama et al.,2000) and with 4-hydroxytamoxifen (Schoenlein et al.,2007). Mifepristone also blocked the growth of MCF-7 sublines made resistant to 4-hydroxytamoxifen (Gaddy et al.,2004) and was lethal to MDA-MB-231 cells that are devoid of estrogen and progesterone receptors (Liang et al.,2003). In p53/BRCA1-deficient mice, mifepristone prevented the formation of breast tumors (Poole et al.,2006), indicating its efficacy not only impairing the growth of established mammary tumors but also inhibiting mammary tumorigenesis. In mice with spontaneous lung cancer or leukemia, mifepristone was also found to improve longevity and quality of life (Check et al.,2009; Check et al.,2010b). Most recently, case studies of patients with widely metastatic thymic, renal, colon, or pancreatic cancers no longer responding to chemotherapy, reported that chronic daily treatment with 200 mg mifepristone had a significant improvement in their qualities of life (Check et al.,2010a).

4. Mifepristone in ovarian cancer therapeutics

The action of antiprogestins on ovarian cancer has received limited attention. First in 1996, it was revealed that the antiprogestin mifepristone arrested OVCAR-3 and A2780 ovarian cancer cells at the G1 phase of the cell cycle (Rose&Barnea,1996). In a small clinical trial conducted with patients having recurrent epithelial ovarian cancer whose tumors had become resistant to standard chemotherapy, mifepristone administration showed promising

effects against some of the tumors (Rocereto et al.,2000). Years later, it was reported that mifepristone enhanced the toxic effect of cisplatin on COC1 ovarian cancer cells *in vitro* and in xenografted immunosuppressed mice (Liu et al.,2003; Qin&Wang,2002).
These initial studies indicated an anti-ovarian cancer activity of mifepristone, yet the molecular target(s) involved in mediating such an effect remained obscure. In 2007, we described some molecular mediators of growth inhibition induced by mifepristone as a single agent in ovarian cancer cells, and further defined its efficacy in an *in vivo* preclinical setting (Goyeneche et al.,2007). We also proved that cytostatic doses of mifepristone added after a lethal dose of cisplatin prevents repopulation of remnant ovarian cancer cells surviving a platinum insult (Freeburg et al.,2009b). We showed that cell cultures exposed to mifepristone after cisplatin had a remarkable increase in the percentage of cells expressing the cell death marker cleaved poly (ADP-ribose) polymerase (PARP) and the mitotic marker phospho-histone H3 suggesting that mifepristone potentiates cisplatin lethality and that the cells likely die as a consequence of mitotic failure (Freeburg et al.,2009b). We also reported that the effect of mifepristone in ovarian cancer cells is independent of p53 functionality and platinum sensitivity (Freeburg et al.,2009a), making mifepristone an even more interesting chemotherapeutic candidate for ovarian cancer as the majority of tumors in relapsing patients are platinum resistant and p53 mutant (Ozols,2006b). Finally, we have shown in ovarian cancer cells that mifepristone potentiates the lethality of otherwise sub-lethal doses of cisplatin, and synergizes with cisplatin growth inhibiting ovarian cancer cells of different genetic backgrounds and platinum sensitivities (Gamarra-Luques&Telleria,2010).

4.1 Mifepristone-induced cytostasis vs. lethality in ovarian cancer cells

Antiprogestin mifepristone is toxic towards ovarian cancer cells, with cytostasis manifested at lower micromolar concentrations and lethality taking place when the compound is used at higher micromolar doses (Freeburg et al.,2009a; Goyeneche et al.,2007; Goyeneche et al.,2011; Tieszen et al.,2011). When mifepristone was used at doses up to 20 μM, the effect was limited to cytostasis demonstrated by the reversibility of the growth inhibition observed when the drug was removed from the culture media, in association with the lack of measurable cell death (Goyeneche et al.,2007). In all ovarian cancer cell lines we investigated, concentrations of mifepristone 30 μM or higher were lethal (Freeburg et al.,2009a; Goyeneche et al.,2011; Tieszen et al.,2011). This lethality was illustrated by the reduced viability of the cells, the increase in cellular particles with hypodiploid fragmented DNA content, and the cleavage of the cell death associated caspase, caspase-3, in parallel with the cleavage of the widely accepted marker of cell death and a substrate for caspase-3, PARP (Scovassi&Poirier,1999). The lethality of concentrations of mifepristone over 40 μM towards ovarian cancer cells was first suggested in OVCAR-3 and A2780 cells (Rose&Barnea,1996). Yet, our studies demonstrate that the lethality of mifepristone monotherapy towards ovarian cancer cells is related to a caspase-associated apoptotic process.
The dose-dependent cytostatic and lethal effects of mifepristone towards ovarian cancer cells, which we globally refer to as cytotoxicity, occur also in breast cancer cells. In the MCF-7 breast cancer cell line the combination of mifepristone and antiestrogen 4-hydroxytamoxifen had greater cytostatic and lethal activities than either monotherapy, whereas the lethality of the treatment was associated with genomic DNA fragmentation and cleavage of PARP (Schoenlein et al.,2007). In addition, it has been shown that MCF-7 cells made resistant to 4-hydroxytamoxifen also respond to mifepristone monotherapy undergoing apoptotic death (Gaddy et al.,2004); finally, although at higher concentrations,

mifepristone was also cytotoxic to progesterone receptor- and estrogen receptor-negative MDA-MB-231 breast cancer cells (Liang et al.,2003; Tieszen et al.,2011).

4.2 The inhibition of ovarian cancer growth by mifepristone occurs regardless of histopathological classification, platinum sensitivity, or p53 genetic background

Ovarian cancer is very heterogeneous from histopathological and genetic viewpoints (Cannistra,2004; Despierre et al.,2010). Furthermore, mutations of the p53 tumor suppressor gene occur at extremely high frequencies in ovarian cancer (Havrilesky et al.,2003), whereas most recurrent patients with ovarian cancer are platinum-resistant, consequently being left with therapeutic alternatives that have very disappointing outcomes (DiSaia&Bloss,2003; Herzog,2006; Vasey,2003). Thus, if the histopathological and genetic backgrounds, sensitivity to platinum, and p53 status of the ovarian cancer cells would not condition their response to the growth inhibition activity of mifepristone, such findings would have pronounced clinical relevance.

We showed that the cytostatic effect of mifepristone displayed similar potency among the ovarian cancer cells representing various histopathological origins (Freeburg et al.,2009a; Goyeneche et al.,2007; Tieszen et al.,2011), such as clear cell adenocarcinoma (SK-OV-3), papillary ovarian adenocarcinoma (Caov-3 cells), glandular with mixed differentiation (IGROV-1), undifferentiated (A2780), and endometrioid (OV2008) cells (Shaw et al.,2004).

We proved that the growth inhibition induced by mifepristone occurred irrespective of the p53 background of the ovarian cancer cell lines studied, with IC_{50s} ranging between ~ 7 to 12 μM (Freeburg et al.,2009a; Goyeneche et al.,2007) in p53 wild type cells [e.g. OV2008, OV2008/C13, A2780, and IGROV-1; (Casalini et al.,2001; Fraser et al.,2003; Sasaki et al.,2000; Siddik et al.,1998)], p53 mutant cells [A2780/CP70 and Caov-3 (Lu et al.,2001; Reid et al.,2004; Yaginuma&Westphal,1992)], or p53 null cells [SK-OV-3; (O'Connor et al.,1997; Yaginuma&Westphal,1992)].

We observed that mifepristone displayed similar growth inhibition potency among SK-OV-3, OV2008, and Caov-3 cell lines (Goyeneche et al.,2007), which have different sensitivities to platinum agents. OV2008 cells were reported as being highly sensitive to cisplatin (Katano et al.,2002), SK-OV-3 cells were originally obtained from a patient with intrinsic resistance to clinically achievable doses of cisplatin and considered, *in vitro*, as semi-resistant to platinum (Ormerod et al.,1996), whereas Caov-3 cells were shown to be resistant to cisplatin (Arimoto-Ishida et al.,2004; Hayakawa et al.,1999). Furthermore, when we studied the action of mifepristone among ovarian cancer cell line pairs consisting of cisplatin-sensitive parental lines and stable cisplatin-resistant sublines derived by *in vitro* selection with stepwise exposure to cisplatin, the toxicity of mifepristone did not discriminate among the cell lines, as we could not find a correlation between the IC_{50s} for mifepristone and the IC_{50s} for cisplatin obtained for the ovarian cancer cell lines studied (Freeburg et al.,2009a). These results confirm that mifepristone growth inhibits ovarian cancer cells regardless of their sensitivities to cisplatin.

5. Anti-ovarian cancer effect of antiprogestins other than mifepristone: ORG-31710 and CDB-2914 (Ulipristal)

ORG-31710 and CDB-2914 (a.k.a. ulipristal) are two members of a family of selective progesterone receptor modulators with a similar structure to RU-38486, as they all contain a dimethylaminophenyl substitution at the 11β-position that confers antiprogestin activity

(Belanger et al.,1981; Benagiano et al.,2008a; Moller et al.,2008) (Fig. 1). ORG-31710 and CDB-2914, however, were designed with the aim to decrease the antagonistic effect of RU-38486 on the glucocorticoid receptor by substitutions made at the 17α side chain (Moller et al.,2008).

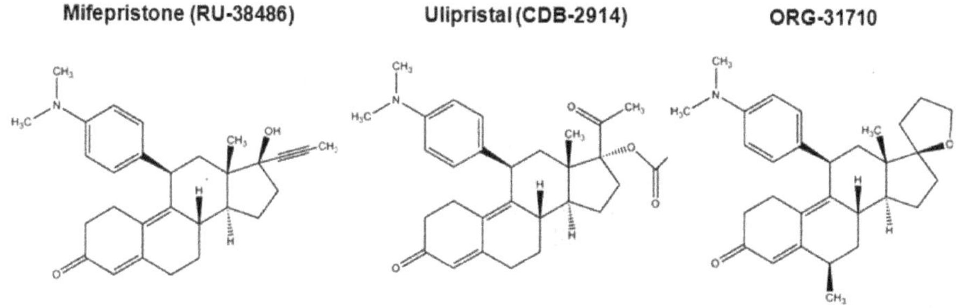

Mifepristone (RU-38486) **Ulipristal (CDB-2914)** **ORG-31710**

Fig. 1. Chemical structure of antiprogestins [Adapted from (Goyeneche et al.,2011)]

Limited information is available on the oncologic value of CDB-2914 and ORG-31710. Both chemicals were effective in rats, reducing the growth of established DMBA-induced breast tumors (Kloosterboer et al.,2000; Wiehle et al.,2007). In cultured human uterine leiomyoma cells, CDB-2914 inhibited cell proliferation down-regulating PCNA expression and inducing apoptosis (Xu et al.,2005). Moreover, a randomized controlled clinical trial revealed that CDB-2914 reduced leiomyoma growth (Levens et al.,2008). ORG-31710, on the other hand, was effective in increasing apoptosis in human periovulatory granulosa cells (Svensson et al.,2001). We have proved that mifepristone, ORG-31710 and CDB-2914, are all cytostatic at lower concentrations and lethal at higher doses towards OV2008 and SK-OV-3 ovarian cancer cells (Goyeneche et al.,2011).

6. Mechanisms of antiproliferation of ovarian cancer cells by antiprogestins

It is apparent that different antiprogestin compounds are cytotoxic to ovarian cancer cells displaying two main effects: (i) a cytostatic effect at lower concentrations blocking cell growth at the G1 phase of the cell cycle; and (ii) a lethal effect at higher doses associated with morphological features of apoptosis and fragmentation of the genomic DNA. The overall toxicity of antiprogestins involves a dose-dependent decline in the activity of the cell cycle regulatory protein cyclin dependent kinase 2 (Cdk-2).

6.1 Cell cycle arrest

Exposure of ovarian cancer cells to concentrations of mifepristone likely to be achieved *in vivo* inhibits their growth by inducing G1 cell cycle arrest without triggering cell death. This is consistent with the dose-dependent tumor growth inhibition achieved by mifepristone monotherapy *in vivo* in nude mice carrying subcutaneous tumors derived from human ovarian cancer cells (Goyeneche et al.,2007).

The growth inhibitory effect of mifepristone on ovarian cancer cells is associated with inhibition of DNA synthesis, down-regulation of the transcription factor E2F1 needed for S phase progression, and inhibition of the activity of Cdk-2. This cell cycle regulatory protein is critical to promote the transition of cells in the cell cycle from G1 to S phase (Conradie et al.,2010). For instance, the activity of Cdk-2 is needed for the stimulation of histone gene transcription (Zhao et al.,2000), which is one of the major events marking the entry into the S phase. To drive cell cycle progression, Cdk-2 should be free of $p21^{cip1}$ and $p27^{kip1}$ binding (Conradie et al.,2010), bound to cyclin E, and allocated to the nucleus to phosphorylate cell cycle regulatory proteins (Brown et al.,2004; Lents et al.,2002). Mifepristone, ORG-31710 and CDB-2914 affect the nucleocytoplasmic trafficking of Cdk inhibitors $p21^{cip1}$ and $p27^{kip1}$, Cdk-2 and its co-factor cyclin E. The antiprogestins also increase $p21^{cip1}$ and $p27^{kip1}$ abundances in both cytoplasm and nuclear compartments in correlation with decreased Cdk-2 and cyclin E nuclear levels, increased cytoplasmic cyclin E, and a remarkable decline in the activity of Cdk-2 in both subcellular compartments (Goyeneche et al.,2007; Goyeneche et al.,2011).

Because Cdk-2 is frequently up-regulated in ovarian tumors as compared to non-cancerous cells (Sui et al.,2001), the potent inhibition of Cdk-2 elicited by antiprogestins may be critically important from a translational therapeutics viewpoint. Moreover, because cytoplasmic localization of Cdk inhibitor $p27^{kip1}$ in ovarian cancer patients has been associated with poor prognosis (Rosen et al.,2005), by promoting an increase in $p27^{kip1}$ in the nucleus, antiprogestins may be able to rescue the tight inhibitory control of Cdk inhibitors on Cdk-2 activity that is mostly lost in ovarian cancer.

The magnitude of inhibition of Cdk-2 activity is related to the growth inhibition potency of the antiprogestins with mifepristone>ORG-31710>CDB-2914 (Goyeneche et al.,2011). Supporting our results, a decline in cyclin E-associated kinase activity (presumably Cdk-2) was reported for T-47D breast cancer cells in response to ORG-31710 in the absence of significant changes in cyclin E and Cdk levels, but in the presence of elevated amounts of $p21^{cip1}$, suggesting that $p21^{cip1}$ contributes to the reduction in Cdk-2 activity after antiprogestin treatment (Musgrove et al.,1997). In ovarian cancer cells, we provide evidence that not only the increased association of $p21^{cip1}$ and $p27^{kip1}$ to Cdk-2 may account for the reduced Cdk-2 activity in the nucleus in response to antiprogestins, but also a reduction in Cdk-2 and cyclin E nuclear levels and redistribution of cyclin E to the cytoplasm, are related variables leading to blunt Cdk-2 nuclear activity needed for the cells to transit from G1 to S phase. A recent study using LNCaP prostate cancer cells revealed that targeting Cdk-2 to the nucleus is sufficient to prevent growth inhibition triggered by 1,25 $(OH)_2$ D3 (Flores et al.,2010), suggesting that antiprogestin-mediated growth inhibition and growth arrest triggered by metabolites of vitamin D may share common molecular intermediaries.

6.2 Cell death

At high concentrations, the antiprogestins mifepristone, ORG-31710 and CDB-2914 blunt the activity of Cdk-2 leading to ovarian cancer cell death in association with morphological features of apoptosis, hypodiploid DNA content, fragmentation of the DNA, and cleavage of the executer caspase substrate PARP (Goyeneche et al.,2011). Such effects may be the consequence of Cdk-2 inhibition. For instance, in addition to regulating cell cycle progression, Cdk-2 is involved in cell survival after DNA damage (Deans et al.,2006; Huang et al.,2006). As a survival factor, Cdk-2 phosphorylates the FOXO1 transcription activator of pro-apoptotic genes, keeping them in the cytoplasm (Huang et al.,2006; Huang&Tindall,2007) . If the activity of Cdk-2 is abolished by an antiprogestin, then FOXO1 may not be retained in the cytoplasm, consequently migrating to the nucleus where it promotes the expression of pro-apoptotic genes (Huang et al.,2006; Huang&Tindall,2007).

The lethality of high concentration antiprogestins has features of apoptosis similar to that of platinum-induced lethality in the same cell lines in terms of nuclear and DNA fragmentation (Goyeneche et al.,2011); however, the molecular mediators of antiprogestin-induced cell death vary among the steroids. Cleavage of the caspase-3 substrate PARP is a commonality among mifepristone, ORG-31710 and CDB-2914. CDB-2914 also causes an up-regulation of PARP which was previously observed in cultured human uterine leiomyoma cells (Xu et al.,2005). In addition, CDB-2914 causes up-regulation of the anti-apoptotic proteins XIAP and Bcl-2, yet cell death still ensues but with less effectiveness than that observed after exposure to high concentrations of mifepristone or ORG-31710, in which both XIAP and Bcl-2 are down-regulated after 3 days of treatment (Goyeneche et al.,2011). Thus, the extended up-regulation of XIAP and Bcl-2 upon CDB-2914 treatment but not after mifepristone or ORG-31710 may account for the reduced cytotoxic potency of CDB-2914. Although with different potencies, high concentrations of antiprogestins lead the cells to cross a cell death threshold or point of no return in which the pro-apoptotic load of the cell surpasses its anti-apoptotic buffering capacity.

6.3 Progesterone receptors are not essential for the growth arrest induced by antiprogestins in ovarian cancer

Because several tumors of both gynecologic and non-gynecologic origin are steroid hormone-dependent and express progesterone receptors, antiprogestins have been investigated as potential anti-cancer therapeutic agents largely based on their capacity to modulate progesterone receptors. However, whether the mechanism(s) through which antiprogestins act to induce cytostasis and lethality in cancer cells actually requires progesterone receptor expression remains obscure.

When targeting cancer cells mifepristone has progesterone-like activity. For example, in T-47D breast cancer cells and HeLa cervical adenocarcinoma cells, mifepristone induced progesterone-regulated reporter genes mainly when the cyclin AMP pathway was activated (Kahmann et al.,1998; Sartorius et al.,1993). In ovarian cancer cells, progesterone blocked cell growth (Syed&Ho,2003; Syed et al.,2007; Syed et al.,2001); likewise, mifepristone also induced cell growth arrest, though with greater potency than synthetic progestins (Goyeneche et al.,2007). These data suggest that the cytostatic effect of mifepristone might be mediated by an agonistic action on progesterone receptors.

Nonetheless, there is ample evidence suggesting that the efficacy of antiprogestins as anti-cancer agents may not require progesterone receptor expression. Liang and colleagues reported that micromolar doses of mifepristone monotherapy were able to inhibit the growth of estrogen receptor- and progesterone receptor-negative MDA-MB-231 breast cancer cells (Liang et al.,2003). In another report mifepristone, instead of blocking growth inhibition induced by progesterone, potentiated progesterone-mediated growth retardation and apoptosis (Moe et al.,2009). Such potentiation of cytotoxicity of progesterone by mifepristone was also observed in progesterone receptor positive MCF-7 breast cancer cells and progesterone receptor negative C4-I cervical carcinoma cells, suggesting that the presence of progesterone receptor is not essential for the anti-growth properties of both progesterone and mifepristone (Fjelldal et al.,2010).

The reported level of expression of progesterone receptors in ovarian cancer cell lines is controversial. Progesterone receptor immuno-reactive proteins A (PR-A) and B (PR-B) were identified in OVCA-429 and OVCA-432 ovarian cancer cells—derived from patients with late-state serous ovarian cancer—at levels higher than those found in immortalized human ovarian surface epithelial cells (Mukherjee et al.,2005). Papillary adenocarcinoma Caov-3 ovarian cells were reported to express progesterone receptor mRNA in one study (Akahira et al.,2002) but not in another report (Hamilton et al.,1984). Similarly, studies in clear adenocarcinoma SK-OV-3 ovarian cells showing some and no expression of progesterone receptor mRNA have been published (Hamilton et al.,1984; Keith Bechtel&Bonavida,2001; McDonnel&Murdoch,2001). We have found low levels of progesterone receptor immuno-reactive proteins in endometrioid OV2008 ovarian cancer cells when compared with MCF-7 breast cancer cells used as positive control (Fig.2A). Moreover, utilizing ten cell lines expanding cancers from the nervous system (meningioma IOMM-Lee cells and glioblastoma U87MG cells), breast (estrogen-responsive MCF-7 and estrogen-unresponsive MDA-MB-231 cells), prostate (androgen-responsive LNCaP and androgen-unresponsive PC-3 cells), bone (osteosarcoma U-2OS and SAOS-2 cells), and ovary (OVCAR-3 and SK-OV-3 cells), and two anti-progesterone receptor antibodies, we failed to detect progesterone receptor immuno-reactive proteins in all but MCF-7 cells, yet all cell lines studied were growth inhibited by mifepristone (Tieszen et al.,2011). Even in MCF-7 cells carrying progesterone receptors, mifepristone reduced their expression, further discouraging the role of these nuclear receptors as mediators of the growth inhibitory effect of mifepristone given that the cytostatic property of mifepristone can be maintained long after the receptors are down-regulated (Tieszen et al.,2011).

These data rule out progesterone receptors as essential mediators of the growth inhibitory effect of antiprogestins. Mainstream literature on the anti-cancer effect of antiprogestin mifepristone assumes that it acts as a progesterone receptor antagonist, implying that the presence of progesterone receptors in the target tissues is a pre-requisite for mifepristone's anti-growth activity. Our work challenges such a dogma (Tieszen et al.,2011), opening the field of study to alternate, non-classical mechanisms whereby antiprogestins operate as cell growth inhibitors without the necessity of nuclear progesterone receptors being present or operational. If these results were translated into the clinic, the presence or absence of classical, nuclear progesterone receptors would not be relevant and would not impact the usage of this drug for cancer therapy.

6.4 Glucocorticoid receptors and the growth inhibitory activity of antiprogestins

Antiprogestins, mainly mifepristone, may drive their anticancer action through glucocorticoid receptors. This is because: (i) mifepristone can bind to glucocorticoid receptors with an affinity similar to that of progesterone receptors (Mao et al.,1992); and (ii) ovarian cancer cells have been reported to express glucocorticoid receptors (Tieszen et al.,2011; Xu et al.,2003). In this regard, we have detected abundant levels of glucocorticoid receptor immuno-reactive proteins alpha (GRα) and beta (GRβ) in SK-OV-3, OVCAR-3, and OV2008 cells [(Tieszen et al.,2011) and (Fig.2B)]. When we cultured OV2008 cells in the presence of the glucocorticoid agonist dexamethasone at concentrations equimolar to cytostatic mifepristone, ORG-31710 or CDB-2914, however, the antiprogestins up-regulated Cdk inhibitors p21^{cip1} and p27^{kip1} and blocked cell growth, but dexamethasone did not, though its activity is demonstrated by the down-regulation of glucocorticoid receptors (Fig.2B). These data suggest that even if antiprogestins bind glucocorticoid receptors in the ovarian cancer cells, they may not trigger receptor transactivation. Supporting our observations with ovarian cancer cells, mifepristone blocked the growth of LNCaP prostate cancer cells that were either androgen-sensitive or -refractory, while competition for glucocorticoid receptors with equimolar doses of mifepristone and hydrocortisone could not reverse the degree of growth inhibition achieved by mifepristone alone (El Etreby et al.,2000b).

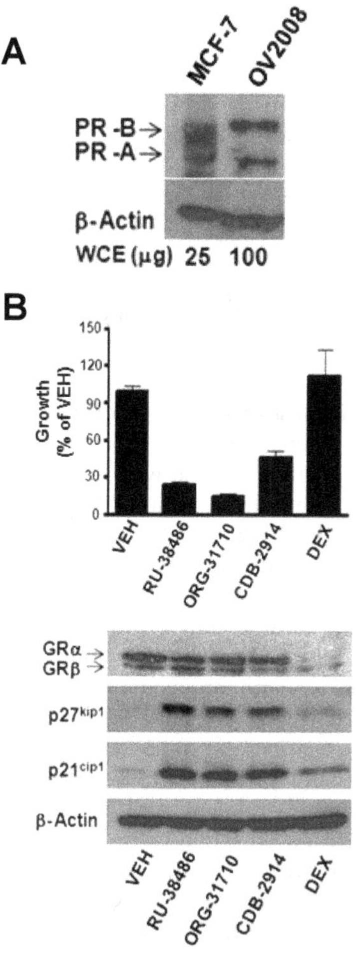

Fig. 2. (A) Expression of progesterone receptor isoforms (PR-A and PR-B) and glucocorticoid receptors (GRα and GRβ) in OV2008 ovarian cancer cells. Whole cell extracts (WCE) from MCF-7 cells were used as positive control for progesterone receptor expression. To detect progesterone receptor proteins in OV2008 cells, we worked with cells growing exponentially and increased the WCE loading 4-fold with respect to MCF-7. (B) Effect of equimolar concentrations of antiprogestins and dexamethasone (DEX) on OV2008 ovarian cancer growth. Cells were exposed to vehicle (VEH), 20 μM mifepristone (RU-38486), ORG-31710, CDB-3914 (ulipristal) or DEX for 72 h. Cell growth (B, upper panel) was analyzed by microcytometry and protein expression (B, lower panel) by Western blot. Bars, mean± SEM.

Mifepristone has potent anti-glucorticoid activity (Baulieu,1991; Benagiano et al.,2008c) . Indeed mifepristone binds GRα with mostly antagonistic activity; yet it may have agonistic potency depending on the concentration of glucocorticoid receptors in the cell (Zhang et al.,2007). Although GRβ has been considered a dominant-negative regulator of GRα (Oakley et al.,1999; Taniguchi et al.,2010; Yudt et al.,2003), it was also reported that mifepristone was the only compound of 57 potential natural and synthetic ligands to bind the GRβ receptor isoform, and that interaction of GRβ with mifepristone led to its nuclear translocation (Lewis-Tuffin et al.,2007). This latter study also found that despite its classification as a dominant-negative isoform lacking transcriptional activity, GRβ was able to regulate gene expression in the absence of GRα, and this activity was modulated by the interaction with mifepristone. A more recent study also reported intrinsic transcriptional activity of GRβ independent of GRα, but neither found an association between mifepristone binding and nuclear translocation of GRβ, nor could detect modulation of GRβ transcriptional activity by mifepristone (Kino et al.,2009), adding controversy to the actual activity of mifepristone on GRβ. This evidence and our results encourage performing more studies to underscore a role, if any, for either isoform of the glucocorticoid receptor on the anti-growth activity of the antiprogestin mifepristone.

6.5 Other potential targets of antiprogestins when operating as cell growth inhibitors

A possibility exists that antiprogestins may have an effect that does not involve specific hormone receptors. In this regard, mifepristone was shown to have a potent antioxidant activity reflected at micromolar concentrations and likely caused by the dimethylamino phenyl side chain of the molecule (Parthasarathy et al.,1994). Furthermore, the growth inhibitory action of mifepristone in endometrial cells and macrophages was attributed, at least in part, to the antioxidant property of the compound (Murphy et al.,2000; Roberts et al.,1995). A putative antioxidant effect of mifepristone on ovarian cancer cells could be interesting in the context of G1 arrest associated with $p21^{cip1}$ upregulation, because $p21^{cip1}$ can be induced in response to some antioxidants in a p53 independent manner (Liberto&Cobrinik,2000; Liu et al.,1999). We have shown that growth arrest caused by mifepristone is associated with $p21^{cip1}$ increase in p53 wild type OV2008 cells and in p53 null SK-OV3 cells, opening the possibility for mifepristone acting as an antioxidant to drive G1 arrest through a p53-independent up-regulation of $p21^{cip1}$.

Another potential target of antiprogestin action is the ubiquitin-proteasome system (UPS). This idea is based on the following facts: (i) to transition from G1 to S phase and to commit to DNA synthesis, the cells must degrade the Cdk-2 inhibitors $p27^{kip1}$ and $p21^{cip}$ via the Skp1-Cullin-F-box protein/Skp2 (SCF^{Skp2}) E3 ubiquitin ligase complex (Bornstein et al.,2003; Tsvetkov et al.,1999). This requires the Cdk-2-dependent phosphorylation of $p27^{kip1}$ on Thr187 (Tsvetkov et al.,1999) and $p21^{cip1}$ on Ser130 (Bornstein et al.,2003); (ii) antiprogestins have a dual effect blocking Cdk-2 activity and triggering the accumulation of $p21^{cip1}$ and $p27^{kip1}$, and these Cdk-2 inhibitors rely on the UPS for their disappearance to enforce the orderly progression of the cell cycle from G1 to the S phase; (iii) there are remarkable similarities in the behavior of antiprogestins and proteasome inhibitors in inducing $p21^{cip1}$ and $p27^{kip1}$ accumulation before triggering caspase-associated lethality (Bazzaro et al.,2006; Freeburg et al.,2009a; Goyeneche et al.,2007). It is therefore possible that antiprogestins induce G1 growth arrest by interfering with the proteasome-mediated degradation of $p27^{kip1}/p21^{cip1}$, leading to Cdk-2 inhibition. It is also reasonable that the sustained levels of $p27^{kip}$ and $p21^{cip1}$ in response to cytostatic doses of antiprogestins are the consequence of a reduced recognition of the Cdk inhibitors by the UPS. Because ovarian cancer cells function with high activity of the UPS (Bazzaro et al.,2006), this proteolytic machinery may be degrading Cdk inhibitors at a high rate, causing the reduced basal levels we found in ovarian cancer cells, thus favoring their proliferation. Antiprogestins may mitigate this process.

An additional potential mechanism mediating the anti-cell growth activity of antiprogestins is the induction of stress of the endoplasmic reticulum. A recent study showed that mifepristone induced an atypical unfolded protein response (UPR) in non-small lung cell carcinoma cells (Dioufa et al.,2010). The role of the endoplasmic reticulum responding to antiprogestins triggering the UPR, which could lead to either survival or death depending on the concentration of antiprogestins, is a provoking hypothesis that should be explored.

The newly discovered progesterone receptor membrane component 1 (PGRMC1) (Gellersen et al.,2009; Rohe et al.,2009) or the family of membrane PRs (mPRα, β, γ, δ, ε) (Dressing et al.,2011; Gellersen et al.,2009; Thomas et al.,2007) may also mediate the anti-tumor effect of antiprogestins. For instance, PGRMC1 expression increases while cognate, nuclear progesterone receptor decreases in advanced stages of ovarian cancer, and overexpression of PGRMC1 interferes with the lethality of cisplatin, suggesting a survival role for PGRMC1 in ovarian cancer development (Peluso et al.,2008). In a panel of ovarian cancer cell lines expressing mPRα, mPRβ, and mPRγ, but not cognate nuclear progesterone receptors, exposure to progesterone mediated the expression of pro-apoptotic proteins via activation of JNK and p38 MAPKs (Charles et al.,2010). Given that at micromolar concentrations the antiprogestin mifepristone operates as an agonist on both mPRα and mPRγ when expressed in yeast (Smith et al.,2008), it is conceivable that antiprogestins carrying a similar structure (Fig.1) may mediate antiproliferation of cancer cells acting as agonists of mPRs.

7. Strategy to utilize antiprogestins in ovarian cancer therapeutics

7.1 Blockage of ovarian cancer re-growth after platinum therapy

We validated an *in vitro* model of ovarian cancer cell repopulation taking place among courses of lethal cisplatin therapy. Using this *in vitro* model system, we demonstrated that intertwining cytostatic concentrations of the antiprogestin mifepristone in between courses of cisplatin treatment is an efficacious strategy to prevent repopulation of ovarian cancer cells leading to a better treatment outcome; in addition, we found that chronic exposure to mifepristone after cisplatin enhances the killing efficacy of this cross-linking agent (Freeburg et al.,2009b). In this study, although the majority of the cells in the culture succumbed to the lethality of cisplatin, there were isolated cells that survived the treatment. These cells, because of their scarcity in the culture plate, may be easily missed in routine cell cultures if long-term follow-up is not conducted. When such a population of remnant cells that escaped the toxicity of platinum was exposed to cisplatin-free medium, the cells relapsed and repopulated the culture. We were able to document the relapse of highly sensitive OV2008 cells after three rounds of cisplatin treatment. The OV2008 cells repopulating after cisplatin incorporated more BrdUrd into their DNA when compared with exponentially growing, untreated cells, suggesting that an increased number of cells synthesizing DNA may be a product of accelerated cell repopulation (Kim&Tannock,2005). When antiprogestin mifepristone was utilized chronically in between cisplatin treatment intervals, the cells that survived the treatment did not synthesize DNA, did not repopulate, and had a very poor clonogenic survival capacity, suggesting a permanent DNA damage to the cells not compatible with their survivability.

The nature of the cells that escape the lethality of cisplatin remains to be determined. There is a possibility that cisplatin is killing only the population of differentiated cancer cells representing the bulk of the culture, but not the scarce tumor initiating cells with the capacity to regenerate the culture, and that appear to be resistant to most common DNA damaging agents (Kvinlaug&Huntly,2007). The presence of tumor initiating cells in ovarian cancer cell lines, however, has yet to be confirmed.

Alternatively, antiprogestins may block repopulation of cells after cisplatin by interfering with a cellular process termed reverse polyploidy or neosis (Erenpreisa&Cragg,2007; Illidge et al.,2000; Sundaram et al.,2004). Cancer cells develop the capacity to escape DNA damage caused by pharmacological doses of platinum agents by reverse polyploidy, leading to the formation of diploid, rapid proliferating cells with increased platinum resistance (Puig et al.,2008). Thus, it is feasible that antiprogestins, when used chronically, block post-platinum repopulation by preventing reverse polyploidy. This hypothesis is based on the observation that OV2008 cells repopulating after cisplatin exposure show giant cells together with a nascent population of small cells (Freeburg et al.,2009b) that may originate from the likely polyploid, giant progenitors. Cultures treated with antiprogestins after platinum do not show this small pool of repopulating cells and instead display an overall reduced number of cells, with predominance of a giant phenotype that ends up committing suicide as marked by cleaved PARP positivity (Freeburg et al.,2009b).

7.2 Potentiation of platinum induced lethality by antiprogestins

We proved that intertwining cytostatic concentrations of antiprogestin mifepristone in between courses of lethal cisplatin-based chemotherapy not only resulted in an efficacious strategy to prevent repopulation of cancer cells in between lethal platinum treatment intervals, but it also potentiated the killing efficacy of cisplatin (Freeburg et al.,2009b).

When ovarian cancer cells are exposed to only mifepristone therapy, the cell cycle is arrested in the G1 phase (Goyeneche et al.,2007; Rose&Barnea,1996). However, when antiprogestin mifepristone is added after cisplatin, the cells tend to accumulate at the S and/or G2/M phases rather than in G1 (Gamarra-Luques&Telleria,2010). This phenomenon may provide the rationale for the potentiation of platinum therapy by the antiprogestin. It is known that cisplatin treatment leads to a transitory S or G2 cell cycle arrest, which is utilized by the cells as an opportunity to repair any damaged DNA; however, if the DNA damage is significant and the DNA repair mechanisms cannot operate, the cells usually trigger their own demise (Sorenson et al.,1990). Thus, mifepristone may be a disruptor of the DNA damage and repair pathways operating after cisplatin exposure. Consequently the cells would enter an unscheduled mitosis with damaged DNA, which usually would trigger a cell death mechanism due to mitotic failure (Vakifahmetoglu et al.,2008). Partial support for this hypothesis is that cells receiving the combination treatment of cisplatin followed by mifepristone show an elevated percentage of cells allocated to the M phase of the cell cycle suggested by 6-fold overexpression of the mitotic marker, phospho-histone H3, when compared to cisplatin-only treated cultures (Freeburg et al.,2009b). This result, together with the data showing that the cultures receiving cisplatin followed by mifepristone express 4-fold more cleaved PARP compared with cultures receiving only cisplatin (Freeburg et al.,2009b), indicate that cells chronically exposed to mifepristone after receiving lethal platinum therapy not only are unable to repopulate, but are also likely to die transiting into an unscheduled mitosis that could trigger cell death (i.e. mitotic death).

Mifepristone may be interfering with early steps in the DNA damage response pathway that lead to a failure of cells to arrest in the G2 phase when challenged with cisplatin. This rationale is supported by data generated utilizing the Chk-1 kinase inhibitor UCN-01 (7-hydroxystaurosporine), which as a single agent is able to induce G1 growth arrest in non-small-cell lung carcinoma similar to the effect observed in ovarian cancer cells treated with mifepristone alone (Goyeneche et al.,2007). When UCN-01 was used after cisplatin, however, the combination was synergistic in terms of growth inhibition likely by reducing the time cells spend in the S or G2 phases to operate the DNA damage check point in order to allow repair the DNA damage induced by platinum (Mack et al.,2003).

We demonstrated that the cytostatic effect of mifepristone in ovarian cancer cells associates with an abrupt reduction in the activity of Cdk-2 (Goyeneche et al.,2007). In addition to its role in the cell cycle and cell survival previously stated, Cdk-2 has been implicated in DNA repair. For instance, the DNA repair machinery is dysfunctional in Cdk-2 deficient cells, and cells lacking the DNA repair component of BRCA1 are prone to cell death in response to Cdk-2 inhibition (Deans et al.,2006). This role played by Cdk-2 in the DNA repair process provides the rationale for a synergistic interaction of Cdk-2 inhibition and DNA damaging agents in the killing of cancer cells and could also explain the potentiation by mifepristone of platinum-induced lethality of ovarian cancer cells.

Another hypothesis as to how antiprogestin mifepristone can facilitate the lethal effect of cisplatin is based upon its capacity to abrogate the expression of the E2F1 transcription factor (Goyeneche et al.,2007). E2F1 is needed to regulate the expression of genes involved in the nucleotide excision DNA repair pathway (NER) (Berton et al.,2005), which is a major mechanism needed to repair ~90% of the platinum-DNA intrastrand crosslinks (Cepeda et al.,2007; Helleday et al.,2008; Kelland,2007; Rabik&Dolan,2007). Because in ovarian cancer increased expression of the endonuclease ERCC1 (excision repair cross-complementing-1) involved in NER has been correlated with cisplatin resistance (Li et al.,2000), and antisense RNA against ERCC1 sensitizes ovarian cancer cells to the lethality of cisplatin (Selvakumaran et al.,2003), it is possible that mifepristone potentiates cisplatin lethality by interfering with the functionality of the NER pathway. Antiprogestins may also dysregulate the homologous recombination DNA repair pathway responsible to repair the ~10% DNA interstrand crosslinks induced by platinum agents; this avenue is of relevance as it is apparent that despite the majority of cisplatin binds DNA via intrastrand crosslinks, it is the low percentage of DNA interstrand crosslinks which causes most of its lethality (Wang&Lippard,2005; Wang et al.,2011).

8. Clinical relevance of repurposing antiprogestins for ovarian cancer treatment

Based upon the evidence presented earlier in this chapter, antiprogestins—of which mifepristone and ulipristal are approved by the United States Food and Drug administration for reproductive medicine—can be re-purposed for another modality-of-use as part of the chemotherapeutic armamentarium for ovarian cancer patients. The translation of antiprogestin therapy to the clinic may have an impact in two manners: (i) adding an antiprogestin between rounds of platinum-based therapy should prevent the repopulation of ovarian cancer cells that escape the lethality of the platinum derivative, and improve treatment success in a synergistic manner when followed by antiprogestin maintenance therapy (compare models in Figs.3A vs.3B); and (ii) working as a single, cytostatic agent, a prototypical antiprogestin may be used for chronic maintenance therapy following lethal platinum agents to delay or avoid disease recurrence in a similar manner anti-estrogens are used to treat some cohorts of breast cancer patients (Osipo et al.,2004) (compare models in Figs.3A vs.3C).

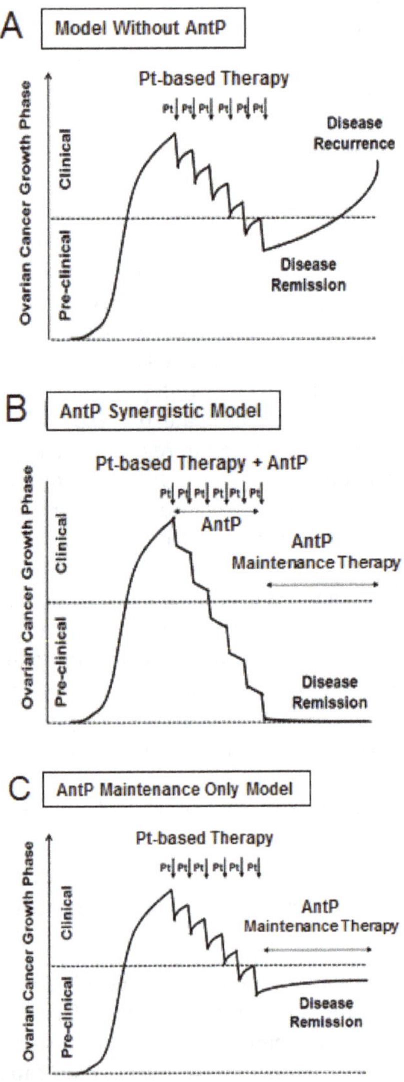

Fig. 3. Clinical translational impact of the use of antiprogestins (AntP) in the context of platinum (Pt) based chemotherapy for ovarian cancer

9. Conclusions

We have described a novel modality of action of antiprogestins acting as cytotoxic agents towards ovarian cancer, displaying a cytostatic effect at lower concentrations blocking cell growth at the G1 phase of the cell cycle, and a lethal effect at higher doses in association with morphological features of apoptosis and fragmentation of the genomic DNA. We have distinguished between lethal and cytostatic actions of these synthetic steroids, and provided evidence that Cdk-2 is involved as a downstream target of the anti-cancer effect of the drugs. Moreover, the remarkable increase in the number of dying cells when antiprogestin mifepristone followed cisplatin exposure (Freeburg et al.,2009b; Gamarra-Luques&Telleria,2010) raises hope that adding antiprogestins to the platinum-based chemotherapeutic schedule in ovarian cancer should allow reducing either the number of platinum cycles or the dose of platinum without losing efficacy in terms of inhibition of tumor growth, yet reducing unwanted side effects. Consequently, the scheduling of antiprogestins between and/or after courses of platinum-based therapy for human ovarian cancer has reasonable potential for improving treatment success, extending the quality and quality of life of patients suffering from this disease.

We have provided data supporting the feasibility for re-repurposing or re-repositioning of antiprogestins originally designed to operate as antiglucocorticoid or antiprogestins, to chronically treat ovarian cancer patients, as it is currently done with antiestrogen therapy for breast cancer. In particular, the emergent role of ORG-31710 and CDB-2914 having far less antiglucocorticoid effects than mifepristone but maintaining its anti-ovarian cancer properties is promising for translation to the clinic.

10. Acknowledgement

This research was supported by award number K22CA121991 and ARRA Supplement K22CA121991-S1 from the National Cancer Institute, the National Institutes of Health (NIH). The authors would like to thank Mr. Nahuel Telleria for editing the manuscript.

11. References

Akahira, J., Suzuki, T., Ito, K., Kaneko, C., Darnel, A. D., Moriya, T., Okamura, K., Yaegashi, N.&Sasano, H. (2002). Differential expression of progesterone receptor isoforms A and B in the normal ovary, and in benign, borderline, and malignant ovarian tumors. *Jpn J Cancer Res* 93(7): 807-815.

Arimoto-Ishida, E., Ohmichi, M., Mabuchi, S., Takahashi, T., Ohshima, C., Hayakawa, J., Kimura, A., Takahashi, K., Nishio, Y., Sakata, M., Kurachi, H., Tasaka, K.&Murata, Y. (2004). Inhibition of phosphorylation of a forkhead transcription factor sensitizes human ovarian cancer cells to cisplatin. *Endocrinology* 145(4): 2014-2022.

Baulieu, E. E. (1991). The antisteroid RU486: its cellular and molecular mode of action. *Trends Endocrinol Metab* 2(6): 233-239.

Bazzaro, M., Lee, M. K., Zoso, A., Stirling, W. L., Santillan, A., Shih Ie, M.&Roden, R. B. (2006). Ubiquitin-proteasome system stress sensitizes ovarian cancer to proteasome inhibitor-induced apoptosis. *Cancer Res* 66(7): 3754-3763.

Belanger, A., Philibert, D.&Teutsch, G. (1981). Regio and stereospecific synthesis of 11 beta-substituted 19-norsteroids. Influence of 11 beta-substitution on progesterone receptor affinity - (1). *Steroids* 37(4): 361-382.

Benagiano, G., Bastianelli, C.&Farris, M. (2008a). Selective progesterone receptor modulators 1: use during pregnancy. *Expert Opin Pharmacother* 9(14): 2459-2472.

Benagiano, G., Bastianelli, C.&Farris, M. (2008b). Selective progesterone receptor modulators 2: use in reproductive medicine. *Expert Opin Pharmacother* 9(14): 2473-2485.

Benagiano, G., Bastianelli, C.&Farris, M. (2008c). Selective progesterone receptor modulators 3: use in oncology, endocrinology and psychiatry. *Expert Opin Pharmacother* 9(14): 2487-2496.

Berton, T. R., Mitchell, D. L., Guo, R.&Johnson, D. G. (2005). Regulation of epidermal apoptosis and DNA repair by E2F1 in response to ultraviolet B radiation. *Oncogene* 24(15): 2449-2460.

Bornstein, G., Bloom, J., Sitry-Shevah, D., Nakayama, K., Pagano, M.&Hershko, A. (2003). Role of the SCFSkp2 ubiquitin ligase in the degradation of p21Cip1 in S phase. *J Biol Chem* 278(28): 25752-25757.

Brown, K. A., Roberts, R. L., Arteaga, C. L.&Law, B. K. (2004). Transforming growth factor-beta induces Cdk2 relocalization to the cytoplasm coincident with dephosphorylation of retinoblastoma tumor suppressor protein. *Breast Cancer Res* 6(2): R130-139.

Bukowski, R. M., Ozols, R. F.&Markman, M. (2007). The management of recurrent ovarian cancer. *Semin Oncol* 34(2 Suppl 2): S1-15.

Cannistra, S. A. (2004). Cancer of the ovary. *N Engl J Med* 351(24): 2519-2529.

Casalini, P., Botta, L.&Menard, S. (2001). Role of p53 in HER2-induced proliferation or apoptosis. *J Biol Chem* 276(15): 12449-12453.

Cepeda, V., Fuertes, M. A., Castilla, J., Alonso, C., Quevedo, C.&Perez, J. M. (2007). Biochemical mechanisms of cisplatin cytotoxicity. *Anticancer Agents Med Chem* 7(1): 3-18.

Charles, N. J., Thomas, P.&Lange, C. A. (2010). Expression of membrane progesterone receptors (mPR/PAQR) in ovarian cancer cells: implications for progesterone-induced signaling events. *Horm Canc* 1(4): 167-176.

Check, J. H., Dix, E., Cohen, R., Check, D.&Wilson, C. (2010a). Efficacy of the progesterone receptor antagonist mifepristone for palliative therapy of patients with a variety of advanced cancer types. *Anticancer Res* 30(2): 623-628.

Check, J. H., Sansoucie, L., Chern, J., Amadi, N.&Katz, Y. (2009). Mifepristone treatment improves length and quality of survival of mice with spontaneous leukemia. *Anticancer Res* 29(8): 2977-2980.

Check, J. H., Sansoucie, L., Chern, J.&Dix, E. (2010b). Mifepristone treatment improves length and quality of survival of mice with spontaneous lung cancer. *Anticancer Res* 30(1): 119-122.

Conradie, R., Bruggeman, F. J., Ciliberto, A., Csikasz-Nagy, A., Novak, B., Westerhoff, H. V.&Snoep, J. L. (2010). Restriction point control of the mammalian cell cycle via the cyclin E/Cdk2:p27 complex. *FEBS J* 277(2): 357-367.

Deans, A. J., Khanna, K. K., McNees, C. J., Mercurio, C., Heierhorst, J.&McArthur, G. A. (2006). Cyclin-dependent kinase 2 functions in normal DNA repair and is a therapeutic target in BRCA1-deficient cancers. *Cancer Res* 66(16): 8219-8226.

Despierre, E., Lambrechts, D., Neven, P., Amant, F., Lambrechts, S.&Vergote, I. (2010). The molecular genetic basis of ovarian cancer and its roadmap towards a better treatment. *Gynecol Oncol* 117(2): 358-365.

Dioufa, N., Kassi, E., Papavassiliou, A. G.&Kiaris, H. (2010). Atypical induction of the unfolded protein response by mifepristone. *Endocrine* 38(2): 167-173.

DiSaia, P. J.&Bloss, J. D. (2003). Treatment of ovarian cancer: new strategies. *Gynecol Oncol* 90(2 Pt 2): S24-32.

Dressing, G. E., Goldberg, J. E., Charles, N. J., Schwertfeger, K. L.&Lange, C. A. (2011). Membrane progesterone receptor expression in mammalian tissues: A review of regulation and physiological implications. *Steroids* 76(1-2): 11-17.

Eisinger, S. H., Fiscella, J., Bonfiglio, T., Meldrum, S.&Fiscella, K. (2009). Open-label study of ultra low-dose mifepristone for the treatment of uterine leiomyomata. *Eur J Obstet Gynecol Reprod Biol* 146(2): 215-218.

El Etreby, M. F., Liang, Y., Johnson, M. H.&Lewis, R. W. (2000a). Antitumor activity of mifepristone in the human LNCaP, LNCaP-C4, and LNCaP-C4-2 prostate cancer models in nude mice. *Prostate* 42(2): 99-106.

El Etreby, M. F., Liang, Y.&Lewis, R. W. (2000b). Induction of apoptosis by mifepristone and tamoxifen in human LNCaP prostate cancer cells in culture. *Prostate* 43(1): 31-42.

El Etreby, M. F., Liang, Y., Wrenn, R. W.&Schoenlein, P. V. (1998). Additive effect of mifepristone and tamoxifen on apoptotic pathways in MCF-7 human breast cancer cells. *Breast Cancer Res Treat* 51(2): 149-168.

Erenpreisa, J.&Cragg, M. S. (2007). Cancer: a matter of life cycle? *Cell Biol Int* 31(12): 1507-1510.

Fedele, L.&Berlanda, N. (2004). Emerging drugs for endometriosis. *Expert Opin Emerg Drugs* 9(1): 167-177.

Fjelldal, R., Moe, B. T., Orbo, A.&Sager, G. (2010). MCF-7 cell apoptosis and cell cycle arrest: non-genomic effects of progesterone and mifepristone (RU-486). *Anticancer Res* 30(12): 4835-4840.

Flores, O., Wang, Z., Knudsen, K. E.&Burnstein, K. L. (2010). Nuclear targeting of cyclin-dependent kinase 2 reveals essential roles of cyclin-dependent kinase 2 localization and cyclin E in vitamin D-mediated growth inhibition. *Endocrinology* 151(3): 896-908.

Fraser, M., Leung, B. M., Yan, X., Dan, H. C., Cheng, J. Q.&Tsang, B. K. (2003). p53 is a determinant of X-linked inhibitor of apoptosis protein/Akt-mediated chemoresistance in human ovarian cancer cells. *Cancer Res* 63(21): 7081-7088.

Freeburg, E. M., Goyeneche, A. A., Seidel, E. E.&Telleria, C. M. (2009a). Resistance to cisplatin does not affect sensitivity of human ovarian cancer cell lines to mifepristone cytotoxicity. *Cancer Cell Int* 9: 4.

Freeburg, E. M., Goyeneche, A. A.&Telleria, C. M. (2009b). Mifepristone abrogates repopulation of ovarian cancer cells in between courses of cisplatin treatment. *Int J Oncol* 34(3): 743-755.

Gaddy, V. T., Barrett, J. T., Delk, J. N., Kallab, A. M., Porter, A. G.&Schoenlein, P. V. (2004). Mifepristone induces growth arrest, caspase activation, and apoptosis of estrogen receptor-expressing, antiestrogen-resistant breast cancer cells. *Clin Cancer Res* 10(15): 5215-5225.

Gamarra-Luques, C. D.&Telleria, C. M. (2010). Enhancement of the lethality of platinum-based therapy by antiprogestin mifepristone in ovarian cancer. *Cancer Epidemiology Biomarkers & Prevention* 19(10): Supplement 1, A113

Gellersen, B., Fernandes, M. S.&Brosens, J. J. (2009). Non-genomic progesterone actions in female reproduction. *Hum Reprod Update* 15(1): 119-138.

Gordon, A. N., Tonda, M., Sun, S.&Rackoff, W. (2004). Long-term survival advantage for women treated with pegylated liposomal doxorubicin compared with topotecan in a phase 3 randomized study of recurrent and refractory epithelial ovarian cancer. *Gynecol Oncol* 95(1): 1-8.

Goyeneche, A. A., Caron, R. W.&Telleria, C. M. (2007). Mifepristone inhibits ovarian cancer cell growth *in vitro* and *in vivo*. *Clin Cancer Res* 13(11): 3370-3379.

Goyeneche, A. A., Seidel, E. E.&Telleria, C. M. (2011). Growth inhibition induced by antiprogestins RU-38486, ORG-31710, and CDB-2914 in ovarian cancer cells involves inhibition of cyclin dependent kinase 2. *Invest New Drugs* [Published ahead of print].

Grunberg, S. M., Weiss, M. H., Russell, C. A., Spitz, I. M., Ahmadi, J., Sadun, A.&Sitruk-Ware, R. (2006). Long-term administration of mifepristone (RU486): clinical tolerance during extended treatment of meningioma. *Cancer Invest* 24(8): 727-733.

Grunberg, S. M., Weiss, M. H., Spitz, I. M., Ahmadi, J., Sadun, A., Russell, C. A., Lucci, L.&Stevenson, L. L. (1991). Treatment of unresectable meningiomas with the antiprogesterone agent mifepristone. *J Neurosurg* 74(6): 861-866.

Hamilton, T. C., Behrens, B. C., Louie, K. G.&Ozols, R. F. (1984). Induction of progesterone receptor with 17 beta-estradiol in human ovarian cancer. *J Clin Endocrinol Metab* 59(3): 561-563.

Han, S.&Sidell, N. (2003). RU486-induced growth inhibition of human endometrial cells involves the nuclear factor-kappa B signaling pathway. *J Clin Endocrinol Metab* 88(2): 713-719.

Havrilesky, L., Darcy, M., Hamdan, H., Priore, R. L., Leon, J., Bell, J.&Berchuck, A. (2003). Prognostic significance of p53 mutation and p53 overexpression in advanced epithelial ovarian cancer: a Gynecologic Oncology Group Study. *J Clin Oncol* 21(20): 3814-3825.

Hayakawa, J., Ohmichi, M., Kurachi, H., Ikegami, H., Kimura, A., Matsuoka, T., Jikihara, H., Mercola, D.&Murata, Y. (1999). Inhibition of extracellular signal-regulated protein kinase or c-Jun N-terminal protein kinase cascade, differentially activated by cisplatin, sensitizes human ovarian cancer cell line. *J Biol Chem* 274(44): 31648-31654.

Helleday, T., Petermann, E., Lundin, C., Hodgson, B.&Sharma, R. A. (2008). DNA repair pathways as targets for cancer therapy. *Nat Rev Cancer* 8(3): 193-204.

Herzog, T. J. (2006). The current treatment of recurrent ovarian cancer. *Curr Oncol Rep* 8(6): 448-454.

Ho, P. C., Yu Ng, E. H.&Tang, O. S. (2002). Mifepristone: contraceptive and non-contraceptive uses. *Curr Opin Obstet Gynecol* 14(3): 325-330.

Huang, H., Regan, K. M., Lou, Z., Chen, J.&Tindall, D. J. (2006). CDK2-dependent phosphorylation of FOXO1 as an apoptotic response to DNA damage. *Science* 314(5797): 294-297.

Huang, H.&Tindall, D. J. (2007). CDK2 and FOXO1: a fork in the road for cell fate decisions. *Cell Cycle* 6(8): 902-906.

Illidge, T. M., Cragg, M. S., Fringes, B., Olive, P.&Erenpreisa, J. A. (2000). Polyploid giant cells provide a survival mechanism for p53 mutant cells after DNA damage. *Cell Biol Int* 24(9): 621-633.

Jemal, A., Siegel, R., Ward, E., Murray, T., Xu, J., Smigal, C.&Thun, M. J. (2006). Cancer statistics, 2006. *CA Cancer J Clin* 56(2): 106-130.

Jurado, R., Lopez-Flores, A., Alvarez, A.&Garcia-Lopez, P. (2009). Cisplatin cytotoxicity is increased by mifepristone in cervical carcinoma: an in vitro and in vivo study. *Oncol Rep* 22(5): 1237-1245.

Kahmann, S., Vassen, L.&Klein-Hitpass, L. (1998). Synergistic enhancement of PRB-mediated RU486 and R5020 agonist activities through cyclic adenosine 3', 5'-monophosphate represents a delayed primary response. *Mol Endocrinol* 12(2): 278-289.

Katano, K., Kondo, A., Safaei, R., Holzer, A., Samimi, G., Mishima, M., Kuo, Y. M., Rochdi, M.&Howell, S. B. (2002). Acquisition of resistance to cisplatin is accompanied by changes in the cellular pharmacology of copper. *Cancer Res* 62(22): 6559-6565.

Keith Bechtel, M.&Bonavida, B. (2001). Inhibitory effects of 17beta-estradiol and progesterone on ovarian carcinoma cell proliferation: a potential role for inducible nitric oxide synthase. *Gynecol Oncol* 82(1): 127-138.

Kelland, L. (2007). The resurgence of platinum-based cancer chemotherapy. *Nat Rev Cancer* 7(8): 573-584.

Kettel, L. M., Murphy, A. A., Morales, A. J.&Yen, S. S. (1994). Clinical efficacy of the antiprogesterone RU486 in the treatment of endometriosis and uterine fibroids. *Hum Reprod* 9 Suppl 1: 116-120.

Kim, J. J.&Tannock, I. F. (2005). Repopulation of cancer cells during therapy: an important cause of treatment failure. *Nat Rev Cancer* 5(7): 516-525.

Kino, T., Manoli, I., Kelkar, S., Wang, Y., Su, Y. A.&Chrousos, G. P. (2009). Glucocorticoid receptor (GR) beta has intrinsic, GRalpha-independent transcriptional activity. *Biochem Biophys Res Commun* 381(4): 671-675.

Kloosterboer, H. J., Deckers, G. H., Schoonen, W. G., Hanssen, R. G., Rose, U. M., Verbost, P. M., Hsiu, J. G., Williams, R. F.&Hodgen, G. D. (2000). Preclinical experience with two selective progesterone receptor modulators on breast and endometrium. *Steroids* 65(10-11): 733-740.

Kvinlaug, B. T.&Huntly, B. J. (2007). Targeting cancer stem cells. *Expert Opin Ther Targets* 11(7): 915-927.

Lents, N. H., Keenan, S. M., Bellone, C.&Baldassare, J. J. (2002). Stimulation of the Raf/MEK/ERK cascade is necessary and sufficient for activation and Thr-160 phosphorylation of a nuclear-targeted CDK2. *J Biol Chem* 277(49): 47469-47475.

Levens, E. D., Potlog-Nahari, C., Armstrong, A. Y., Wesley, R., Premkumar, A., Blithe, D. L., Blocker, W.&Nieman, L. K. (2008). CDB-2914 for uterine leiomyomata treatment: a randomized controlled trial. *Obstet Gynecol* 111(5): 1129-1136.

Lewis-Tuffin, L. J., Jewell, C. M., Bienstock, R. J., Collins, J. B.&Cidlowski, J. A. (2007). Human glucocorticoid receptor beta binds RU-486 and is transcriptionally active. *Mol Cell Biol* 27(6): 2266-2282.

Li, D.-Q., Wang, Z.-B., Bai, J., Zhao, J., Wang, Y., Hu, K.&Du, Y.-H. (2004). Effects of mifepristone on proliferation of human gastric adenocarcinoma cell line SGC-7901 in vitro. *World Journal of Gastroenterology* 10(18): 2628-2631.

Li, Q., Yu, J. J., Mu, C., Yunmbam, M. K., Slavsky, D., Cross, C. L., Bostick-Bruton, F.&Reed, E. (2000). Association between the level of ERCC-1 expression and the repair of cisplatin-induced DNA damage in human ovarian cancer cells. *Anticancer Res* 20(2A): 645-652.

Liang, Y., Eid, M. A., El Etreby, F., Lewis, R. W.&Kumar, M. V. (2002). Mifepristone-induced secretion of transforming growth factor beta1-induced apoptosis in prostate cancer cells. *Int J Oncol* 21(6): 1259-1267.

Liang, Y., Hou, M., Kallab, A. M., Barrett, J. T., El Etreby, F.&Schoenlein, P. V. (2003). Induction of antiproliferation and apoptosis in estrogen receptor negative MDA-231 human breast cancer cells by mifepristone and 4-hydroxytamoxifen combination therapy: a role for TGFbeta1. *Int J Oncol* 23(2): 369-380.

Liberto, M.&Cobrinik, D. (2000). Growth factor-dependent induction of p21(CIP1) by the green tea polyphenol, epigallocatechin gallate. *Cancer Lett* 154(2): 151-161.

Liu, M., Wikonkal, N. M.&Brash, D. E. (1999). Induction of cyclin-dependent kinase inhibitors and G(1) prolongation by the chemopreventive agent N-acetylcysteine. *Carcinogenesis* 20(9): 1869-1872.

Liu, Y., Wang, L. L.&Deng, Y. (2003). Enhancement of antitumor effect of cisplatin against human ovarian carcinoma cells by mifepristone in vivo. *Di Yi Jun Yi Da Xue Xue Bao* 23(3): 242-244.

Lu, X., Errington, J., Curtin, N. J., Lunec, J.&Newell, D. R. (2001). The impact of p53 status on cellular sensitivity to antifolate drugs. *Clin Cancer Res* 7(7): 2114-2123.

Mack, P. C., Gandara, D. R., Lau, A. H., Lara, P. N., Jr., Edelman, M. J.&Gumerlock, P. H. (2003). Cell cycle-dependent potentiation of cisplatin by UCN-01 in non-small-cell lung carcinoma. *Cancer Chemother Pharmacol* 51(4): 337-348.

Mao, J., Regelson, W.&Kalimi, M. (1992). Molecular mechanism of RU 486 action: a review. *Mol Cell Biochem* 109(1): 1-8.

Martin, V. R. (2007). Ovarian cancer: an overview of treatment options. *Clin J Oncol Nurs* 11(2): 201-207.

Matsuda, Y., Kawamoto, K., Kiya, K., Kurisu, K., Sugiyama, K.&Uozumi, T. (1994). Antitumor effects of antiprogesterones on human meningioma cells in vitro and in vivo. *J Neurosurg* 80(3): 527-534.

McDonnel, A. C.&Murdoch, W. J. (2001). High-dose progesterone inhibition of urokinase secretion and invasive activity by SKOV-3 ovarian carcinoma cells: evidence for a receptor-independent nongenomic effect on the plasma membrane. *J Steroid Biochem Mol Biol* 78(2): 185-191.

Modesitt, S. C.&Jazaeri, A. A. (2007). Recurrent epithelial ovarian cancer: pharmacotherapy and novel therapeutics. *Expert Opin Pharmacother* 8(14): 2293-2305.

Moe, B. G., Vereide, A. B., Orbo, A.&Sager, G. (2009). High concentrations of progesterone and mifepristone mutually reinforce cell cycle retardation and induction of apoptosis. *Anticancer Res* 29(4): 1053-1058.

Moller, C., Hoffmann, J., Kirkland, T. A.&Schwede, W. (2008). Investigational developments for the treatment of progesterone-dependent diseases. *Expert Opin Investig Drugs* 17(4): 469-479.

Mukherjee, K., Syed, V.&Ho, S. M. (2005). Estrogen-induced loss of progesterone receptor expression in normal and malignant ovarian surface epithelial cells. *Oncogene* 24(27): 4388-4400.

Murphy, A. A., Morales, A. J., Kettel, L. M.&Yen, S. S. (1995). Regression of uterine leiomyomata to the antiprogesterone RU486: dose-response effect. *Fertil Steril* 64(1): 187-190.

Murphy, A. A., Zhou, M. H., Malkapuram, S., Santanam, N., Parthasarathy, S.&Sidell, N. (2000). RU486-induced growth inhibition of human endometrial cells. *Fertil Steril* 74(5): 1014-1019.

Musgrove, E. A., Lee, C. S., Cornish, A. L., Swarbrick, A.&Sutherland, R. L. (1997). Antiprogestin inhibition of cell cycle progression in T-47D breast cancer cells is accompanied by induction of the cyclin-dependent kinase inhibitor p21. *Mol Endocrinol* 11(1): 54-66.

Naora, H.&Montell, D. J. (2005). Ovarian cancer metastasis: integrating insights from disparate model organisms. *Nat Rev Cancer* 5(5): 355-366.

Narvekar, N., Cameron, S., Critchley, H. O., Lin, S., Cheng, L.&Baird, D. T. (2004). Low-dose mifepristone inhibits endometrial proliferation and up-regulates androgen receptor. *J Clin Endocrinol Metab* 89(5): 2491-2497.

O'Connor, P. M., Jackman, J., Bae, I., Myers, T. G., Fan, S., Mutoh, M., Scudiero, D. A., Monks, A., Sausville, E. A., Weinstein, J. N., Friend, S., Fornace, A. J., Jr.&Kohn, K. W. (1997). Characterization of the p53 tumor suppressor pathway in cell lines of the National Cancer Institute anticancer drug screen and correlations with the growth-inhibitory potency of 123 anticancer agents. *Cancer Res* 57(19): 4285-4300.

Oakley, R. H., Jewell, C. M., Yudt, M. R., Bofetiado, D. M.&Cidlowski, J. A. (1999). The dominant negative activity of the human glucocorticoid receptor beta isoform. Specificity and mechanisms of action. *J Biol Chem* 274(39): 27857-27866.

Ormerod, M. G., O'Neill, C., Robertson, D., Kelland, L. R.&Harrap, K. R. (1996). cis-Diamminedichloroplatinum(II)-induced cell death through apoptosis in sensitive and resistant human ovarian carcinoma cell lines. *Cancer Chemother Pharmacol* 37(5): 463-471.

Osipo, C., Liu, H., Meeke, K.&Jordan, V. C. (2004). The consequences of exhaustive antiestrogen therapy in breast cancer: estrogen-induced tumor cell death. *Exp Biol Med (Maywood)* 229(8): 722-731.

Ozols, R. F. (2006a). Challenges for chemotherapy in ovarian cancer. *Ann Oncol* 17 Suppl 5: v181-187.

Ozols, R. F. (2006b). Systemic therapy for ovarian cancer: current status and new treatments. *Semin Oncol* 33(2 Suppl 6): S3-11.

Parthasarathy, S., Morales, A. J.&Murphy, A. A. (1994). Antioxidant: a new role for RU-486 and related compounds. *J Clin Invest* 94(5): 1990-1995.

Pectasides, D., Psyrri, A., Pectasides, M.&Economopoulos, T. (2006). Optimal therapy for platinum-resistant recurrent ovarian cancer: doxorubicin, gemcitabine or topotecan? *Expert Opin Pharmacother* 7(8): 975-987.

Peluso, J. J., Liu, X., Saunders, M. M., Claffey, K. P.&Phoenix, K. (2008). Regulation of ovarian cancer cell viability and sensitivity to cisplatin by progesterone receptor membrane component-1. *J Clin Endocrinol Metab* 93(5): 1592-1599.

Philibert, D., Moguilewsky, M., Mary, I., Lecaque, D., Tournemine, C., Secchi, J.&Deraedt, R. (1985). Pharmacological profile of RU486 in animals. *The Antiprogesterone Steroid RU486 and Human Fertility Control.* E. E. Baulieu and S. J. Segal. NY, Plenum Press.

Poole, A. J., Li, Y., Kim, Y., Lin, S. C., Lee, W. H.&Lee, E. Y. (2006). Prevention of Brca1-mediated mammary tumorigenesis in mice by a progesterone antagonist. *Science* 314(5804): 1467-1470.

Puig, P. E., Guilly, M. N., Bouchot, A., Droin, N., Cathelin, D., Bouyer, F., Favier, L., Ghiringhelli, F., Kroemer, G., Solary, E., Martin, F.&Chauffert, B. (2008). Tumor cells can escape DNA-damaging cisplatin through DNA endoreduplication and reversible polyploidy. *Cell Biol Int* 32(9): 1031-1043.

Qin, T. N.&Wang, L. L. (2002). Enhanced sensitivity of ovarian cell line to cisplatin induced by mifepristone and its mechanism. *Di Yi Jun Yi Da Xue Xue Bao* 22(4): 344-346.

Rabik, C. A.&Dolan, M. E. (2007). Molecular mechanisms of resistance and toxicity associated with platinating agents. *Cancer Treat Rev* 33(1): 9-23.

Reid, T., Jin, X., Song, H., Tang, H. J., Reynolds, R. K.&Lin, J. (2004). Modulation of Janus kinase 2 by p53 in ovarian cancer cells. *Biochem Biophys Res Commun* 321(2): 441-447.

Roberts, C. P., Parthasarathy, S., Gulati, R., Horowitz, I.&Murphy, A. A. (1995). Effect of RU-486 and related compounds on the proliferation of cultured macrophages. *Am J Reprod Immunol* 34(4): 248-256.

Rocereto, T. F., Saul, H. M., Aikins, J. A., Jr.&Paulson, J. (2000). Phase II study of mifepristone (RU486) in refractory ovarian cancer. *Gynecol Oncol* 77(3): 429-432.

Rohe, H. J., Ahmed, I. S., Twist, K. E.&Craven, R. J. (2009). PGRMC1 (progesterone receptor membrane component 1): a targetable protein with multiple functions in steroid signaling, P450 activation and drug binding. *Pharmacol Ther* 121(1): 14-19.

Rose, F. V.&Barnea, E. R. (1996). Response of human ovarian carcinoma cell lines to antiprogestin mifepristone. *Oncogene* 12(5): 999-1003.

Rosen, D. G., Yang, G., Cai, K. Q., Bast, R. C., Jr., Gershenson, D. M., Silva, E. G.&Liu, J. (2005). Subcellular localization of p27kip1 expression predicts poor prognosis in human ovarian cancer. *Clin Cancer Res* 11(2 Pt 1): 632-637.

Sartorius, C. A., Tung, L., Takimoto, G. S.&Horwitz, K. B. (1993). Antagonist-occupied human progesterone receptors bound to DNA are functionally switched to transcriptional agonists by cAMP. *J Biol Chem* 268(13): 9262-9266.

Sasaki, H., Sheng, Y., Kotsuji, F.&Tsang, B. K. (2000). Down-regulation of X-linked inhibitor of apoptosis protein induces apoptosis in chemoresistant human ovarian cancer cells. *Cancer Res* 60(20): 5659-5666.

Schneider, C. C., Gibb, R. K., Taylor, D. D., Wan, T.&Gercel-Taylor, C. (1998). Inhibition of endometrial cancer cell lines by mifepristone (RU 486). *J Soc Gynecol Investig* 5(6): 334-338.

Schoenlein, P. V., Hou, M., Samaddar, J. S., Gaddy, V. T., Thangaraju, M., Lewis, J., Johnson, M., Ganapathy, V., Kallab, A.&Barrett, J. T. (2007). Downregulation of retinoblastoma protein is involved in the enhanced cytotoxicity of 4-hydroxytamoxifen plus mifepristone combination therapy versus antiestrogen monotherapy of human breast cancer. *Int J Oncol* 31(3): 643-655.

Scovassi, A. I.&Poirier, G. G. (1999). Poly(ADP-ribosylation) and apoptosis. *Mol Cell Biochem* 199(1-2): 125-137.

Selvakumaran, M., Pisarcik, D. A., Bao, R., Yeung, A. T.&Hamilton, T. C. (2003). Enhanced cisplatin cytotoxicity by disturbing the nucleotide excision repair pathway in ovarian cancer cell lines. *Cancer Res* 63(6): 1311-1316.

Shaw, T. J., Senterman, M. K., Dawson, K., Crane, C. A.&Vanderhyden, B. C. (2004). Characterization of intraperitoneal, orthotopic, and metastatic xenograft models of human ovarian cancer. *Mol Ther* 10(6): 1032-1042.

Siddik, Z. H., Mims, B., Lozano, G.&Thai, G. (1998). Independent pathways of p53 induction by cisplatin and X-rays in a cisplatin-resistant ovarian tumor cell line. *Cancer Res* 58(4): 698-703.

Smith, J. L., Kupchak, B. R., Garitaonandia, I., Hoang, L. K., Maina, A. S., Regalla, L. M.&Lyons, T. J. (2008). Heterologous expression of human mPRalpha, mPRbeta and mPRgamma in yeast confirms their ability to function as membrane progesterone receptors. *Steroids* 73(11): 1160-1173.

Sorenson, C. M., Barry, M. A.&Eastman, A. (1990). Analysis of events associated with cell cycle arrest at G2 phase and cell death induced by cisplatin. *J Natl Cancer Inst* 82(9): 749-755.

Spitz, I. M. (2006). Progesterone receptor antagonists. *Curr Opin Investig Drugs* 7(10): 882-890.

Steinauer, J., Pritts, E. A., Jackson, R.&Jacoby, A. F. (2004). Systematic review of mifepristone for the treatment of uterine leiomyomata. *Obstet Gynecol* 103(6): 1331-1336.

Sui, L., Dong, Y., Ohno, M., Sugimoto, K., Tai, Y., Hando, T.&Tokuda, M. (2001). Implication of malignancy and prognosis of p27(kip1), Cyclin E, and Cdk2 expression in epithelial ovarian tumors. *Gynecol Oncol* 83(1): 56-63.

Sundaram, M., Guernsey, D. L., Rajaraman, M. M.&Rajaraman, R. (2004). Neosis: a novel type of cell division in cancer. *Cancer Biol Ther* 3(2): 207-218.

Svensson, E. C., Markstrom, E., Shao, R., Andersson, M.&Billig, H. (2001). Progesterone receptor antagonists Org 31710 and RU 486 increase apoptosis in human periovulatory granulosa cells. *Fertil Steril* 76(6): 1225-1231.

Syed, V.&Ho, S. M. (2003). Progesterone-induced apoptosis in immortalized normal and malignant human ovarian surface epithelial cells involves enhanced expression of FasL. *Oncogene* 22(44): 6883-6890.

Syed, V., Mukherjee, K., Godoy-Tundidor, S.&Ho, S. M. (2007). Progesterone induces apoptosis in TRAIL-resistant ovarian cancer cells by circumventing c-FLIPL overexpression. *J Cell Biochem* 102(2): 442-452.

Syed, V., Ulinski, G., Mok, S. C., Yiu, G. K.&Ho, S. M. (2001). Expression of gonadotropin receptor and growth responses to key reproductive hormones in normal and malignant human ovarian surface epithelial cells. *Cancer Res* 61(18): 6768-6776.

Taniguchi, Y., Iwasaki, Y., Tsugita, M., Nishiyama, M., Taguchi, T., Okazaki, M., Nakayama, S., Kambayashi, M., Hashimoto, K.&Terada, Y. (2010). Glucocorticoid receptor-beta and receptor-gamma exert dominant negative effect on gene repression but not on gene induction. *Endocrinology* 151(7): 3204-3213.

Thomas, P., Pang, Y., Dong, J., Groenen, P., Kelder, J., de Vlieg, J., Zhu, Y.&Tubbs, C. (2007). Steroid and G protein binding characteristics of the seatrout and human progestin membrane receptor alpha subtypes and their evolutionary origins. *Endocrinology* 148(2): 705-718.

Tieszen, C. R., Goyeneche, A. A., Brandhagen, B. N., Ortbahn, C. T.&Telleria, C. M. (2011). Antiprogestin mifepristone inhibits the growth of cancer cells of reproductive and non-reproductive origin regardless of progesterone receptor expression. *BMC Cancer* 11(1): 207.

Tsvetkov, L. M., Yeh, K. H., Lee, S. J., Sun, H.&Zhang, H. (1999). p27(Kip1) ubiquitination and degradation is regulated by the SCF(Skp2) complex through phosphorylated Thr187 in p27. *Curr Biol* 9(12): 661-664.

Vakifahmetoglu, H., Olsson, M.&Zhivotovsky, B. (2008). Death through a tragedy: mitotic catastrophe. *Cell Death Differ* 15(7): 1153-1162.

Vasey, P. A. (2003). Resistance to chemotherapy in advanced ovarian cancer: mechanisms and current strategies. *Br J Cancer* 89 Suppl 3: S23-28.

Wang, D.&Lippard, S. J. (2005). Cellular processing of platinum anticancer drugs. *Nat Rev Drug Discov* 4(4): 307-320.

Wang, Q. E., Milum, K., Han, C., Huang, Y. W., Wani, G., Thomale, J.&Wani, A. A. (2011). Differential contributory roles of nucleotide excision and homologous recombination repair for enhancing cisplatin sensitivity in human ovarian cancer cells. *Mol Cancer* 10: 24.

Wiehle, R. D., Christov, K.&Mehta, R. (2007). Anti-progestins suppress the growth of established tumors induced by 7, 12-dimethylbenz(a)anthracene: comparison between RU486 and a new 21-substituted-19-nor-progestin. *Oncol Rep* 18(1): 167-174.

Wilailak, S.&Linasmita, V. (2004). A study of pegylated liposomal Doxorubicin in platinum-refractory epithelial ovarian cancer. *Oncology* 67(3-4): 183-186.

Xu, M., Song, L.&Wang, Z. (2003). Effects of Dexamethasone on glucocorticoid receptor expression in a human ovarian carcinoma cell line 3AO. *Chin Med J (Engl)* 116(3): 392-395.

Xu, Q., Takekida, S., Ohara, N., Chen, W., Sitruk-Ware, R., Johansson, E. D.&Maruo, T. (2005). Progesterone receptor modulator CDB-2914 down-regulates proliferative cell nuclear antigen and Bcl-2 protein expression and up-regulates caspase-3 and poly(adenosine 5'-diphosphate-ribose) polymerase expression in cultured human uterine leiomyoma cells. *J Clin Endocrinol Metab* 90(2): 953-961.

Yaginuma, Y.&Westphal, H. (1992). Abnormal structure and expression of the p53 gene in human ovarian carcinoma cell lines. *Cancer Res* 52(15): 4196-4199.

Yokoyama, Y., Shinohara, A., Takahashi, Y., Wan, X., Takahashi, S., Niwa, K.&Tamaya, T. (2000). Synergistic effects of danazol and mifepristone on the cytotoxicity of UCN-01 in hormone-responsive breast cancer cells. *Anticancer Res* 20(5A): 3131-3135.

Yudt, M. R., Jewell, C. M., Bienstock, R. J.&Cidlowski, J. A. (2003). Molecular origins for the dominant negative function of human glucocorticoid receptor beta. *Mol Cell Biol* 23(12): 4319-4330.

Zhang, S., Jonklaas, J.&Danielsen, M. (2007). The glucocorticoid agonist activities of mifepristone (RU486) and progesterone are dependent on glucocorticoid receptor levels but not on EC50 values. *Steroids* 72(6-7): 600-608.

Zhao, J., Kennedy, B. K., Lawrence, B. D., Barbie, D. A., Matera, A. G., Fletcher, J. A.&Harlow, E. (2000). NPAT links cyclin E-Cdk2 to the regulation of replication-dependent histone gene transcription. *Genes Dev* 14(18): 2283-2297.

12

Sexuality After Ovarian Cancer Therapy

Juliane Farthmann and Annette Hasenburg
University Hospital, Dept. of Gynecology, Freiburg
Germany

1. Introduction

Patients who are diagnosed with cancer are mainly concerned about the chance of being cured. Long-term aspects of quality of life seem second rate at this moment due to the fear of death and sickness and the patient´s urgent desire to survive. Interests or aims in life, which were important before the diagnosis of a life threatening disease can be completely changed. Doctors tend to concentrate on the necessary therapeutic steps and do not want to overrun the patient with assumed "unimportant" information e.g. the influence of the disease and treatment on sexual function.

Approximately 10% of patients get confronted with ovarian cancer when they are premenopausal (Edmondson et al. 2001). Also for older patients an active sexual life can be important and might be impaired by the disease and therapy (Braehler et al. 1994).

Sexuality can imply different things to different people, the extent to which patients are affected varies significantly, and health care professionals should assess each patient carefully according to her needs (Jefferies et al. 2004, Aerts et al. 2009).

In an evaluation by Stead, although most health care professionals thought that the majority of women with ovarian cancer would experience a sexual problem, only one out of four doctors and one of five nurses discussed sexual topics with their patients. Reasons for not addressing these problems included embarrassment, lack of knowledge of the topic, lack of experience discussing the topic and lack of resources, such as professionals with training in sexual medicine to provide support, if needed (Stead et al. 2003, Hasenburg et al. 2011).

Important elements of quality of life may be affected by ovarian cancer. The impact of the disease on sexuality is determined by multiple factors. Not only can the diagnosis and treatment of ovarian cancer cause sexual problems, but also psychological distress, vulnerable body image and an altered relationship with a partner can diminish overall sexual well-being (Sadovsky et al. 2009).

For example, 62% of patients complain of dyspareunia and 75% of orgasmic dysfunction after therapy for ovarian cancer (Taylor et al. 2004). The significance of radical pelvic and para-aortal lymph node dissection with regard to sexual arousal disorders is not yet well defined. Depending on the patient´s individual history and present circumstances in life (married, single etc.) these effects can differ considerably.

A small percentage of patients desire pregnancy. They are especially affected. Only in selected cases a fertility preserving therapy can be offered. Patients with borderline tumors of the ovary have a much better overall survival but often still need a bilateral salpingo-oophorectomy with long-term consequences (GCP Guideline on ovarian cancer 2007, in German).

This chapter will elucidate the impact of ovarian cancer and the necessary therapy on women´s quality of life and sexuality and will give helpful recommendations how treating physicians can include this aspect. The aim of this article is to call attention to the subject of sexual function in cancer patients and to provide management strategies. The general and disease-specific changes of sexual function caused by oncologic therapies are outlined.

2. Ovarian cancer (OC) therapy

Apart from the psychological aspects of the diagnosis, there are many physical changes due to OC therapy. OC still being the most aggressive tumor of the female genital tract is a very severe threat to the woman´s life and in many cases it cannot be cured. Due to the lack of screening possibilities, OC in most cases is diagnosed at an advanced stage (Jemal et al. 2010). State of the art treatment includes optimal tumor debulking with a following combination therapy of taxol and carboplatinum (GCP Guideline on ovarian cancer 2007, in German). Overall survival with this therapy has been mostly unchanged over the years and is the worst among gynaecological tumors (Jemal et al. 2010). In advanced stages the five year survival does not exceed 40% (Hanker et al. 2010) Therapy is long and strenuous but it is the only chance for cure. After relapse, many patients have to live with ovarian cancer as a chronic disease for many years, but most of the time they are under therapy. Therefore, aspects of quality of life are of major importance.

2.1 Surgical therapy: Influence on sexuality

It is widely accepted that the radicality of the surgical approach increases the chance of the patient to be cured (Bristow et al. 2002). Optimal tumor debulking should be the goal of every surgery. The surgical approach for OC comprises a longitudinal laparotomy from the symphysis to the xyphoid, hysterectomy, bilateral salpingoophorectomy, infragastric omentectomy, pelvic and paraaortal lymphadenectomy and, if necessary bowel resection etc. (GCP Guideline on ovarian cancer 2007, in German). The operation results in a sudden onset of menopause in premenopausal patients, but also has negative side effects on the sexuality of postmenopausal patients. Thus, prior to therapy, it is important to inform the patient about all possible side effects including those on sexual function. Many patients will experience the side effects of their therapy without prior counselling in the course of their disease.

After therapy of ovarian cancer, 75% of patients have difficulties to reach orgasm (Taylor et al. 2004). It has not been clarified whether this results from the severity of the disease, the chemotherapy or from the pelvic and para-aortic lymphadenectomy. The latter could cause damage to the autonomic nerves, comparable to prostate cancer surgery in men (Madeb et al. 2007). A current study from the "AGO-Ovar" (working group on gynecological oncology) is supposed to resolve this question: the LION-PAW study, a substudy of the LION Study (Lymphadenectomy In Ovarian Neoplasm) - (PAW = Pleasure Ability of Women), has the aim to clarify to which extent a radical lymphadenectomy affects the women's sexual function (ClinicalTrials.gov Identifier: NCT00712218).

If the patient seems to be dissatisfied with her sexual life, it has to be evaluated whether she suffers from a hypoactive sexual desire disorder (HSDD, American Psychiatric Association, 1987), which is defined as a deficiency or absence of sexual fantasies and desire for sexual activity. There is little initiative on the patient´s side, and sexual intercourse is rare. Stead (2003) and Taylor (2004) reported a prevalence of HSDD between 47% and 67% in clinical studies of ovarian cancer patients. Interestingly, Raboch et al. (1985) even saw a decrease of libido of 42% and of sexual intercourse of 30% in women after hysterectomy and salpingo-ophorectomy for benign causes. Therefore it seems that sexual problems are mainly influenced by the salpingo-oophorectomy and the following loss of hormone production and are not only due to the diagnosis of cancer.

A large study about sexual activity in patients after ovarian cancer therapy was performed by Taylor et al. (2004) at the MD Anderson Cancer Center. Patients who contacted the center during or after ovarian cancer therapy filled in the Sexual Activity Questionnaire (SAQ). This questionnaire comprises questions about pleasure, arousal, orgasm or sexual activity in general. 50% of the 233 women, who were included, were sexually active at least once a month, especially if they were married ($p < 0.001$) and under 56 years of age ($p< 0.001$) and did not receive cancer specific therapy at this time. Identification with the own body also had a positive impact on sexual activity ($p < 0.004$). 80% of the sexually active women reported vaginal dryness, 40% very strong. 62% complained about pain or discomfort during intercourse. 75% had problems with orgasm, a third of the women almost always. Correlating these results with the physical performance status of the women, lower sexual activity correlated with low performance status and depressive disorders. Regarding vaginal dryness and problems with penetration there was no difference whether the patients were currently under therapy or not. Those patients who were sexually inactive had the following reasons for being inactive: 44% missing partner, 38% lack of interest, 23% physical problems, 10% suffered from the fatigue syndrome (Taylor et al. 2004).

Aerts et al. showed in a retrospective study of fifty women after pelvic surgery for gynaecological cancer that significantly more patients reported sexual problems than controls (83% vs 20%), including decreased desire and impaired vaginal lubrication. Pelvic surgery was specifically related to changed intensity of orgasm, reduced vaginal sensitivity and elasticity, dyspareunia and vaginal narrowing and shortening (Aerts et al 2009, Hasenburg et al. 2011).

2.2 Chemotherapy: Influence on sexuality

Chemotherapy or, in advanced stages, anti-hormonal therapy are a very important part of ovarian cancer therapy. Side effects such as the fatigue syndrome in at least 10% of the women or coexisting depressive disorders are common in 21-25% of the patients and may additionally affect the sexual life of a patient (Taylor et al. 2004, Arden-Close et al. 2008, Reich et al. 2008). Other side effects are nausea and vomiting, weight loss, and also pain (Oskay-Oezcelik et al. 2010). Obviously, in this situation, sexual life becomes less important. But even if the woman does not suffer from a lack of desire, a changed body image due to a long scar on her abdomen or more importantly alopecia may make her feel less attractive. Also with her long-term partner she may be uncomfortable and afraid to present herself.

3. Special patient groups

3.1 The premenopausal patient

Cancer affecting young women prior to completing family planning represents a struggle for the patient and her partner as well as for the caring physician. Cancer treatment does not only impair sexual function and body image, but also the reproductive function with a premature menopause, e.g. the onset of menopause before the age of 40 (Beckmann et al. 2006). Women who are premenopausal at the time of diagnosis are especially affected as the physical changes are more pronounced than in older patients. A sudden onset of menopause has a much higher occurrence of depression, hot flashes and other postmenopausal symptoms than in the natural course of menopause (Gupta et al. 2006). Patients may experience premature menopause including symptoms such as mood swings, hot flashes, libido loss and insufficient lubrication. Therefore, a hormone replacement therapy should be recommended (Michaelson-Cohen et al 2009).

A fertility conserving approach is possible for selected patients with early stage ovarian cancer and with germ cell tumors of the ovary (Gershenson et al. 2007, Wright et al. 2009). However, young patients are often faced with the fact that fertility cannot be preserved and the wish to have children cannot be fulfilled. Aims in life have to be changed and the whole concept of life has to be reconsidered. In this situation sexuality at first sight is out of focus.

Especially for women, who were either planning to have children or had not given family planning much thought yet, especially if they were single at the time of diagnosis, it is the clinician's responsibility to communicate the cancer-associated issues but also the consequences the therapeutic interventions may have on the patient's fertility. A multidisciplinary approach is necessary and the patient should be advised to visit a fertility centre prior to therapy initiation. Information about different fertility preservation options and contact data of fertility centres can be obtained from the network FertiPROTEKT (www.fertiprotekt.de, in German).

The emotional and physical impact of loss of fertility can be complex and long lasting for women, who are experiencing high levels of distress, menopausal symptoms, and changes in sexual function persisting into survivorship. Alternative family-building strategies like adoption have to be explored before and/or during treatment (Carter et al. 2010). Especially for these patients psycho-oncological counselling should be offered (Hasenburg et al. 2011).

3.2 Borderline tumors of the ovary (BOT)

Patients with borderline tumors of the ovary have a much better prognosis and a higher chance of being cured than patients with ovarian cancer. Therefore, the long-term aspects of therapy are especially important. Most of the patients do not receive chemotherapy, but in most cases both ovaries and the uterus have to be removed (Cadron et al. 2009). For some cases, a fertility preserving operation is possible, but close follow-up is necessary.

3.3 Palliation

Even with the therapeutic progress for ovarian cancer during the last decade, most patients with advanced disease cannot be cured and often live in a palliative situation for months and years. They receive chemotherapy with the possible side effects of fatigue syndrome, sleeping disorders, nausea and vomiting, depression etc. which are additionally aggravated by the consuming disease itself.

The idea of palliation is to maintain quality of life with all aspects as long as possible. Just because a patient has a life threatening disease does no imply that she does not longer wish to live her sexual feelings or to convey expressions of her sexuality (Jefferies et al. 2004).

The importance of sexuality even in a palliative situation was recently described by Vitrano et al. (2011). 65 patients admitted to an acute pain relief or palliative care unit were asked about the role of sexuality in their lives. The patients had a mean Karnofsky index of 58 (range 40-70) and a mean well-being sensation of 5.67 (range 2-10). In summary, 60% of patients did not feel to be less attractive with their disease, 30% of patients felt a little, and only 10% very much less attractive. Most patients (86.4%) considered a dialogue about sexuality and to face such an issue with skilled people as important. About half of the patients (47%) reported that sexuality was very important for their psychological well-being. Only 7.6% of patients had satisfactory sexual intercourse, 15.2% had little activity, 39.4% had an insufficient activity, and 37.8% did not have any activity. A significant relationship was observed with age (p= 0.002), Karnofsky status (p = .024), and well-being (p = .004). Only 12.1% of patients were sexually satisfied, 12.1% experienced a mild satisfaction, 30.3% had insufficient satisfaction, and 45.5% had no sexual satisfaction. Only 3% of patients had a satisfactory frequency of intercourse, 45.5% had a low or limited frequency, and 51.5% had no sexual intercourse. For 50% of the patients emotional aspects were very important and for 12.1% important. The emotional aspects had a relevant role in sexuality, possibly as a surrogate of impaired physical activity (Vitrano et al. 2011). This survey clearly shows the ongoing importance of maintaining sexual life, even in a palliative situation.

Understanding palliation "as making life easier" and more valuable for a person with a non-curable disease, is an important mission.

4. Changes due to therapy (surgery and chemotherapy)

4.1 Impairment of body image

Treatment of ovarian cancer is multimodal, which makes it necessary to differentiate between the side effects of the various therapeutic interventions. Stigmata may be obvious to others like alopecia, scars, a preternatural anus or a urostomy. These can greatly alter the patient's body image and self-esteem. The patient's situation before the disease - whether the integrity of the body has been an important aspect for the woman - may have an impact on the coping process.

Somatic and psychological problems of sexual dysfunction are difficult to differentiate and are inter-dependent. If the patient manages to accept the disease and the associated physical changes, it is easier for her to return to a satisfactory quality of life including sexual function. The mental situation of the patient can be especially impaired, if there had been psychological injuries or traumata in the past, which can be reactivated during her course of the disease, especially if there is a lack of help by the partner, family or friends (Hasenburg 2008).

A partner can often be affected by helplessness and passivity. Due to false considerations, the couple might not talk about these issues, thus, a vicious circle may develop (see Fig. 1). On the other hand, the disease can be used as a chance to intensify the relationship (Rowland et al. 2009).

4.2 Psychological problems

A co-existing depression should be thoroughly assessed. Approximately one out of four cancer patients has any type of depression and at least half of those are willing to accept professional help or referral for this issue (Curry et al. 2002, Passik et al. 1998).

It might be difficult to differentiate between a fatigue syndrome or depressive symptoms. Patients suffering from depression should be offered antidepressive therapy. Some of the antidepressive agents can induce a lack of desire, but a severe depression can also impair sexual functioning. Specific pharmacotherapy may be necessary and the depression should not be treated with hormones alone. Often it is sufficient to take the antidepressive medication for a few weeks and both the mental situation as well as the sexual desire can improve over the course of treatment. If overall well-being increases, sexual life and the relationship may experience benefit (Hasenburg et al. 2008).

4.3 Partnership

There is some information about the effect of a cancer diagnosis or other severe illnesses on relation- and partnerships. Bhatti et al. (2011) reported about the impact of chronic diseases on major life changing decisions like marriage, divorce, childbearing etc. It is suggested that the poor health from a spouse at a young age may cause marriage breakup over time.

For a couple with early stage disease and the option of fertility sparing surgery, the decision to intend to have a child is difficult due to the fear of recurrence (Bhatti et al. 2011).

Glantz et al. (2009) described that the risk of being abandoned by the partner after surviving a severe disease is especially higher for women (20.8%) than for men (2.9%). When counselling a patient with cancer, the partner should not be neglected, who often does not know how to support his wife. This may lead to misunderstandings, and a vicious cycle. As reported by Hasenburg et al. (2011) women with gynaecological cancer often report being fearful of signalling (unintentionally) a desire for sexual intimacy, when they are merely attempting to create emotional proximity in their partner relationship. In order to avoid this miscommunication, women distance themselves from their wish for emotional intimacy, often resulting in an increased sense of loneliness during illness and the period of recovery, and hence reduced quality of life. Most women would also have appreciated their partner being informed about the possible side-effects on sexuality and partner relationship (Corney et al. 1994). Raising the topic of psychological, relational and sexual functioning by health care providers could help to ease the way for a more freely flowing discussion of this topic between health professionals, patients and their partners and could give patients the opportunity to improve their coping strategies and reduce anxiety (Janda et al. 2004).

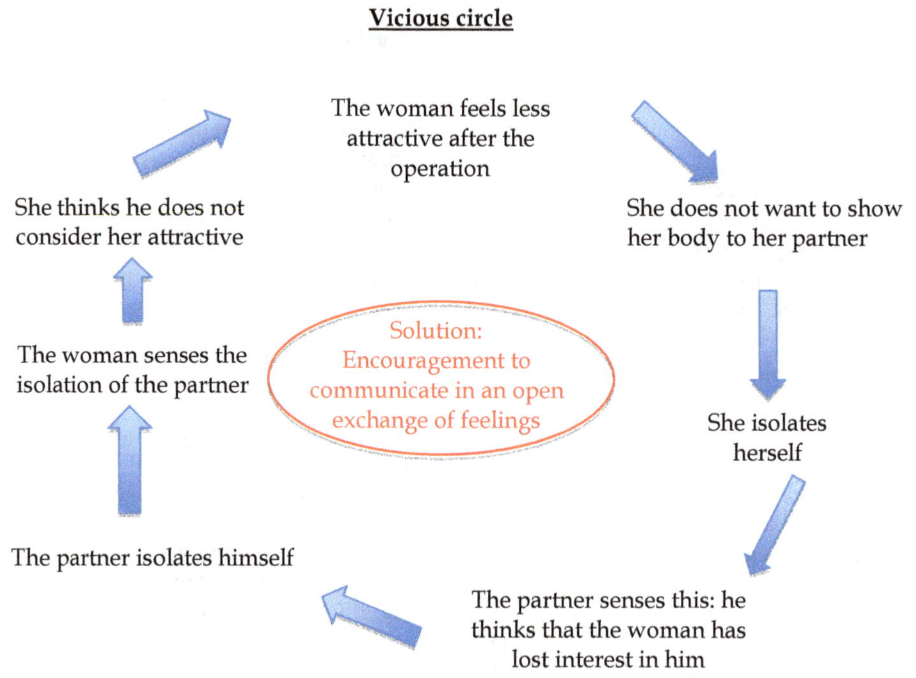

Vicious circle

The woman feels less attractive after the operation

She does not want to show her body to her partner

She isolates herself

The partner senses this: he thinks that the woman has lost interest in him

The partner isolates himself

The woman senses the isolation of the partner

She thinks he does not consider her attractive

Solution: Encouragement to communicate in an open exchange of feelings

Fig. 1. Vicious cycle.

The aspect of sexual minority women (SMW) like patients with homosexual relationships should not be ignored. There has been some research in this field, and the review of Boehmer et al. (2009) indicated that partnerships of SMW are not directly comparable with heterosexual ones. It seems that SMW may experience less disruption in their sexual relationships like fewer sexual problems such as decreased lubrication, reduced quality and quantity of orgasm, impaired body image, and experience more understanding and supportive partners compared to heterosexual women (Boehmer et al. 2009). However, in SMW there can be problems to obtain information and support from medical professionals with respect to sexual functioning. Sexual functioning may be worse among subgroups of sexual minority women (Boehmer et al. 2009). For example, Mc Gregor found that internalized homophobia was associated with a higher level of distress in lesbians with breast cancer (Mc Gregor et al. 2001).

5. What can the physician do?

Counselling ovarian cancer patients about sexuality, the first step is to evaluate the patient´s sexual life before the onset of the disease. Cancer and cancer treatment can exacerbate former sexual function problems and can also create new ones. As sexual dysfunction may be present in healthy individuals, these issues can often be overlooked initially. Awareness of these potential problems will help the patient to adapt to post treatment difficulties such as fatigue syndrome, and body image impairment by the above mentioned reasons. A pretreatment discussion of sexuality and intimacy provides a baseline for comparison with the subsequent re-evaluation during and after treatment (Grzankowski 2011).

People have different opinions about what is normal, so the doctor has to evaluate whether the patient has been satisfied with her sexual life in the past. Questions like "Has anything changed in your sexuality after the diagnosis of your disease?" are very helpful to ascertain if there is any need to go deeper into this topic. Asking "How were your sexual desires recently? How was it on your partner´s side?" also help to start talking. For some patients the cancer diagnosis can even be used as an excuse to refrain from being sexually active, they therefore refuse professional help (Hasenburg et al. 2011).

According to the Pfizer Global Study (2002) 80% of cancer patients would like to have more information about the impact of their illness and subsequent therapy on their sexuality. 91% of the cancer patients were afraid to ask their treating physician about sexual problems, and even 97% of the doctors did not inform their patients about possible sexual dysfunction. These findings emphasize that there is a great need for intensive training in communication skills. Physicians have to learn how to actively approach this distressing issue. Furthermore they have to be aware that the way of addressing sexual problems and counselling might be influenced by their own sexual experience (Hasenburg et al. 2008). When talking about sexuality issues, the doctor should try to find the patients language and wording, so that it is easier for her to talk about these problems. Medical technical terms should be avoided, if possible.

For women, sexuality might stand for intimacy and tenderness, instead for sexual intercourse only. The treating physician has to identify the special problem for each woman and can help her to cope with losing sexual and erotic potency (Hasenburg et al. 2008).

It is of major importance to sensitize physicians working with ovarian cancer patients to the issues of quality of life and sexuality. Each patient has to be informed about the long-term consequences of the disease and the scheduled therapy. Although sexuality is a taboo subject, the potential long-term consequences of oncological therapy on sexual function, possibly on fertility and quality of life have to be considered and discussed with the patient. Patients need to understand that problems in sexual function do not imply a general failure of the person.

The doctor has a role-model function and should address these issues frankly, making it clear to the patient that sexuality is an important aspect of quality of life. A special training in sexual medicine may be helpful but it is not mandatory.

5.1 Hormone Replacement Therapy (HRT)

The role of hormone replacement therapy is often controversially discussed (Jefferies et al. 2004, Mørch et al. 2009). After ovarian cancer therapy, premenopausal patients are likely to suffer from premature onset of menopause, while postmenopausal patients may suffer from libido loss. Sudden onset of menopause can cause more severe symptoms such as postoperative depressive episodes, hot flashes, mood changes and long-term consequences such as osteoporosis or sexual dysfunction due to sudden hormone deprivation than the gradually beginning menopause. This implies that in these patients a hormone replacement therapy should be considered and discussed even prior to surgery.

In older patients a reduction of desire can be due to the lack of androgens after bilateral salpingo-oophorectomy. The stromal cells and the hilar interstitial cells in the ovaries are essential for the synthesis of androgens (testosterone and androstendione) which, among other factors, preserve a woman's libido after menopause (Fogle et al. 2007). Thus, the side effects of cancer treatment on the gonads can hurt all age groups. Androgens can be replaced by transdermal testosterone substitution (Buster et al. 2005, Davis et al. 2008). In the study of Shifren et al. (2009) a significant rise in sexual interest and activity could be shown after androgen replacement for women after hysterectomy and bilateral salpingo-oophorectomy for benign disease. However, oncological safety is yet unclear and androgen replacement can not be recommended up to now.

Estrogen substitution is important to ameliorate hot flashes, osteoporosis, vaginal dryness and other postmenopausal symptoms. The largest study on this topic from Sweden on 649 patients with OC and 150 with borderline tumors of the ovary, aged between 50 and 74 years showed that neither pre- nor postoperative HRT affected overall survival, nor the kind of HRT administered (multivariate hazard ratio = 0.57; 95%-CI: 0.42-0.78), (Mascarenhas et al. 2006). In a second study of postmenopausal patients with ovarian cancer, HRT treatment was also not associated with an increased risk of recurrence (Michaelson-Cohen et al. 2009).

As an alternative to orally administered HRT, estradiol can be substituted with oestrogen patches or a vaginal ring (Estring®). The systemic effects with the latter are reduced while local oestrogen effects are sufficient (Henriksson et al. 1996). Serum levels are higher with oestrogen patches than with the vaginal ring (Gupta et al. 2008). In ovarian cancer, there is no contraindication for local oestrogen therapy (GCP Guideline on ovarian cancer 2007, in German).

If the quality of life is reduced due to oestrogen deprivation secondary to ovarian cancer, hormone therapy with sex steroids can be initiated after a careful risk-benefit assessment

(Michaelson-Cohen et al. 2009). In patients with an endometrioid histology, low-dose-oestrogens should be combined with a progesterone therapy (GCP Guideline on ovarian cancer 2007, in German).

5.2 Alternatives for HRT

For patients suffering from postmenopausal symptoms with a contraindication against HRT or who refuse HRT, there are alternative therapeutic options. The main symptoms need to be identified, so these can specifically be addressed.

There is a great choice of herbal and homeopathic medicines with a significant placebo effect leading to a reduction of postmenopausal symptoms in up to 20% of the patients (Tempfer et al. 2007). However, alternative drugs should not be taken without medical advice. The risks and side effects of these medications have not been completely investigated. Food supplements containing isoflavone in soy or red clover could slightly improve hot flashes (GCP guideline on hormone replacement therapy by the German Society of Gynecology & Obstetrics, in German; Wuttke et al. 2008, Haimov-Kochmann et al. 2008).

In order to prevent osteoporosis in premenopausal patients with a sudden onset of menopause vitamin D (1000 IE/d), a daily supplement of calcium (1500mg/d), physical exercise and abstinence from nicotine are recommended (GCP guideline on osteoporosis 2009, in German). In patients with preexisting osteoporosis bisphosphonates should be administered (Reid 2009).

5.3 Pharmaceutical alternatives

If hot flashes and sleep disorders persist, antidepressants can be an option (selective serotonin reuptake inhibitors, SSRI) (Bordeleau et al. 2010). With e.g. 75 mg venlafaxine daily a reduction of hot flashes of approximately 60% was observed compared to 20% with placebo (Pachman et al. 2010). Another possibility are anticonvulsive (e.g. gabapentin) or antihypertensive agents (clonidin, methyldopa) (Hall et al. 2011).

A survey of the medications showed the following reductions of hot flashes (Sideras et al. 2010):

- Venlafaxine: 33% reduction of symptoms; 37.5 bis 75mg/d
- Paroxetine: 41% reduction of symptoms; 20mg/d
- Fluoxetine: 13% reduction of symptoms; 20mg/d
- Sertraline: 3 to 18% reduction of symptoms, 50mg/d
- Gabapentin: 45 to 50% reduction of symptoms, 900mg/d

5.4 Vaginal dilators

Patients who have undergone surgical shortening of the vagina, radiation therapy of the pelvis or brachy-therapy should be informed about the available treatment options for vaginal strictures or adhesions to preserve the patient's ability for cohabitation. These include the use of vaginal dilators or bepanthen tampons which can be combined with oestrogen-containing lotions or lubricants. Treatment can be initiated four to six weeks after therapy (GCP Guideline on diagnosis and therapy of cervical cancer 2008, in German). It is important to use the vaginal dilators regularly (e.g. Dilator Set®), even if the patient is not in a relationship, because dilatation becomes increasingly difficult with time. Accompanying pelvic floor muscle training can be recommended and results in gain over muscle identification, control and strength (Derzko et al. 2007). Possible fears of the patient such as manipulating her own genitals or resuming of sexual intercourse should be actively discussed.

6. Conclusion

The potential impact of ovarian cancer therapy such as surgery, chemotherapy or even radiation therapy on sexual function and fertility needs to be discussed with each patient. Even for women in a palliative setting, sexuality and intimacy should be an issue.

Impaired sexual function after treatment of ovarian cancer is a common problem and represents a significant limitation of quality of life. While for younger patients infertility and early postmenopausal symptoms may be of major concern, postmenopausal women might consider the loss of the remaining androgen function of the ovaries as most striking. The significance of radical pelvic and para-aortic lymphadenectomy for sexual function remains unclear.

Local or systemic oestrogen therapy subsequent to treatment of ovarian cancer is considered an adequate treatment of postmenopausal symptoms. Apart from symptomatic therapy, physical interventions (e.g. physiotherapy) and physical activity should be included as supportive actions. For patients with an underlying depressive condition an antidepressive medication should be taken into account, even if only for a limited time.

Health care providers have a model function when discussing therapy-induced changes of sexual function and should regard sexuality as an essential element of quality of life. Therefore, the possible treatment side effects, including therapeutic or preventive options, and the quality of life after cancer must be discussed with the patient prior to therapy initiation. By understanding that sexuality is an important and normal aspect of life and not a "luxury issue" even for patients with a non-curable disease, treating physicians can support their patients and help them to maintain a good or at least acceptable quality of life.

7. GCP guidelines

1. Interdisciplinary guideline of the German Cancer society and the German Society of Gynecology and Obstetrics on diagnosis and therapy of malignant ovarian tumors. In German, 2007. www.awmf.org/leitlinien/detail/ll/032-035.html
2. Interdisciplinary guideline of the German Cancer society and the German Society of Gynecology and Obstetrics on diagnosis and therapy of cervical cancer. In German, 2008. www.awmf.org/leitlinien/detail/ll/032-033.html
3. Interdisciplinary guideline of the German Osteoporosis Society on prophylaxis, diagnosis and therapy of osteoporosis. In German, 2009. ww.awmf.org/leitlinien/detail/ll/034-003.html
4. Interdisciplinary guideline of the German Society of Gynecology and Obstetrics on hormone therapy in peri- and postmenopausal women. In German, 2009. ww.awmf.org/leitlinien/detail/ll/ 015-062.html

8. References

[1] Aerts L, Enzlin P, Verhaeghe J et al. Sexual and psychological functioning in women after pelvic surgery for gynaecological cancer. European journal of gynaecological oncology. 2009;30: 652-6.

[2] Arden-Close E, Gidron Y, Moss-Morris R. Psychological distress and its correlates in ovarian cancer: a systematic review. Psychooncology. 2008 Nov;17(11):1061-72. Review.

[3] Bhatti Z, Salek M, Finlay A. Chronic diseases influence major life changing decisions: a new domain in quality of life research. J R Soc Med. 2011 Jun;104(6):241-50.

[4] Buster JE, Kingsberg SA, Aguirre O et al. Testosterone patch for low sexual desire in surgically menopausal women: a randomized trial. Obstet Gynecol 2005; 105: 944-952.

[5] Boehmer U, Potter J, Bowen DJ. Sexual functioning after cancer in sexual minority women. Cancer J. 2009 Jan-Feb;15(1):65-9.

[6] Bordeleau L, Pritchard KI, Loprinzi CL, Ennis M, Jugovic O, Warr D, Haq R, Goodwin PJ. Multicenter, randomized, cross-over clinical trial of venlafaxine versus gabapentin for the management of hot flashes in breast cancer survivors. J Clin Oncol. 2010 Dec 10;28(35):5147-52. Epub 2010 Nov 8.

[7] Brähler E, Unger U. Sexual activity in advanced age in the context of gender, family status and personality aspects-results of a representative survey. Z Gerontol. 1994 Mar-Apr;27(2):110-5.

[8] Bristow RE, Tomacruz RS, Armstrong DK, Trimble EL, Montz FJ. Survival effect of maximal cytoreductive surgery for advanced ovarian carcinoma during the platinum era: a meta-analysis. J Clin Oncol. 2002 Mar 1;20(5):1248-59.

[9] Cadron I, Leunen K, Van Gorp T, Amant F, Neven P, Vergote I. Management of borderline ovarian neoplasms. J Clin Oncol. 2007 Jul 10;25(20):2928-37. Review.

[10] Carter J, Goldfrank D, Schover LR. J Sex Med. Simple strategies for vaginal health promotion in cancer survivors. 2011 Feb;8(2):549-59. doi: 10.1111/j.1743-6109.2010.01988.x. Epub 2010 Aug 16.

[11] Carter J, Chi DS, Brown CL, Abu-Rustum NR, Sonoda Y, Aghajanian C, Levine DA, Baser RE, Raviv L, Barakat RR. Cancer-related infertility in survivorship. Int J Gynecol Cancer. 2010 Jan;20(1):2-8. Review.

[12] Corney RH, Crowther ME, Everett H et al. Psychosexual dysfunction in women with gynaecological cancer following radical pelvic surgery. British journal of obstetrics and gynaecology. 1993;100: 73-8.

[13] Curry C, Cossich T, Matthews JP et al. Uptake of psychosocial referrals in an outpatient cancer setting: improving service accessibility via the referral process. Support Care Cancer. 2002;10: 549-55.

[14] Davis SR, Moreau M, Kroll R, Bouchard C, Panay N, Gass M, Braunstein GD, Hirschberg AL, Rodenberg C, Pack S, Koch H, Moufarege A, Studd J; APHRODITE Study Team. Testosterone for low libido in postmenopausal women not taking estrogen. N Engl J Med. 2008 Nov 6;359(19):2005-17.

[15] Derzko C, Elliott S, Lam W. Management of sexual dysfunction in postmenopausal breast cancer patients taking adjuvant aromatase inhibitor therapy. Curr Oncol. 2007 Dec;14 Suppl 1:S20-40.

[16] Edmondson RJ, Monaghan JM. The epidemiology of ovarian cancer. Int J Gynecol Cancer. 2001 Nov-Dec;11(6):423-9. Review.

[17] Fogle RH, Stanczyk FZ, Zhang X, Paulson RJ. Ovarian androgen production in postmenopausal women. J Clin Endocrinol Metab. 2007 Aug;92(8):3040-3. Epub 2007 May 22.

[18] Gershenson DM. Management of ovarian germ cell tumors. J Clin Oncol 2007; 25: 2938–2943.

[19] Glantz MJ, Chamberlain MC, Liu Q, Hsieh CC, Edwards KR, Van Horn A, Recht L. Gender disparity in the rate of partner abandonment in patients with serious medical illness. Cancer. 2009 Nov 15;115(22):5237-42.

[20] Grzankowski KS, Carney M. Quality of life in ovarian cancer. Cancer Control. 2011 Jan;18(1):52-8. Review.

[21] Gupta P, Sturdee DW, Palin SL, et al. Menopausal symptoms in women treated for breast cancer: the prevalence and severity of symptoms and their perceived effects on quality of life. Climacteric 2006;9(1):49–58.

[22] Gupta P, Ozel B, Stanczyk FZ, Felix JC, Mishell DR Jr. The effect of transdermal and vaginal estrogen therapy on markers of postmenopausal estrogen status. Menopause. 2008 Jan-Feb;15(1):94-7.

[23] Hall E, Frey BN, Soares CN. Non-hormonal treatment strategies for vasomotor symptoms: a critical review. Drugs. 2011 Feb 12;71(3):287-304. Review.

[24] Hanker LC, Kaufmann M. Problematik des Ovarialkarzinoms: oft zu spät erkannt, oft untertherapiert. Gyn (15) 2010.

[25] Hasenburg A, Amant F, Aerts L, Pascal A, Achimas-Cadariu P, Kesic V. Psycho-Oncology: Structure and profiles of European centres treating patients with gynecological cancer. Int J Gynecol Cancer 2011, accepted.

[26] Hasenburg A, Gabriel B, Einig E-M. Sexualität nach Therapie eines Ovarialkarzinoms. Geburtsh Frauenheilk 2008; 68: 994-997.

[27] Henriksson L, Stjernquist M, Boquist L et al. A one year multi-center study of efficacy and safety of a continuous, low dose estradiol releasing vaginal ring (Estring) in postmenopausal women with symptoms and signs of urogenital aging. Am J Obstet Gynecol 1996; 174: 85–92.

[28] Janda M, Obermair A, Cella D et al. Vulvar cancer patients' quality of life: a qualitative assessment. Int J Gynecol Cancer. 2004;14: 875-81.

[29] Jefferies H, Groves J. In: Gynecologic Cancer: Controversies in Management. Edited by David Gershenson, McGuire and Gore von Churchill Livingstone. 2004, ISBN 0-443-07142-X.

[30] Jemal A, Siegel R, Xu J, Ward E. Cancer statistics, 2010. CA Cancer J Clin. 2010 Sep-Oct;60(5):277-300. Epub 2010 Jul 7. Erratum in: CA Cancer J Clin. 2011 Mar-Apr;61(2):133-4.

[31] Madeb R, Golijanin D, Knopf J, Vicente I, Erturk E, Patel HR, Joseph JV. Patient-reported validated functional outcome after extraperitoneal robotic-assisted nerve-sparing radical prostatectomy. JSLS. 2007 Oct-Dec;11(4):443-8. Review.

[32] Mascarenhas C, Lambe M, Bellocco R, Bergfeldt K, Riman T, Persson I, Weiderpass E. Use of hormone replacement therapy before and after ovarian cancer diagnosis and ovarian cancer survival. Int J Cancer. 2006 Dec 15;119(12):2907-15.

[33] McGregor BA, Carver CS, Antoni MH, et al. Distress and internalized homophobia among lesbian women treated for early stage breast cancer. Psychol Women Quart. 2001;25:1–9.

[34] Michaelson-Cohen R, Beller U. Managing menopausal symptoms after gynecological cancer. Curr Opin Oncol. 2009 Jul 7. [Epub ahead of print].

[35] Mørch LS, Løkkegaard E, Andreasen AH, Krüger-Kjaer S, Lidegaard O. Hormone therapy and ovarian cancer. JAMA. 2009 Jul 15;302(3):298-305.

[36] Oskay-Oezcelik G, Neubert S, Munstedt K, Liebrich K, Hanker LC, Lorenz R, Wimberger P, Mahner S, Hindenburg HJ, Sehouli J. What do primary and recurrent ovarian cancer (OC) patients expect from their doctors? Final results of a german survey in 676 patients. A Study of The North-Eastern German Society of Gynaecological Oncology (NOGGO). ASCO 2010.

[37] Pachman DR, Jones JM, Loprinzi CL. Management of menopause-associated vasomotor symptoms: Current treatment options, challenges and future directions. Int J Womens Health. 2010 Aug 9;2:123-35.

[38] Passik SD, Dugan W, McDonald MV et al. Oncologists' recognition of depression in their patients with cancer. J Clin Oncol. 1998;16: 1594-600.

[39] Raboch J, Boudnik V, Raboch Jr J. Sex life following hysterectomy. Geburtsh Frauenheilk 1985; 45: 48–50

[40] Reid DM. Prevention of osteoporosis after breast cancer. Maturitas. 2009 Sep 20;64(1):4-8. Epub 2009 Aug 25.

[41] Sadovsky R, Basson R, Krychman M et al. Cancer and sexual problems. The journal of sexual medicine. 2009;7: 349-73.

[42] Shifren JL, Braunstein GD, Simon JA et al. Transdermal testosterone treatment in women with impaired sexual function after oophorectomy. N Engl J Med 2000; 343: 682–688

[43] Sideras K, Loprinzi CL. Nonhormonal management of hot flashes for women on risk reduction therapy. J Natl Compr Canc Netw. 2010 Oct;8(10):1171-9.

[44] Sitruk-Ware R. Estrogen therapy during menopause. Practical treatment recommendations. Drugs 1990; 39: 203–217.

[45] Stead ML, Brown JM, Fallowfield L, Selby P. Lack of communication between healthcare professionals and women with ovarian cancer about sexual issues. Br J Cancer 2003; 88: 666–671

[46] Taylor C. Predictors of sexual functioning in ovarian-cancer patients. J of Clin Oncol 2004; 22: 881–889.

[47] Vitrano V, Catania V, Mercadante S. Sexuality in patients with advanced cancer: a prospective study in a population admitted to an acute pain relief and palliative care unit. Am J Hosp Palliat Care. 2011 May;28(3):198-202.

[48] Wright JD, Shah M, Mathew L, Burke WM, Culhane J, Goldman N, Schiff PB, Herzog TJ. Fertility preservation in young women with epithelial ovarian cancer. Cancer. 2009 Sep 15;115(18):4118-26.

13

Quality of Life of Patients with Ovarian Cancer

Wei-Chu Chie[1] and Elfriede Greimel[2]
[1]*Institute of Epidemiology and Preventive Medicine, College of Public Health, National Taiwan University*
[2]*Department of Obstetrics and Gynaecology, Medical University Graz, Graz*
[1]*Taiwan*
[2]*Austria*

1. Introduction

1.1 Current status of ovarian cancer

Ovarian cancer is one of the leading female cancers around the world (International Agency for Research on Cancer, 2011). Up to now, there is no effective method of early detection (US Task Force of Preventive Services, 2011). When detected, the stages are usually advanced, and patients have poor prognosis and poor health-related quality of life (HRQoL). Patient-reported outcomes have been recommended as endpoints of clinical trials by the U.S. Food and Drug Administration (FDA) (2011). Therefore, besides improving survival, a better HRQoL is a major goal for the development of methods for new detection and treatments.

1.2 The impacts of the disease

Patients with ovarian cancer share general functioning and systemic problems with patients with other cancers (Cella et al., 1993; Cain et al., 1998; Base-Enquist et al., 2001; Aaronson et al., 1993). Regarding disease-specific problems, abdominal / gastrointestinal symptoms because of the space-occupying nature of the tumor and the malignant ascites from the tumor in the pelvic and abdominal cavity are most important issues (Cain et al., 1998; Base-Enquist et al., 2001; Cull et al., 2001; Greimel et al., 2003a, 2003b). The disease recurs easily. Patients may suffer repeating debulking surgeries and chemotherapies that affect their HRQoL.

1.3 The impacts of the treatments

The standard treatment of this disease is debulking (cytoreduction) surgery followed by platinum-based chemotherapy (du Bois at al., 2005), while a new approach of neoadjuvant chemotherapy followed by debulking surgery (Brisow & Chi, 2006). These treatments, no matter which comes first, can improve survival and improve HRQoL of patients by reducing tumor size and ascites, and also patients' psychological distress. But they may also have negative impacts on HRQoL of patients because of the adverse effects of chemotherapy and surgery.

1.4 Other important aspects of HRQoL

The life-threatening nature of the illness can also cause psychological distress (Cull et al., 2001; Greimel et al., 2003a, 2003b). As all other gynecological cancers, patients with ovarian cancer suffer from body image concerns and problems in sexual life (Cain et al., 1998; Base-Enquist et al., 2001; Cull et al., 2001; Greimel et al., 2003a, 2003b).

2. Domains of HRQoL affected by disease and treatments of ovarian cancer

2.1 Disease-related problems

2.1.1 General functioning and systemic symptoms

General functioning including physical, emotional, social, etc. (Cella et al., 1993; Aaronson et al., 1993) and ability of getting around (independence) are major issues in this category (Cain et al., 1998; Base-Enquist et al., 2001). Weight loss is also seen as a disease-related systemic symptom for advanced tumor (Cain et al., 1998; Base-Enquist et al., 2001).

2.1.2 Abdominal (gastrointestinal) symptoms

Abdominal (gastrointestinal) symptoms are major disease-related HRQoL problems of patients with ovarian cancer. These symptoms may include abdominal swelling, fullness, pain or cramps, indigestion, change of bowel habit, etc. Abdominal pain and bowel habit change can also arise from treatment (Cain et al., 1998; Base-Enquist et al., 2001; Cull et al., 2001; Greimel et al., 2003a, 2003b).

2.2. Treatment-related problems

2.2.1 Urological and gynecological symptoms

The urological or gynecological symptoms are not as common as other gynecological cancers, and they are usually caused by treatment. Urinary frequency and dry vagina are often complained of (Cull et al., 2001; Greimel et al., 2003a, 2003b).

2.2.2 Chemotherapy side effects

Chemotherapy can cause nausea and vomiting, poor appetite (Cella et al., 1993; Cain et al., 1998; Base-Enquist et al., 2001; Aaronson et al., 1993), hair loss (Cain et al., 1998; Base-Enquist et al., 2001; Cull et al., 2001; Greimel et al., 2003a, 2003b), peripheral neuropathy including numbness and weakness, other sensory change, skin problems and muscle pain (Cull et al., 2001; Greimel et al., 2003a, 2003b). Urinary frequency can also be attributed to chemotherapy (Cull et al., 2001; Greimel et al., 2003a, 2003b).

2.2.3 Termination of reproductive ability and menopausal symptoms

For women of reproductive age, both surgical treatment and chemotherapy can cause early menopause and the termination of reproductive ability (Cain et al., 1998; Base-Enquist et al., 2001). Menopausal symptoms caused by hormonal depletion, including hot flush (flash) and night sweats, are also experienced by these patients (Cull et al., 2001; Greimel et al., 2003a, 2003b).

2.3 Other important aspects in HRQoL

2.3.1 Body image and psychological problems

Like all other gynecological cancer, ovarian cancer per se and its treatment can cause body image and psychological problems. For the body image problems, patients may feel less attractive, less like a woman, dissatisfied with body or appearance, etc. (Cain et al., 1998; Base-Enquist et al., 2001; Cull et al., 2001; Greimel et al., 2003a, 2003b). For the psychological problem, patients may have negative emotions (Cella et al., 1993; Aaronson et al., 1993), or suffer from burdens of and worries about disease or treatment (Cull et al., 2001; Greimel et al., 2003a, 2003b).

2.3.2 Sexuality

Like all other gynecological cancers, sexuality is negatively affected. Issues include interest in sex, real sexual activity and enjoyment (Cain et al., 1998; Base-Enquist et al., 2001; Cull et al., 2001; Greimel et al., 2003a, 2003b). Dry vagina during intercourse, a result of hormonal depletion, can also be classified in this category (Cull et al., 2001; Greimel et al., 2003a, 2003b).

3. Existing instruments for assessment of HRQoL

We have at present two systems of disease-specific instruments for assessment of HRQoL of patients with ovarian cancer: the Functional Assessment of Cancer Therapy (FACT) and the European Organisation for Research and Treatment of Cancer (EORTC). Both have a generic core questionnaire, the FACT-G and the EORTC QLQ-C30, and a disease-specific supplementary questionnaire, the FACT-O and the EORTC QLQ-OV28.

3.1 The FACT system: FACT-G and FACT-O

3.1.1 The scale structure of the FACT system

The FACT-G was developed as a general measure for HRQoL of patients with cancer in 1987 (Cella et al., 1993) and validated in patients with different cancers before the development of ovarian specific scale (Weitzner et al., 1995; Cella, 1995; List at al., 1996; Brady at al., 1997; Esper at al., 1997; Yellen at al., 1997; McQuellon et al., 1997; Ward at al., 1999). The instrument contains four domains and 27 questions: physical well-being (PWB), 7 questions; social / family well-being (SWB), 7 questions; emotional well-being (EWB), 6 questions; and functional well-being (FWB), 7 questions (Cella et al., 1993). Each question has 5 options: 0 (not at all), 1 (a little bit), 3 (quite a bit), and 4 (very much). All item scores are recoded to make a high score corresponding to better HRQoL. It can be seen either as a disease-specific instrument vs. other diseases or a generic instrument for all patients with cancer. An ovarian cancer-specific subscale (OCS) was developed in 1998 using the same option format (Cain et al., 1998) and was reported to have good reliability and validity in 2001 (Base-Enquist et al., 2001). The questionnaire contains one domain, originally 12 questions: stomach swelling, losing weight, vomiting, hair loss, stomach cramping, and concerns about fertility (negative questions); bowel control, good appetite, appearance, getting around, feel like a woman, and interested in sex (positive questions, reverse coded). One question (concerns about fertility) was deleted because most patients are beyond childbearing age. The two instruments are used together when assessing HRQoL of patients with ovarian cancer. The score of each scale is a summation of recoded question scores within each scale. The total score is a summation of all scores of all 38 (27 and 11) questions together.

3.1.2 Reliability and validity of the FACT system in patients with ovarian cancer

Reliability and validity of the FACT-O with FACT-G were reported by Base-Enquist et al. (2001). The internal consistency (Cronbach's alpha) coefficient of the 11 questions in FACT-O was 0.92, and test-retest correlation coefficient of the total FACT-O score was 0.81. The correlation coefficients between the total FACT-O score, subscale scores of FACT-G, and subscale scores of other related instruments were as expected (good convergent and divergent validity). The scores of subscales of the FACT-G and the total FACT-O score were significantly different in different performance and treatment status, and were sensitive to changes of performance status. According to the validation results, the FACT-O is a reliable and valid instrument used with the FACT-G in assessment of ovarian cancer-specific HRQoL as a whole for patients with ovarian cancer.

3.2 The EORTC system: QLQ-C30 and QLQ-OV28

3.2.1 The scale structure of the EORTC system

The development of the EORTC QLQ-C30 can be traced back in 1986. The questionnaire was designed for the measurement of general HRQoL issued for patients with cancer (Aaronson et al., 1993). It can also be seen either as a disease-specific instrument vs. other diseases or a generic instrument for all patients with cancer. The questionnaire contains 30 questions belonging to five functional scales (physical, role, emotional, social, and cognitive), nine symptom scales (fatigue, nausea and vomiting, pain, dyspnea, sleep disturbance, appetite loss, constipation, and diarrhea), financial difficulty in the past week, and one global health status (overall health and quality of life) scale. Each question has 4 options: 1 (not at all), 2 (a little), 3 (quite a bit), and 4 (very much). Each scale is scored separately. There is no total score. All scale scores are transformed into 0-100 from a recoded summation of item scores in each scale. For all functional scales, a higher score represents a better HRQoL. For all symptom scales and financial difficulty, a higher score means a poorer HRQoL. Previous studies showed good reliability and validity for different cancer diagnoses (Bjordal & Kaasa, 1992; Aaronson et al., 1993; Hjermstad et al., 1995; Groenvold et al., 1997; Kobayashi et al., 1998).

The EORTC QLQ-OV28 was designed as a supplement to the EORTC QLQ-C30 for the use in ovarian cancer clinical trials and related studies (Cull et al., 2001; Greimel et al., 2003a, 2003b). It contains seven subscales and 28 questions - abdominal / gastrointestinal symptoms (7 questions: abdominal pain, feeling bloated, clothes too tight, changed bowel habit, flatulence, fullness when eating, indigestion), peripheral neuropathy (4 questions: tingling, numbness, and weakness), other chemotherapy side-effects (7 questions: hair loss and upset by hair loss, taste change, muscle pain, hearing problem, urinary frequency, and skin problem), hormonal / menopausal (2 questions: hot flushes and night sweat), body image (2 questions: less attractive, dissatisfied with body), attitude to disease and treatment (3 questions: disease burden, treatment burden, and worry about future), and sexual function (4 questions: interest in sex, sexual activity, enjoyment of sex, and dry vagina). Each scale is scored separately as that of the EORTC QLQ-C30. For symptom scales, a higher score means a poorer HRQoL. For function scales (body image and sexual function), a higher score represent a better HRQoL. In addition to the cross-cultural validation of the EORTC, Chie et al. (2010) reported the translation and validation of the EORTC QLQ-OV28 in Taiwan and found a relatively low importance of body image, menopausal, and sexuality problems because of low emphasis on attractiveness and avoidance of sexual activity after having cancer.

3.2.2 Reliability and validity of the EORTC system in patients with ovarian cancer

Greimel et al. (2003b) reported the result of cross-cultural validation of the EORTC QLQ-OV28 used with the EORTC QLQ-C30. The internal consistency (Cronbach's alpha) coefficients of all subscales except body image (0.58) were above 0.70 (ranging from 0.77 to

0.90). There was no scaling error except the subscale of other chemotherapy side effects (5/42). The intraclass correlation coefficients for test-retest of all subscales ranged from 0.74 to 0.94. The correlation coefficients between subscales of the EORTC QLQ-OV28 and EORTC QLQ-C30 were as expected. For responsiveness, scores of abdominal symptoms, peripheral neuropathy, other chemotherapy side effects, and disease burden responded significantly after treatment. For sensitivity (known-groups comparison), subscale scores differed most significantly between patients with primary and recurrent tumors. According to the validation report, the EORTC QLQ-OV28 is a reliable and valid multi-dimensional instrument used with the EORTC QLQ-C30 for the assessment of HRQoL of multiple aspects for patients with ovarian cancer.

3.3 Comparison of scale structures of the two systems

The comparison of the two sets of instruments is shown in Tables 1 and 2. The functional scales of the FACT-G and the EORTC QLQ-C30 are similar. Both include physical, mental or emotional, social, and role or functional subscales. The FACT-G emphasizes familial functioning, while the EORTC QLQ-C30 includes cognitive functioning. Both have an overall measure for HRQoL: the FACT-G uses a summation of all scores, while the EORTC QLQ-C30 measures it separately. The EORTC QLQ-C30 also has symptom and financial difficulty subscales. The FACT-G includes some symptoms in physical or function subscales (Table 1). The contents of the FACT-O and the EORTC QLQ-OV28 are similar. However, the FACT-O has only one overall scale for ovarian cancer, while the EORTC QLQ-OV28 has seven subscales covering problems of different organ-systems or aspects of HRQoL (Table 2).

FACT		EORTC	
Physical	Energy	**Physical**	Strenuous activity
	Nausea		Long walk
	Family needs		Short walk
	Pain		Stay in chair
	Side effects		Self-care
	Feel ill		
	Bed-ridden		
Social /family	Close to friends	**Social**	Interfere with family life
	Family support		With social activities
	Friends' support		
	Family comm. illness		
	Close to partner		
	Sexual life		
Emotional	Feel sad	**Emotional**	Tense
	Satisfied with coping		Worry
	Losing hope		Irritable
	Feel nervous		Depressed
	Worry / dying	**Cognitive**	Concentration
	Worry / getting worse		Remembering

FACT		EORTC	
Functional	Able to work Work fulfilling Enjoy life Sleep well Enjoy pleasure	**Role**	Limited work Limited leisure
	Content with QOL	**Overall**	Health QOL
Symptoms		Pain, Fatigue, Nausea & vomiting Dyspnea, Sleep, Appetite, constipation, diarrhea	
Other scale(s)		Financial difficulty	

Table 1. Comparison of FACT-G and the EORTC QLQ-C30.

FACT	EORTC	
FACT-O (one scale) Stomach swelling, losing weight, bowel control, vomiting, hair loss, good appetite, appearance, getting around, feel like a woman, stomach cramping, interested in sex, concerns about fertility (deleted)	**GI symptoms**	Abdominal pain, Feeling bloated, Clothes tight, Changed bowel habit, Flatulence, Fullness when eating, Indigestion
	Peripheral neuropathy	Tingling, Numbness, Weakness
	Other chemotherapy side effects	Hair loss & upset, Taste change, Muscle pain, Hearing problem, Urinary frequency, Skin problem
	Attitude to disease	Disease burden, Treatment burden, Worry about future
	Sexual function	Interest in sex, Sexual activity, Sex enjoyment, Dry vagina

Table 2. Comparison of FACT-O and the EORTC QLQ-OV28.

4. Equivalence of the FACT and the EORTC systems

Are the results of the two systems equivalent? Hozner et al. (2006) reported a study on 737 patients with different cancers for the equivalence of the FACT-G and the EORTC QLQ-C30, the core content of the two systems. Both classical test theory and Rasch measurement model were used. Three of the four subscales common to the two systems are equating: physical, emotional, and role / functional, but not the social / family subscale. A converting table was generated according to the results. No such study was conducted for the FACT-O and the EORTC QLQ-OV28 because the FACT-O has only one subscale, therefore the two site-specific questionnaires have no common subscales to study.

5. Application of two systems in assessing HRQoL of patients with ovarian cancer undergoing different treatments across different cultures

5.1 The application of the FACT system

The two systems of instruments measuring HRQoL of patients with ovarian cancer were used in clinical trials and non-trial clinical studies. The FACT system was more widely used because the FACT-O was developed earlier than the EORTC QLQ-OV28. The FACT-O has been applied in studies assessing palliative chemotherapy for advanced ovarian cancer (using EORTC QLQ-C30 and FACT-O) (Doyle et al., 2001), general chemotherapy (Le et al., 2004), adjuvant and salvage chemotherapy for advanced ovarian cancer (Le et al., 2005), interval cytoreduction in advanced ovarian cancer (Wenzel et al., 2005), active coping (Canada et al., 2006), Thallidomide therapy (Gordinier et al., 2007), phase I/II gemcitabine and doxirubicine (Goff et al., 2003)] and phase II gemicitabine and topotecan trials for platinum-refractory ovarian cancers (Goff et al., 2008), and factors for decreased QoL (von Gruenigen et al., 2009). In summary, the FACT-O and FACT-G scores became better when there was response to treatment, active coping can improve HRQoL, and factors causing decreased HRQoL can be detected and managed in advance.

5.2 The application of the EORTC system

The use of the EORTC QLQ-OV28 with the EORTC QLQ-C30 was less common because it was developed later than the FACT-O. The two questionnaires were first used in a study assessing HRQoL for patients after pelvic exenteration in 2004 (Roos et al., 2004) where more physical, social, and sexual problems, especially for young patients were reported after surgery. A comparison of HRQoL of patients with early vs. advanced ovarian cancer (Mirabeau-Beale et al., 2009) found comparable HRQoL in two groups. A clinical trial of neoadjuvant platinum-based chemotherapy followed by (interval) debulking surgery vs. standard care of primary debulking surgery followed by platinum-based chemotherapy in stage IIIC or IV ovarian cancer used the two questionnaires did not detect any difference between the two arms in HRQoL (Vergote et al., 2010). The EORTC QLQ-C30 alone without the EORTC QLQ-OV28 has been used in a randomized trial of cisplatin / paclitaxel vs. carboplatin / paclitaxel and found patients undergoing carboplatin / paclitaxel treatment had better HRQoL (Greimel et al., 2006). Another study using the EORTC QLQ-C30 assessing the HRQoL of long-term survivors of ovarian cancer found long-term survivors had better HRQoL scores before treatment than short-term survivors, and long-term survivors had significant improvement of HRQoL in emotional and global health scores 1 year after treatment and remained stable. The scores of all domains but dyspnea were comparable with women without cancer (Greimel et al., 2011).

5.3 A comparison of the two systems in HRQoL assessment

A review article in 2010 commented after comparing all generic and specific questionnaires for HRQoL of patients with gynecologic cancers that there is little evidence that disease-, symptom- or treatment-specific instruments are more responsive or sensitive than generic or cancer-specific questionnaires, and a superior quality and quantity data reported for the FACT system compared with the EORTC system (Luckett et al., 2010). Nordin and Greimel on behalf of the EORTC Quality of Life Gynecology Group (2010) responded in a letter that such comments are not substantiated and provided examples of good results of cross-cultural validation. In addition to the cross-cultural nature, the multi-dimensional structure of the EORTC system may also help clinical researchers and practitioners conduct more detailed assessment of different aspects of HRQoL of patients.

6. Future development

Ovarian cancer is an important gynecological cancer which affects the survival and HRQoL of patients (International Agency for Research on Cancer, 2011). The keys to improve both survival and HRQoL are methods of early detection (US Task Force of Preventive Services, 2011) and effective treatment (du Bois at al., 2005; Brisow & Chi, 2006). We expect breakthroughs in both early detection and effective treatment in the near future. Patient-reported outcomes have been recommended as endpoints of clinical trials by the U.S. Food and Drug Administration (FDA) (2011). To evaluate the effectiveness of these methods, HRQoL is an essential primary endpoint. Two systems of HRQoL assessment, i.e. the FACT and the EORTC systems are available. Both cover major issues of HRQoL and show good reliability and validity in previous reports and are used widely around the world in clinical trials and clinical studies. Therefore, we expect that the assessment of HRQoL of patients can be routinely included in clinical researches and practice, to understand and further improve patients' HRQoL.

7. Conclusions

Ovarian cancer is one of the leading female cancers around the world. There is no effective method of early detection. When detected, the stages are usually advanced, and patients have poor health-related quality of life (HRQoL). The standard treatments of this disease including debulking surgery and chemotherapy can improve survival and may have either positive or negative impacts on HRQoL of patients. The disease recurs easily. Patients may suffer repeating debulking surgeries and chemotherapies that affect their HRQoL. In this chapter, we introduced and reviewed the scale structures, psychometric properties and clinical validities of existing instruments - the FACT system and the EORTC system for the assessment of HRQoL for patients with ovarian cancer, and report the results of their application in clinical trials and observational studies. We hope that HRQoL can be emphasized and routinely assessed for all patients with ovarian cancer in future clinical researches and practice.

8. References

Aaronson NK, Ahmedzai A, Berman B, et al. (1993). The European Organization for Research and Treatment of Cancer QLQ-C30: a quality-of-life instrument for use in international clinical trials in oncology. *Journal of the National Cancer Institute* Vol.85, No.3, (March 1993), pp. 365-376, ISSN 0027-8874.

Basen-Enquist K, Bodurka-Bevers D, Fitzderald MA, et al. (2001). Reliability and validity of the Functional Assessment of Cancer Therapy-Ovarian. *Journal of Clinical Oncology* Vol.19, No.6, (March 2001), pp. 1809-1817, ISSN 0732-183X.

Bjordal K, Kaasa S. (1992). Psychometric validation of the EROTC Core Quality of Life Questionnaire, 30-item version and a diagnosis-specific module for head and neck cancer patients. *Acta Oncologica* Vol.31, No.3, (March 1992), pp. 311-321, ISSN 0284-186X.

Brady MJ, Cella DF, Mo F, et al. (1997). Reliability and validity of the Functional Assessment of Cancer Therapy-Breast quality-of-life instrument. *Journal of Clinical Oncology* Vol.15, No.3, (March 1997), pp.974-986, 1809-1817, ISSN 0732-183X.

Brisow RE, Chi DS. (2006). Platinum-based neoadjuvant chemotherapy and interval surgical cytoreduction for advanced ovarian cancer: a meta-analysis. *Gynecologic Oncology* Vol.103, No.3, (December 2006), pp.1070-1076, ISSN 0090-8258.

Cain JM, Wenzel LB, Monk BJ, et al. (1998). Palliative care and quality of life considerations in the management of ovarian cancer. In: *Ovarian cancer-controversies in management.* Gershenson DM, McGuire WP (eds). New York, NY, Churchill Livingston, pp 281-307, ISBN 978-0443078040.

Canada AL. Parker PA, de Moor JS, et al. (2006). Active coping mediates the association between religion / spirituality and quality of life in ovarian cancer. *Gynecologic Oncology* Vol.101, No.1 (April 2006), pp. 102-107, ISSN 0090-8258.

Cella D, Tulsky DS, Gray G, et al. (1993). The Functional Assessment of Cancer Therapy Scale: development and validation of the general measure. *Journal of Clinical Oncology* Vol.11, No.4, (April 1993), pp. 570-579, ISSN 0732-183X.

Cella DF. (1995). Reliability and validity of the Functional Assessment of Cancer Therapy-Lung (FACT-L) quality of life instrument. *Lung Cancer* Vol.12, No.3, (June 1995), pp.199-220, ISSN 0169-5002.

Chie WC, Lan CY, Chiang C, Chen CA. (2010). Quality of life of patients with ovarian cancer in taiwan: validation and application of the Taiwan Chinese version of the EORTC QLQ-OV28, brief report. *Psycho-Oncology* Vol.19, No.7, (July 2010), pp. 782-785, ISSN 1099-1611.

Cull A, Howat S, Greimel E, et al. (2001). Development of a European Organisation for Research and Treatment of Cancer questionnaire module to assess the quality of life of ovarian cancer patients in clinical trials: a progress report. *European Journal of Cancer* Vol.37, No.1, (January 2001), pp. 47-53, ISSN 0959-8049.

Doyle C, Crump M, Pintile M, Oza AM. (2001). Does palliative chemotherapy palliate? Evaluation of expectation, outcomes, and cost in women receiving chemotherapy for advanced ovarian cancer. *Journal of Clinical Oncology* Vol.19, No.6, (February 2001), pp. 1266-1274, ISSN 0732-183X.

du Bois A, Quinn M, Thigpen T, et al. (2005). 2004 Consensus Statements on the management of ovarian cancer: final document of the 3rd International Gynecologic Cancer Intergroup Ovarian cancer Consensus conference (GCIC CCCC 2004). *Ann Oncol* Vol.16, No.suppl 8, (October 2005), pp.ivvv7-ivvv12, ISSN 0923-7534.

Esper P, Mo F, Chodak G, et al. (1997). Measuring quality of life in men with prostate cancer using the Functional Assessment of Cancer Therapy-Prostate instrument. *Urology* Vol.50, No.6, (December 1997), pp. 920-928. ISSN 0090-4295.

Goff BA, Thompson T, Greer BE, Jacobs A, Storer B. (2003). Treatment of recurrent platinum-resistent ovarian or peritoneal cancer with gemcitabine and doxorubicin. A phase I/II trial of the the Puget Sound Oncology Consortium. *American Journal of Obstetrics and Gynecology* Vol.188, No.6. (June 2003), pp. 1556-1564, ISSN 0002-9378.

Goff BA, Holmberg LA, Veljovich D, Kurland BF. (2008). Treat of recurrent or persistent platinum-refractory ovarian, fallopian tube, or primary peritoneal cancer with gemcitabine and topotecan. A phase II trial of the Puget Sound Oncology Consortium. *Gynecologic Oncology* Vol.110, No.2, (August 2008), pp. 146-151, ISSN 0090-8258.

Gordinier ME, Dizon DS, Weitzen S, et al. (2007). Oral thalidomide as palliative chemotherapy in women with advanced ovarian cancer. *Journal of Palliative Medicine* Vol.10, No.1, (February 2007), pp. 61-65, ISSN 1096-6218.

Greimel ER, Bottomley A, Cull A, et al. (2003a). An international field study of the reliability and validity of a disease-specific questionnaire module (the QLQ-OV28) in assessing the quality of life of patients with ovarian cancer. *European Journal of Cancer* Vol.39, No.10, (July 2003), pp.1402-1408, ISSN 0959-8049.

Greimel ER, Bottomley A, Cull A, et al. (2003b). Cooridgendum to "An international field study of the reliability and validity of a disease-specific questionnaire module (the QLQ-OV28) in assessing the quality of life of patients with ovarian cancer": [European Journal of Cancer 39: 1402-1408.]. *European Journal of Cancer* Vol.39, No.17, (November 2003), pp. 2570, ISSN 0959-8049.

Greimel E, Bjelic-Radisic V, Pfisterer J. et al. (2006). Randomised study of the Arbeitsgemeinschaft Gynaekologische Onkologie Ovarian Cancer Study Group comparing quality of life in patients with ovarian cancer treated with cisplatin/paclitaxel versus carboplatin/paclitaxel. *Journal of Clinical Oncology* Vol.24, No.4, (February 2006), pp.579-585, ISSN 0732-183X.

Greimel E, Daghofer F Petru E. (2011). Prospective assessment of quality of life in long-term ovarian cancer survivors. *International Journal of Cancer* Vol.128, No.12 (June 2011), pp. 3005-3011, ISSN 1097-0215.

Groenvold, M, Klee MC, Sprangers MAG, Aaronson NK. (1997). Validation of the EORTC QLQ-C30 quality of life questionnaire through combined qualitative and quantitative assessment of patient-observer agreement. *Journal of Clinical Epidemiology* Vol.50, No.4, (April 1997), pp. 441-450, ISSN 0895-4356.

Hjermstad MJ, Fossa SD, Bjordal K, Kaasa S. (1995). Test/retest study of the European Organization for Research and Treatment of Cancer Core Quality-of-Life Questionnaire. *Journal of Clinical Oncology* Vol.13, No.5, (May 1995), pp. 1249-1254, ISSN 0732-183X.

Hozner B, Bode RK, Hahn EA, et al. (2006). Equating EORTC QLQ-C30 and FACT-G scores and its use in oncological research. *European Journal of Cancer* Vol.42, No.18, (December 2006), pp. 3169-3177, ISSN 0959-8049.

International Agency for Research on Cancer. (2011). Available from http://globocan.iarc.fr/factsheets/populations/factsheet.asp?uno=900#WOMEN

Kobayashi K, Takeda F, Teramukai S, et al. (1998). A cross-validation of the European Organization for Research and Treatment of Cancer QLQ-C30 (EORTC QLQ-C30) for Japanese with lung cancer. *European Journal of Cancer* Vol.34, No.6, (May 1998), pp. 810-815, ISSN 0959-8049.

Le T, Leis A, Pahwa P, et al. (2004). Quality of life evaluation in patients with ovarian cancer during chemotherapy treatment. *Gynecologic Oncology* Vol.92, No.3, (March 2004), pp. 839-844 , ISSN 0090-8258.

Le T, Hopkins L, Fung MFK. (2005). Quality of life assessment during adjuvant and salvage chemotherapy for advance stage epithelial ovarian cancer. *Gynecologic Oncoogyl* Vol.98, No.1, (July 2005), pp. 39-44, ISSN 0090-8258.

List MA, D'Antionio LL, Cella DF, et al. (1996). The Performance Status Scale for head and neck cancer patients and the Functional Assessment of Cancer Therapy -Head and Neck Scale. *Cancer* Vol.77, No.11, (June 1996), pp.2294-2301, ISSN 1097-0142.

Luckett T, King M, Butow P. et al. (2010). Assessing health-related quality of life in gynecologic oncology. A systematic review or questionnaires and their ability to detect clinically important difference and change. *International Journal of Gynecological Cancer* Vol.20, No.4, (May 2010), pp. 664-684, ISSN 1525-1438.

McQuellon RP, Russell GB, Cella DF, et al. (1997). Quality of life measurement in bone marrow transplantation: development of the Functional Assessment of Cancer Therapy-Bone Marrow Transplant (FACT-BMT) scale. *Bone Marrow Transplantation* Vol.19, No.4, (February 1997), pp. 357-368, ISSN 0268-3369.

Mirabeau-Beale KL, Kornblith AB, Penson T, et al. (2009). Comparison of the quality of life of early and advanced stage ovarian cancer survivors. *Gynecologic Oncology* Vol.114, No.2, (August 2009), pp. 353-359, ISSN 0090-8258.

Nordin AJ, Greimel E on behalf of the EORTC Quality of Life Gynecology Group. (2010). Assessing health-related quality of life in gynecologic oncology (letter). *International Journal of Gynecological Cancer* Vol.20, No.8, (November 2010), p. 1301, ISSN 1525-1438.

Roos EJ, de Graeff A, van Eijkeren MA, Boon TA, Heintz APM. (2004). Quality of life after pelvic extenteration. *Gynecologic Oncology* Vol.93, No.3, (June 2004), pp. 610-614, ISSN 0090-8258.

U.S. Food and Drug Administration. (July 2011). Available from http://www.fda.gov/Drugs/GuidanceComplianceRegulatoryInformation/Guidances/default.htm

The US Task force of preventive services. (July 2011). Available from http://www.uspreventiveservicestaskforce.org/uspstf/uspsovar.htm

Vergote I, Trope CG, Amant F, et al. (2010). Neoadjuvant chemotherapy or primary surgery in stage IIIc or IV ovarian cancer. *New England Journal of Medicine* Vol.363, No.10, (September 2010), pp.943-953, ISSN 0028-4793.

von Gruenigen VE, Huang HQ, Gil KM, et al. (2009). Assessment of factors that contribute to decreased quality of life in Gynecologic Oncology Group ovarian cancer trials. *Cancer* Vol.115, No.20, (October 2009), pp. 4857-4864, ISSN 1097-0142.

Ward WL, Hahn EA, Mo F, et al. (1999). Reliability and validity of the Functional Assessment of Cancer Therapy-Colorectal (FACT-C) Scale quality of life instrument. *Quality of Life Research* Vol. 8, No.3, (May 1999), pp.181-195, ISSN 0962-9343.

Weitzner MA, Meyers CA, Gelke CK, et al. (1995). The Functional Assessment of Cancer Therapy (FACT) Scale: development of a brain subscale and revalidation of the general version (FACT-G) in patients with primary brain tumors. *Cancer* Vol.75, No.5, (March 1995), pp. 1151-1161, ISSN 1097-0142.

Wenzel L, Huang HQ, Monk BJ, Rrose PG, Cella D. (2005). Quality of life comparison in a randomized controlled trial of interval secondary cytoreduction in advanced ovarian carcinoma: a Gynecologic Oncology Group study. *Journal of Clinical Oncology* Vol.23, No.24, (August 2005), pp. 5605-5612, ISSN 0732-183X.

Yellen SB, Cella DF, Webster K, et al. (1997). Measuring fatigue and other anemia-related symptoms with the Functional Assessment of Cancer Therapy (FACT) measurement system. *Journal of Pain and Symptom Management* Vol.13, No.2 (February 1997), pp. 63-74, ISSN 0885-3924.

14

Intraperitoneal Radionuclide Therapy – Clinical and Pre-Clinical Considerations

J. Elgqvist[1], S. Lindegren[2] and P. Albertsson[1]
[1]*Department of Oncology, Sahlgrenska Academy, University of Gothenburg*
[2]*Department of Radiation Physics, Sahlgrenska Academy, University of Gothenburg*
Sweden

1. Introduction

For early stage (stage I) epithelial ovarian cancer (EOC) surgery may be the sole curative therapy. However, the vast majorities of cases are diagnosed in more advanced stages and need a multimodal treatment strategy. Therefore, in stage II and higher, surgery with a cytoreductive intent, (i.e. to remove as much as possible the macroscopic disease from the peritoneal surfaces in adjunct to bilateral salpingo-oophorectomy) is not curative by itself, but has to be supplemented by cytotoxic therapy. This is mainly administered as intravenously (i.v.) chemotherapy or sometimes as intraperitoneal (i.p.) chemotherapy. Although there are trials using whole abdominal or moving-strip external beam radiotherapy as adjuvant therapy (Einhorn et al., 2003) or i.p. radiotherapy with colloid preparations of ^{198}Au or ^{32}P (Rosenhein et al., 1979; Varia et al., 2003) these have so far not presented results to merit a place in the normal therapeutic arsenal, and long term toxicity from normal tissues is a major concern.

Despite extensive cytoreductive surgery and modern chemotherapy, with complete remissions (CR) at second look laparotomy (SLL) and normalisation of the serum marker cancer antigen 125 (CA-125), approximately 70% of the patients in stage III recur and will eventually succumb to their disease. The recurrence pattern is normally the development of ascites due to progression of treatment resistant cells growing as peritoneal microscopic deposits. From this incurable situation the progression is dominated by a continuous accumulation of ascites with intestinal adhesions and bowel obstructions. This progression can often be temporarily halted by palliative chemotherapy, or in special occasions, local external beam radiotherapy, but will in any event, eventually lead to a great deal of suffering and pain from above the abdominal cavity pathology.

Since the negative impact on survival and the suffering associated with uncontrolled spread in the abdominal cavity, efforts have been directed to develop more effective local treatments. Such a local more aggressive treatment strategy has proven effective as chemotherapy injected locally in the peritoneal cavity (i.p.) could show as a reduction in recurrences and a decrease in mortality, although at the expense of clearly increased toxicity (Jaaback & Johnson, 2009). The use of ^{90}Y, conjugated to a monoclonal antibody (mAb) and studied in a large prospective randomised controlled study, unfortunately did not demonstrate a benefit (Oei et al., 2007; Verheijen et al., 2006).

These negative results on overall survival of i.p. radioimmunotherapy (RIT) using the β-emitter ^{90}Y, conjugated to a mAb, are a concern (Verheijen et al., 2006), even if a decreased local i.p. recurrence has been seen (Oei et al., 2007). A number of important issues relating to this trial including the physical properties of the used nuclide will be discussed in depth, which might give clues to optimization of future trials of intraperitoneal RIT.

2. Radionuclides

In targeted radionuclide therapy the cytotoxic effect is mediated by a radionuclide, brought to the target by the targeting construct (Elgqvist et al., 2010). Below is a list of the radionuclides used, in both animal and clinical studies. The list includes a presentation of their physical characters, and in which studies they have been used.

^{225}Ac (Actinium-225). ^{225}Ac decays with a half-life of 10 days and emits four α-particles in a serial decay. The α-particle emitted from ^{225}Ac has an energy of 5.8 MeV (mean linear energy transfer [LET] ≈ 120 keV/μm) and the daughters are ^{221}Fr ($T_{½}$ = 4.8 min, E = 6.3 MeV, mean LET ≈ 118 keV/μm), ^{217}At ($T_{½}$ = 32.3 ms, E = 7.1 MeV, mean LET ≈ 109 keV/μm), and ^{213}Bi ($T_{½}$ = 45.6 min, E = 8.4 MeV, mean LET ≈ 99 keV/μm). The α-decays are accompanied by gamma(γ)-radiation, enabling scintigraphy and dosimetry. ^{225}Ac has been used in one animal study (Borchardt et al., 2003).

^{211}At (Astatine-211). ^{211}At (an α-particle emitter) is cyclotron produced via the nuclear reaction ^{207}Bi(α,2n)^{211}At. ^{211}At decays with a half-life of 7.2 hours in 2 ways: (*i*) via emission of an α-particle (E = 5.9 MeV) to ^{207}Bi, or (*ii*) via an electron capture process to ^{211}Po. ^{207}Bi decays with a half-life of 31.6 y to ^{207}Pb (stable). ^{211}Po decays with a half-life of 0.5 s to ^{207}Pb via α-particle emission (E = 7.4 MeV). The 5.9- and 7.4-MeV α-particles have a mean LET of ~122 and ~106 keV/μm and a particle range in tissue of ~48 and ~70 μm, respectively. The decays are accompanied by γ-radiation, enabling scintigraphy and dosimetry. ^{211}At has been used in animal studies (Andersson et al., 1999, 2000a, 2000b, 2001; Bäck et al., 2005; Elgqvist et al., 2005a, 2005b, 2006a, 2006b, 2006c, 2009a, 2009b; Steffen et al., 2006) and in one clinical study (Andersson et al., 2009).

^{213}Bi (Bismuth-213). ^{213}Bi (an α-particle emitter) is available via a generator based technology due to its relatively long-lived parent radionuclide, ^{225}Ac. ^{213}Bi decays with a half-life of 45.6 min to ^{209}Bi (stable) during which it emits an α-particle of 8.4 MeV (mean LET and particle range in tissue: ~99 keV/μm and ~89 μm, respectively). The α-particle emission is accompanied by γ-radiation. ^{213}Bi has been used in animal studies (Knör et al., 2008; Song et al., 2007).

^{90}Y (Yttrium-90). ^{90}Y is chemically similar to the lanthanoids and decays with a half-life of 64 h by the emission of electrons (β) with a maximum energy of ~2.2 MeV (E_{mean} = 933 keV). The emitted electrons have a maximum range in tissue of ~12 mm (mean range ≈ 4 mm) and a mean LET ≈ 0.2 keV/μm. Due to the emission of *Bremsstrahlung,* scintigraphy is feasible. ^{90}Y has been used in one animal study (Buchsbaum et al., 2005) and in clinical studies (Alvarez et al., 2002; Epenetos et al., 2000; Grana et al., 2004; Hird et al., 1990; Hnatowich et al., 1988; Maraveyas et al., 1994; Oei et al., 2007; Rosenblum et al., 1999; Stewart et al., 1990; Verheijen et al., 2006).

^{177}Lu (Lutetium-177). This radionuclide has a half-life of 6.7 d and decays by the emission of $β^-$-particles with a maximum energy of 497 keV (E_{mean} = 133 keV), which have a range in tissue of ~2 mm (mean range ≈ 0.2 mm), and a mean LET < 0.1 keV/μm. It also emits γ-radiation (208 keV). ^{177}Lu can be produced in large scale owing to the high thermal

neutron capture cross-section of ^{176}Lu (2100 barn) using moderate flux reactors. ^{177}Lu has been used in animal studies (Buchsbaum et al., 1999, 2005; Persson et al., 2007; Tolmachev et al., 2007) and in clinical studies (Alvarez et al., 1997; Epenetos et al., 1987; Meredith et al., 1996, 2001).

^{131}I (Iodine-131). ^{131}I has a half-life of 8 d and decays by the emission of β-particles with a maximum energy of 807 keV (E_{mean} = 182 keV, mean LET ≈ 0.1 keV/μm), which have a maximum range in tissue of ~3.6 mm (mean range ≈ 0.4 mm). It emits γ-radiation (364 keV) enabling scintigraphy and dosimetry. ^{131}I has been used in animal studies (Kievit et al., 1996; Molthoff et al., 1992; Turner et al., 1998) and in clinical studies (Buchsbaum et al., 1999; Buijs et al., 1998; Buist et al., 1993; Colcher et al., 1987; Crippa et al., 1995; Epenetos et al., 1987; Mahé et al., 1999; Molthoff et al., 1992, 1997; Muto et al., 1992; Stewart et al., 1989a, 1989b; Van Zanten-Przybysz et al., 2000, 2001).

^{186}Re (Rhenium-186) and ^{188}Re (Rhenium-188). ^{186}Re has a half-life of 3.7 d and decays by emitting β-particles having a maximum energy of 1.07 MeV (mean LET ≈ 0.1 keV/μm), 90% of it delivered within ~1.8 mm. ^{186}Re also emits γ-radiation. ^{186}Re has been used in clinical studies (Breitz et al., 1995; Jacobs et al., 1993). ^{188}Re has a half-life of 17 h and decays by emitting β-particles having a maximum energy of 795 keV (mean LET ≈ 0.1 keV/μm). The emitted γ-radiation enables scintigraphy and dosimetry. ^{188}Re has been used in one clinical study (Macey & Meredith, 1999).

3. Targeting constructs

In developing treatment strategies against EOC based on the concept of targeted radionuclide therapy several candidates as targeting constructs have been evaluated. Below follow a compilation of the main targeting constructs that have been used for bringing the radionuclide to the target, in animal as well as in clinical studies.

HMFG1 is a murine monoclonal antibody (mAb) which is directed to an epitope of the MUC1 gene product. MUC1 is a large, heavily glycosylated mucin (>400 kDa) expressed on the apical surface of the majority of secretory epithelial cells (Gendler, 2001). MUC1 is overexpressed in 90% of adenocarcinomas, including cancers of the ovary (Mukherjee et al., 2003). The extracellular portion of the MUC1 protein mainly consists of a variable number of highly conserved 20 amino acid repeats (Verheijen et al., 2006). HMFG1 has been used in clinical studies (Epenetos, et al., 1987; Verheijen et al., 2006).

HMFG2 is a murine mAb that is directed towards a large mucin-like molecule normally produced by the lactating breast. The mAbs react with similar components expressed by the majority (>90%) of ovarian, breast and other carcinomas (Arklie, et al., 1981). The HMFG2 epitope is generally expressed at a higher level in tumors (Burchell et al., 1983). HMFG2 has been used in one clinical study (Epenetos et al., 1987).

AUA1 is a murine IgG1 mAb that binds to an antigen expressed by a wide range of adenocarcinoma, including the majority (>90%) of carcinomas of the ovary. The antigen is a 40 kDa glycoprotein (Epenetos et al., 1982). AUA1 has been used in one clinical study (Epenetos et al., 1987).

H17E2 is a murine IgG1 mAb that is directed to placental and placental-like alkaline phosphatase (PLAP) (Travers & Bodmer, 1984). This enzyme is expressed as a surface membrane antigen (~67 kDa) of many neoplasms, including 60%–85% of ovarian carcinomas (Benham et al., 1978; Sunderland et al., 1984). H17E2 has been used in one clinical study (Epenetos et al., 1987).

Hu2PLAP is a human IgG1 κ mAb that has the same specificity as the murine H17E2 mAb described above. Hu2PLAP has been used in one clinical study (Kosmas et al., 1998).
H317 is a murine IgG mAb developed after immunisation with syncytiotrophoblast microvilli preparations from term placenta. It is specific for the *L*-phenylalanine inhibitable placental alkaline phosphatase (PLAP). H317 has been used in one clinical study (Kosmas et al., 1998).
Trastuzumab (Herceptin; Genentech, South San Francisco, CA) is a humanized IgG1 mAb that recognizes the extracellular domain of the HER-2/*neu* oncoprotein (Carter et al., 1992). Trastuzumab has been used in one animal study (Borchardt et al., 2003).
Pertuzumab is a human mAb binds to the dimerization domain II of HER-2. Pertuzumab is based on the human immunoglobulin IgG1 κ framework sequences, and is produced in Chinese hamster ovary cells. It has been used in one animal study (Persson et al., 2007).
B72.3 is a murine mAb that has been shown to be immunoreactive with the glycoprotein complex TAG-72 (>200 kDa) with the characteristics of a mucin (Johnson et al., 1986; Thor et al., 1986; Wolf et al., 1989). TAG-72 expression has been shown in the majority of ovarian carcinomas tested (Nuti et al., 1982). B72.3 has been used in clinical studies (Colcher et al., 1987; Rosenblum et al., 1999).
CC49 is a murine mAb is a high-affinity murine product that reacts with the tumor-associated glycoprotein TAG-72, which is expressed by the majority of common epithelial tumors (Schlom et al., 1990). CC49 has been used in one animal study (Buchsbaum et al., 2005) and in clinical studies (Alvarez et al., 1997, 2002; Buchsbaum et al., 1999; Macey et al., 1999; Meredith et al., 1996).
OC125 is a murine mAb that is directed against the tumor marker CA-125, and has been used in clinical studies (Hnatowich et al., 1988; Mahé et al., 1999; Muto et al., 1992).
MOv18 is a murine mAb that recognizes and reacts with a surface antigen, which is a membrane folate-binding glycoprotein of 38 kDa expressed on approximately 90% of all human ovarian carcinomas (Boerman et al., 1991; Campbell et al., 1991; Miotti et al., 1987). MOv18 (murine and in some cases chimeric) has been used in animal studies (Andersson et al., 1999, 2000a, 2000b, 2001) and in clinical studies (Buijs et al., 1998; Buist et al., 1993; Molthoff et al., 1992, 1997; Van Zanten-Przybysz et al., 2000, 2001).
MX35 is a murine IgG1 mAb directed towards a cell-surface glycoprotein of ~95 kDa on OVCAR-3 cells (Welshinger et al., 1997) and is expressed strongly and homogeneously on ~90% of human epithelial ovarian cancers (Rubin et al., 1993). The antigen recognized by MX35 is characterized as the sodium-dependent phosphate transport protein 2b (NaPi2b) (Yin et al., 2008). MX35 F(ab′)2 has been used in animal studies (Bäck et al., 2005; Elgqvist et al., 2006a, 2006b, 2006c, 2009a, 2009b) and in one clinical study (Andersson et al., 2009).
NR-LU-10 is a IgG2b murine mAb that is reactive with a glycoprotein (~40 kDa) expressed on most carcinomas of epithelial origin (Goldrosen et al., 1990; Varki et al., 1984). NR-LU-10 has been used in clinical studies (Breitz et al., 1995; Jacobs et al., 1993).
A5B7 is an anti-CEA IgG1 mAb that has been used in one large-animal model (sheep) study (Turner et al., 1998).
17-1A is a chimeric mAb is directed towards a ~39 kDa membrane-associated pancarcinoma glycoprotein (Edwards et al., 1986; Koprowski et al., 1979). It has been used in one animal study (Kievit et al., 1996).
323/A3 is a murine mAb that is directed to a ~39 kDa membrane-associated pancarcinoma glycoprotein (same as 17-1A) (Edwards et al., 1986; Koprowski et al., 1979). It has been used in one animal study (Johnson et al., 1986).

hCTMO1 is an antibody that was constructed by taking the short hypervariable regions of the murine mAb CTMO1 and grafting them into a human IgG4. It is directed towards a glycoprotein expressed on malignant cells of epithelial origin (Baker et al., 1994; Zotter et al., 1988). hCTMO1 has been used in one clinical study (Davis et al., 1999).

OV-TL 3 is a murine IgG1 mAb that recognizes a cell-surface antigen highly expressed on >90% of ovarian carcinomas (Poels et al., 1986). It has been used in one clinical study (Buist et al., 1995).

139H2 is a IgG1 mAb which binds to a protein determinant of episialin (Hilkens et al., 1988). 139H2 has been used in one animal study (Molthoff et al., 1992).

P-P4D is a targeting construct which is a pseudo-symmetrical covalent dimer of the monomeric peptide P-P4. It has been used in one animal study (Knör et al., 2008).

PAI2 is a targeting construct that is a plasminogen activator inhibitor type 2 and which is a member of the serine protease inhibitor (Serpin) superfamily and forms SDS-stable 1:1 complexes with urokinase plasminogen activator (uPA) (Song et al., 2007). It has been used in one animal study (Song et al., 2007).

Affibody molecules are composed of alpha helices and lack disulfide bridges. Two such molecular constructs, $(Z_{HER2:4})_2$ and $(Z_{HER2:342})_2$ (~15 kDa) have been used in animal studies (Steffen et al., 2006a, 2006b; Tolmachev et al., 2007).

4. Labeling chemistry

In nuclear medicine targeted therapy all to date approved radiopharmaceuticals are based on β-particle emitters. However, an increasing interest has been focused on α-particle emitting radionuclides as they offer several advantages over the most commonly used β-emitters for the treatment of micro-tumors. Unlike medically applied therapeutic radionuclides that decay by medium- to high-energy β-particle emissions leading to low-LET radiation with particle ranges varying from 1 to 10 mm, α-particle emitting radionuclides emit high-LET radiation in a small volume determined by the α-particle ranges of 50–100 µm. Only a few α-emitters fulfill the criteria for endoradiotherapeutic applications, the most studied being ^{211}At, ^{212}Bi, and ^{213}Bi. All these nuclides decay by 100% α-particle emission. Astatine-211 decays in two branches, 58% probability through electron capture to ^{211}Po which in turn decays through an α-particle emission (7.45 MeV) with a half-life of 0.52 seconds to the stable ^{207}Pb. The other branch (42%), resulting in an α-particle of 5.87 MeV, also ends in the stable ^{207}Pb through the daughter ^{207}Bi. The decay of ^{212}Bi is very similar to the decay of ^{213}Bi in terms of half-life and energy emitted ($T_{½}$ for ^{212}Bi = 60.6 min versus $T_{½}$ for ^{213}Bi = 45.6 min, mean E_{α} of both nuclides ≈ 8–8.5 MeV). However, while ^{213}Bi can be isolated as pure nuclide from the $^{225}Ac/^{213}Bi$ generator, ^{212}Bi is obtained *in situ* from the decay of ^{212}Pb. Lead-212 decays to ^{212}Bi with a half-life of 10.6 h.

For stable attachment of metals such as $^{212}Pb/^{212}Bi$ or ^{213}Bi to tumor specific targeting constructs an intermediate bifunctional chelating agent is required. A number of different chelating derivatives have been developed for conjugate labeling of various carrier molecules. Biological targeting constructs such as antibodies and peptides are commonly labeled with metal nuclides via chelating agents based on DTPA (diethylenetriaminepentaacetic acid) or DOTA (1,4,7,10-tetraazacyclododecane-1,4,7,10-tetraacetic acid). Heat sensitive proteins are preferably labeled with the semi rigid open chain DTPA derivatives, e.g. CHX A``DTPA, due to the fast metal coordination reaction kinetics at room temperature. DOTA is a versatile chelating agent which shows strong binding to a number of different metals, and the rigid structure give a metal-complex stronger than that of the corresponding complex to DTPA. However, chelating a metal to DOTA require heat or microwave assisted reaction condition, to be completed in reasonable times and with good yields, and are therefore more suitable for labeling to small molecules and peptides (Cordier et al., 2010).

The most common functional leaving group of the reagent is succinimidyl ester which is directed towards free amines on proteins and peptides, mainly presented on the side chain of lysine. For example, an antibody of IgG class has a molecular weight of approximately 150 kDa, and contains approximately 1200 amino acids, of which a number of lysine is randomly distributed. A lysine directed reagent conjugated to the antibody will therefore be non-specifically distributed in the protein structure, occasionally including the active antigen binding sites. Consequently the antigen binding capacity of the antibody may be affected when using lysine amine binding reagents. Site specific conjugation of antibodies can be achieved by targeting the sulfhydryl group on the side chain of cystein. In antibodies, cystein form disulfide bridges at specific sites within the antibody distant from the antigen binding site. The disulfide bridges can chemically be gently disrupted resulting in conjugate sites for a labelling reagent, e.g. malemido reagents. In this way the antigen binding of the conjugated antibody will not be compromised.

Independent of chelating moiety the procedure for labeling is conjugation of the chelating derivative to the carrier molecule and then labeling to the conjugate. The direct chelating of the metal nuclide to the conjugate is a prerequisite when labeling with metal nuclides with very short half-lives, e.g. ^{213}Bi. The other α-emitting isotope of bismuth ^{212}Bi is generated in the decay of ^{212}Pb. Generally ^{212}Pb or a mixture of ^{212}Pb/^{212}Bi is bound to a DOTA conjugate targeting construct. However, it has been reported that a fraction will be dechelated in the decay of ^{212}Pb, leaving a free fraction of ^{212}Bi (Su et al., 2005).

Compared with the ^{213}Bi, ^{211}At is perhaps the most versatile mainly because of its longer half-life, 7.2 h, which allow time for radiolabeling and quality control, and the time to distribute to the target cancer cells. Astatine is the heaviest element in the halogen family and since its discovery in 1940 (Corşon et al., 1947) it has been proposed for use in nuclear medicine applications. Several research and preclinical studies utilising ^{211}At for therapeutic nuclear medicine applications have been conducted, including the free halide, and ^{211}At-labeled tumor specific targeting constructs (Zalutsky et al., 2000). Many of these studies include tumor specific monoclonal antibodies, as they constitute suitable carrier properties for a number of different malignancies (Anderson et al., 2000b). Encouraging preclinical results have been obtained in radioimmunotherapy with astatinated antibodies and two phase I studies have emerged from these studies (Andersson et al., 2009; Zalutsky et al., 2008). However, ^{211}At requires a medium energy cyclotron for its production which is a major obstacle hampering clinical studies. And of the available cyclotrons having the capacity to produce ^{211}At, only a few of those facilities actually produce ^{211}At. Of the available cyclotrons having the capacity to produce ^{211}At, only a few of those facilities actually produce ^{211}At. In addition, one of the most demanding challenges in ^{211}At-radioimmunotherapy applications has been the development of adequate chemical labeling procedures for the production of ^{211}At-labeled antibodies at clinical levels of activity. Unlike direct iodination of proteins, astatine cannot be stably attached to unmodified antibodies (Visser et al., 1981). A number of different bifunctional labeling reagents for astatination of proteins have therefore been developed in which the common feature involves an electrophilic substitution reaction of organic tin as leaving group in the formation of an aryl-carbon- astatine bond, and a functional group for binding to proteins, commonly N-succinimidyl esters (Wilbur et al., 1989; Yordanov et al., 2001; Zalutsky et al., 1988). The radiochemistry is in general conducted in two steps, labeling of the reagent and conjugation of the labeled reagent to antibody. However, when using this strategy problems with yields and the final quality are frequently occurring, and have been recognised being due to radiolytic effects within the reacting solvents (Pozzi et al., 2007). Especially at high activity concentration conditions the α-particle decay of astatine may during labeling result in a considerable absorbed dose to the reaction solvent which can affect the chemistry, i.e. self-oxidation of astatine, decompose the precursor and/or alter the structural and biological integrity of the antibody. In fact, it has been reported that antibodies can be subjected to a maximum absorbed dose of approximately 1000 Gy without affecting its immunoreactivity (Larsen & Bruland, 1995).

Similar to metal radiolabeling, in which a bifunctional chelate is conjugated to the protein prior to labeling, the ATE reagent can be conjugated to the protein prior to astatination. In this way problems related to absorbed dose to reaction volumes, and dependency on protein concentration, can be avoided. The resulting yield and specific activities can be kept high even at high activity reaction conditions (Lindegren et al., 2008). However, although stable *in vitro* it has been found that the aryl-carbon-astatine bond is not stable *in vivo* when bound to small carrier molecules, e.g. antibody fragments such as F(ab)-fragments and minibodies.

Based on the higher strength of boron-astatine bonds (Kerr, 1977), new bifunctional reagents based on boron-cage structures, *nido*-carborane and *closo*-decaborate(2-) have been developed to increase the *in vivo* stability of astatination of biomolecules (Wilbur et al., 2004, 2009). The rout for synthesis of astatinated antibodies and fragments with the boron-cage reagents is, as the in metal radiolabeling, conjugation of the reagent to the antibody and subsequently direct radiohalogenation of the immunoconjugate. Halogenation yields are therefore generally higher than the yields obtained in two step astatination of the ATE reagents. Greater stability to dehalogenation of the astatinated products labeled via boron-cage chemistry has been confirmed (Wilbur et al., 2004).

5. Animal studies

Several animal studies investigating radionuclide therapy have been performed during the past couple of years. They have been investigating the pharmacokinetics, toxicity and therapeutic efficacy. The studies presented below comprise a selection of these studies using different radionuclides as well as different targeting constructs, and are paragraphed based on which radionuclide have been used, i.e. ^{225}Ac, ^{211}At, ^{213}Bi, ^{90}Y, ^{177}Lu, or ^{131}I. Some of the studies are not in an intraperitoneal setting, but have been mentioned because of their importance and relevance.

5.1 ^{225}Ac-Trastuzumab

One study has investigated the immunoreactivity, internalization, and cytotoxicity using SKOV-3 cells (Borchardt et al., 2003). The immunoreactivity was retained (50%-90%) and the radioimmunocomplex internalized into the cells (50% at 2 h). Various therapies were evaluated, using unlabeled trastuzumab and 8.1, 12.2, or 16.6 kBq of ^{225}Ac-trastuzumab or ^{225}Ac-labeled control antibody. The therapies were given 9 d after tumor inoculation. Groups of control mice and mice administered unlabeled trastuzumab had median survivals of 33, 37 or 44 d, respectively. The median survival was 52–126 d using ^{225}Ac-trastuzumab, and 48-64 d using the ^{225}Ac-control mAb. Some deaths from toxicity occurred at the highest activity levels. The study showed that i.p. administration of ^{225}Ac-trastuzumab extended survival in mice at levels that produce no apparent toxicity. An advantage of ^{225}Ac is that it emits a cascade of α-particles, implying a very high cytotoxic effect if the α-particle emissions occur in close vicinity to the cancer cell nuclei. The disadvantage is that when ^{225}Ac decays it will be separated from its targeting construct, making the remaining emitted α-particles an unspecific irradiation that potentially could lead to both dosimetry and toxicity problems. ^{225}Ac should therefore be used with caution in situations other than for example during intracavitary treatments or when the radioimmunocomplex is relatively rapid internalized into the cancer cells.

5.2 ^{211}At-MOv-18, ^{211}At-MX35 and ^{211}At-Affibody

Astatine-211 is a very promising radionuclide due to its half-life of 7.2 h and short particle range (~70 μm). A drawback is its limited availability due to the fact that it is cyclotron produced, and only a few cyclotrons world-wide produce ^{211}At today. The potential problem with unspecific irradiation (as described above for ^{225}Ac) is negligible due to the fact that the α-particle emanating from the second decay route (from ^{211}Po to ^{207}Pb) occurs with a very short half-life (0.5 seconds), i.e. in close vicinity to the targeted cancer cell (Palm et al., 2004). Andersson et al. have performed studies investigating the pharmacokinetics and therapeutic efficacy of ^{211}At-labeled mAbs (Andersson et al., 1999, 2000a, 2000b, 2001). In one of those studies the purpose was to compare the therapeutic efficacy of ^{211}At-MOv18 and ^{131}I-MOv18 (Andersson et al., 2001). The study used OVCAR-3 cells growing i.p. in mice. Two weeks after the i.p. inoculation of 1 × 10^7 tumor cells twenty mice were treated i.p. with MOv18 labeled with either ^{211}At (310–400 kBq) or ^{131}I (5.1–6.2 MBq). The pharmacokinetics of the labeled antibody in tumor-free animals was studied and the resulting absorbed dose to bone marrow was estimated. When the mice were treated with ^{211}At-MOv18 nine out of ten mice were free of macro- and microscopic tumors compared to three out of ten when ^{131}I-MOv18 was used. The equivalent dose to bone marrow was 2.4–3.1 Sv from ^{211}At-MOv18 and 3.4–4.1 Sv from ^{131}I-MOv18. The study showed that the therapeutic efficacy of ^{211}At-MOv18 was high, and superior to that using ^{131}I-MOv18.

Other studies using ^{211}At-mAbs have also been completed (Bäck et al., 2005; Elgqvist et al., 2005a, 2005b, 2006a, 2006b, 2006c, 2009a, 2009b). In one of those studies the purpose was to estimate the efficacy of RIT using ^{211}At-MX35 F(ab')2 or ^{211}At-Rituximab F(ab')2 (non-specific) against differently sized ovarian cancer deposits on the peritoneum, and to calculate absorbed dose to tumors and critical organs (Elgqvist et al., 2006a). At 1–7 w after inoculation animals were i.p. treated with ~400 kBq ^{211}At-MX35 F(ab')2, ~400 kBq ^{211}At-Rituximab F(ab')2, or unlabeled Rituximab F(ab')2. Eight weeks after each treatment the mice were sacrificed and the presence of tumors and ascites was determined. When given treatment 1, 3, 4, 5, or 7 w after cell inoculation the tumor-free fraction (TFF) was 0.95, 0.68, 0.58, 0.47, 0.26, and 1.00, 0.80, 0.20, 0.20, and 0.0 when treated with ^{211}At-MX35 F(ab')2 or ^{211}At-Rituximab F(ab')2, respectively. The conclusion of the study was that treatment with ^{211}At-MX35 F(ab')2 or ^{211}At-Rituximab F(ab')2 resulted in a TFF of 0.95–1.00 when the tumor radius was ≤30 μm. The TFF was decreased (TFF ≤ 0.20) for the non-specific ^{211}At-Rituximab F(ab')2 when the tumor radius exceeded the range of the α-particles. The tumor specific mAb resulted in a significantly better TFF, for different tumor sizes, explained by a high mean absorbed dose (>22 Gy) from the activity bound to the tumor surface, probably in addition to some contribution from penetrating activity.

Another study (although not i.p.) evaluated the relative biological effectiveness (RBE) of ^{211}At-mAb (Bäck et al., 2005). The endpoint was growth inhibition (GI) of subcutaneous OVCAR-3 xenografts. The animals received i.v. injections of ^{211}At-MX35 F(ab')2 (0.33, 0.65, and 0.90 MBq). External irradiation of the tumors was performed with a ^{60}Co source. To compare the biologic effects of the two radiation qualities, the mean value for GI was plotted for each tumor as a function of its corresponding absorbed dose. Exponential fits of these curves were made, and the absorbed doses required for a GI of 0.37 (D_{37}) were derived, and also the RBE of ^{211}At was determined. Absorbed doses in tumors were 1.35, 2.65, and 3.70 Gy. D_{37} was determined to 1.59 ± 0.08 Gy (mean ± SEM). Tumor growth after irradiation by the ^{60}Co source resulted in a D_{37} of 7.65 ± 1.0 Gy. The RBE of ^{211}At irradiation was calculated to be 4.8 ± 0.7 Gy.
In yet another study (also not i.p.) HER-2 binding affibody molecules were labeled with ^{211}At, using the PAB and a decaborate-based linker, and the biodistribution in tumor bearing mice was investigated (Steffen et al., 2006a). Compared with a previous biodistribution with ^{125}I, the ^{211}At biodistribution using the PAB linker showed higher uptake in lungs, stomach, thyroid and salivary glands, indicating release of free ^{211}At. When the decaborate-based linker was used, the uptake in those organs was decreased, but instead, high uptake in kidneys and liver was found. The conclusion of the study was that affibody molecules have suitable blood-kinetics for targeted radionuclide therapy with ^{211}At, the labeling chemistry however affects the distribution in normal organs to a high degree and needs to be improved to allow clinical use.

5.3 ^{213}Bi-P-P4D and ^{213}Bi-PAI2

Bismuth-213 has a well established chemistry, is available via a generator, and has recently achieved an increased attention. A drawback is its short half-life (45.6 min), which necessitates a rapid specificity, once injected. Using ^{213}Bi in intracavitary or i.p. applications, or using pretargeting techniques, could however overcome this potential problem. A study using ^{213}Bi has been performed by Knör et al. developing peptidic radioligands, which targets cancer cell urokinase receptors (uPAR, CD87) (Knör et al., 2008). DOTA-conjugated, uPAR-directed ligands were synthesised. Biodistribution of ^{213}Bi-P-P4D was analysed in mice 28 d after i.p. inoculation of OV-MZ-6 ovarian tumor cells in the absence or presence of the plasma expander gelofusine. Binding of ^{213}Bi-P-P4D to monocytoid U937 and OV-MZ-6 cells was shown using the natural ligand of uPAR, pro-uPA, or a soluble form of uPAR, suPAR, as competitors. The ^{213}Bi-P-P4D showed superior binding to OV-MZ-6 cells *in vitro*, and accumulation of ^{213}Bi-P-P4D in tumor tissue was shown by biodistribution analysis in mice bearing i.p. OV-MZ-6-derived tumors. Gelofusine reduced the kidney uptake of ^{213}Bi-P-P4D by 50%. In conclusion, ovarian cancer cells overexpressing uPAR were specifically targeted *in vitro* as well as *in vivo* by ^{213}Bi-P-P4D, and the kidney uptake was reduced by gelofusine.
An additional study also using ^{213}Bi has been published by Song et al. in which they investigated the pharmacokinetics, toxicity and *in vivo* stability of ^{213}Bi-PAI2, and also determined if a prior injection of the metal chelator Ca-DTPA or lysine would reduce the toxicity by decreasing the renal uptake (Song et al., 2007). Two different chelators (CHX-A''-DTPA and cDTPA) were used for the preparation of the ^{213}Bi-PAI2 conjugate; for i.p. administration in mice and ear vein injection in rabbits. Neither the mice nor the rabbits displayed any short term toxicity over 13 w at 1,420 MBq/kg and 120 MBq/kg ^{213}Bi-PAI2, respectively. The kidney uptake was markedly decreased (threefold) by blocking with lysine. Nephropathy caused by radiation was observed at 20–30 w in the mice, whereas severe renal tubular necrosis was detected at 13 w in the rabbits. In conclusion, the

nephropathy was the dose-limiting toxicity, and lysine was effective in reducing the uptake in the kidneys. Maximum tolerated doses were 350 and 120 MBq/kg for the mice and rabbits, respectively. The same research group has earlier shown the *in vitro* cytotoxicity and *in vivo* inhibition of tumor growth in breast, prostate, pancreatic, and ovarian cancer (Allen et al., 2003; Li et al., 2002; Qu et al., 2005; Ranson et al., 2002; Song et al., 2006).

5.4 ^{90}Y(or ^{177}Lu)-DOTA-biotin-streptavidin-CC49

Owing to efforts at developing strategies for RIT against ovarian cancer (Alvarez et al., 2002) the same research group also investigated pretargeted RIT in an i.p. tumor model (LS174T) using four CC49 anti-tumor-associated glycoprotein 72 (TAG-72) single-chain antibodies linked to streptavidin as a fusion protein (CC49 fusion protein) (Buchsbaum et al., 2005). A synthetic clearing agent was administered i.v. one day later to produce hepatic clearance of unbound CC49. A low molecular weight radiolabeled reagent composed of biotin conjugated to the chelating agent 7,10-tetra-azacyclododecane-N,N',N'',N'''-tetraacetic acid (DOTA) complexed with ^{111}In-, ^{90}Y-, or ^{177}Lu was injected four hours later. The radiolocalization to tumor sites was superior with i.p. administration of radiolabeled DOTA-biotin as compared to i.v. administration. Imaging and biodistribution studies showed good tumor localization with ^{111}In- or ^{177}Lu-DOTA-biotin. Tumor localization of ^{111}In-DOTA-biotin was 43% ID/g (percentage of injected dose per gram) and 44% ID/g at 4 and 24 hours with the highest normal tissue localization in the kidney with 6% ID/g at 48 and 72 h. ^{90}Y-DOTA-biotin at doses of 14.8–22.2 MBq or ^{177}Lu-DOTA-biotin at doses of 22.2–29.6 MBq produced significant prolongation of survival compared with controls ($p = 0.03$ and $p < 0.01$). The conclusion of the study was that pretargeted RIT using regional administration of CC49 fusion protein and i.p. ^{90}Y- or ^{177}Lu-DOTA-biotin is a therapeutic strategy in the LS174T i.p. tumor model and that this strategy may be applicable to humans. LS174T is a human colon cancer cell line, but as it was used in an i.p. setting in this study together with CC49 (which reacts with the tumor-associated glycoprotein TAG-72, expressed by the majority of common epithelial tumors) we think it is relevant to present the results.

5.5 ^{177}Lu-Pertuzumab and ^{177}Lu-Affibody

Lutethium-177-Pertuzumab has been used for disseminated HER-2-positive micrometastases (Persson et al., 2007), and showed good targeting in mice bearing HER-2-overexpressing xenografts. Absorbed radiation dose in tumors was more than 5 to 7 times higher than that in blood and in any normal organ. ^{177}Lu-Pertuzumab delayed tumor progression compared with controls (no treatment, $p < 0.0001$; Pertuzumab, $p < 0.0001$; and ^{177}Lu-labeled irrelevant mAb, $p < 0.01$). Adverse side effects of the treatment could not be detected. In conclusion, the results support the possibility using ^{177}Lu-Pertuzumab in clinical studies.

In a study by Tolmachev et al. a ^{177}Lu-labeled anti-HER-2 affibody molecule ($Z_{HER2:342}$) targeting xenografts was used (Tolmachev et al., 2007). Due to the small size (~7 kDa) of the affibody molecule rapid glomerular filtration and high renal accumulation occurred. Reversible binding to albumin reduced the renal excretion and uptake though. The affibody molecule $(Z_{HER2:342})_2$ (i.e. dimeric) was fused with the albumin-binding domain (ABD) conjugated with the isothiocyanate derivative of CHX-A''-DTPA and thereafter labeled with ^{177}Lu. Fusion with ABD caused a 25-fold reduction of the renal uptake in comparison with the non-fused dimer molecule $(Z_{HER2:342})_2$. The biodistribution showed high uptake of the conjugate in HER-2-expressing tumors. Treatment of SKOV-3 microxenografts (having a high HER-2 expression) with 17 or 22 MBq ^{177}Lu-CHX-A''-DTPA-ABD-$(Z_{HER2:342})_2$ prevented formation of tumors completely. In LS174T xenografts (having a low HER-2 expression), this treatment resulted in a small but significant increase of the survival. In conclusion, fusion with ABD improved the *in vivo* biodistribution and indicated ^{177}Lu-CHX-A''-DTPA-ABD-$(Z_{HER2:342})_2$ as a candidate for the treatment of disseminated tumors having high HER-2 expression.

5.6 ^{131}I-A5B7

In a large animal study of human tumors in cyclosporin-immunosuppressed sheep, by Turner et al., evaluation and measurement of tumor uptake of ^{131}I-mAbs was done (Turner et al., 1998). Human cancer cells were orthotopically inoculated (~10^7 cells): SKMEL melanoma subcutaneously; LS174T and HT29 colon carcinoma into bowel, peritoneum and liver; and JAM ovarian carcinoma into the ovary and peritoneum. The tumor xenografts grew within 3 w and generally maintained their histological appearance, a few tumor deposits showing some degree of dedifferentiation though. Regional lymph node metastases were shown for xenografts from the melanoma and ovarian carcinoma. An anti-CEA mAb (A5B7) labeled with ^{131}I was administered intravenously. The peak uptake at 5 d in orthotopic tumors in the gut was 0.027% ID/g and 0.034% ID/g in hepatic metastases with tumor-to-blood ratios of 2.0–2.5. The non-specific uptake in melanoma tumors was 0.003% ID/g. In conclusion, the uptake of ^{131}I-mAb in human tumors was comparable to the uptake observed in patients, and this sheep model may therefore be more realistic than mice xenografts for prediction of the efficacy of RIT.

6. Clinical studies

Several clinical protocols have been reported on during the past twenty years, although almost all of them have been small phase I radiopharmaceutical biokinetics and absorbed dose-finding studies (Alvarez et al., 2002; Jacobs et al., 1993; Macey et al., 1999; Meredith et al., 1996, 2001; Van Zanten-Przybysz et al., 2000,2001), or phase I/II studies with no controls or at best matched historical cases (Epenetos et al., 1987, 2000; Hird et al., 1990; Nicholson et l., 1998; Stewart et al., 1989a, 1989b). Tumor stage and degree of advanced disease have varied greatly between, and also within, these studies as have the used targeting constructs and the choice of radionuclide. Albeit, these studies are important as they have provided us with the necessary starting hubs to the scaffold of knowledge that needs to be acquired. The major exception from this is the only randomised phase III study reported by Verheijen et al. (Verheijen et al., 2006). Despite its negative results it still holds as the major publication so far on intraperitoneal (i.p.) radioimmunotherapy for ovarian cancer and also stresses the importance of performing randomized studies. This study was spurred by the positive findings in a non-randomized phase I/II trial (Epenetos et al., 2000; Nicholson et al., 1998), where prolonged disease free and long term survival was described after one i.p. treatment, using ^{90}Y labeled murine HMFG1 antibody, in patients that had received a complete response on standard treatment (surgery and primary chemotherapy). Prior to these reports, a few other small clinical studies using different radionuclides and targeting constructs, had likewise suggested a possibly better treatment effect of i.p. radioimmunotherapy, correlating inversely with size of residual disease; ^{131}I (Epenetos et al., 1987; Crippa et al., 1995; Stewart et al., 1989a, 1989b); and ^{186}Re (Jacobs et al., 1993).

Thus, the Verheijen study (Verheijen et al., 2006) finally recruited 447 patients between February 1998 and January 2003, with ovarian cancer (FIGO stage Ic-IV) to evaluate if a single i.p. infusion of 25 mg of the β-particle emitter ^{90}Y conjugated to the murine HMFG1 antibody could prolong survival in patients in complete clinical response (physical examination and CT-scan and CA-125) after surgical debulking and finishing standard platinum containing chemotherapy and, importantly, with a macroscopically negative second-look laparoscopy. However, contrary to the beliefs from the pre-studies this large prospective randomized study failed to demonstrate any survival benefit. Using Cox proportional hazards analysis of survival, no difference was found, after a median follow-up of 3.5 years 70/224 patients had died in the active treatment arm compared with 61/223 in the control arm. Also time to relapse was similar between groups and 104/224 active treatment patients experienced relapse compared with 98/223 of controls.

Although the study was carefully planned and well conducted and performed one should consider the following points which could have contributed to conceal positive effects of the active treatment. A) Peritoneal adhesions in up to an entire quadrant did not exclude patients in this study, which could potentially result in a significant underdosing of ≤ 25% of the abdominal cavity. Further, the adhesions were assessed by laparoscopy, CT scan or isotope diffusion scan, where only the latter can allow a solid enough assessment of adhesions and to discern between one or two quadrants of adhesions. Importantly, it is unclear if patients (no adhesions versus one quadrant with adhesions) were stratified between each treatment arm. B) A possible skewing of patients with more advanced disease characteristics to the treatment arm is evident, e.g. in the active treatment arm there were 8% more patients with residual disease after initial surgery (44.2% vs. 35.9%) and there were 3% more stage III and IV patients in the treatment arm which also had a higher mean CA-125 level after laparoscopy (never explained). Furthermore, 7% more patients in the standard arm received consolidation chemotherapy (19.7% vs. 12.5%). C) Regarding the radioimmunocomplex and their antigenicity towards the cancer cells one may note that the overall antibody mass of 25 mg may have been insufficient to provide a concentration gradient to help "push" the radiolabeled antibody into the tumors. This can be contrasted to the 250 mg/m^2 of cold antibody used with Zevalin or the 450 mg total antibody dose used with Bexxar. As a multi-center study the radiolabeling process was by necessity performed by each institution and although a radiolabeling efficiency of 95% was confirmed with thin-layer chromatography, a potential loss of affinity of the antibody for the antigen, as a result of the radiolabeling process was not addressed. And lastly; D) The impact of a ≤60% MUC1 staining for 18% of the patients in the treatment arm is grossly unknown.

Although no survival benefit for ^{90}Y-HMFG1 i.p. instillation as consolidation treatment for epithelian ovarian cancer was found, an improved local control of i.p. disease was reported on in a pattern of failure analysis (Oei et al., 2007). Of the 104/224 treatment arm and 98/223 control arm relapses, there were significantly fewer i.p. (40 vs. 69, $p < 0.05$) and more extraperitoneal (47 vs. 13, $p < 0.05$) relapses in the treatment arm. Correspondingly, time to i.p. recurrence was significantly longer (53.4 vs. 46.4 months, $p = 0.0019$) and time to extraperitoneal recurrence was significantly shorter for the treatment arm (51 vs. 63.6 months, $p < 0.001$).

Thus, the main negative result of the Verheijen study balances back somewhat, in that, some treatment effects can be seen locally i.p. with a delaying of local relapses which, however, could not translate into an effect on survival. Bearing in mind the above listed concerns, it is from our research group's perspective (the Targeted Alpha Therapy Group, www.TAT.gu.se), tempting to argue that the failure of the treatment could simply be explained by the choice of radionuclide, i.e. when treating microscopic disease with high energy β-particles emitted from ^{90}Y, the electron will have too long a range in order to deliver high enough energy to the cancer cell nuclei. It has been modelled that high energy β-particle emissions will not deposit large amounts of radiation energy into small microscopic tumor spheroids.

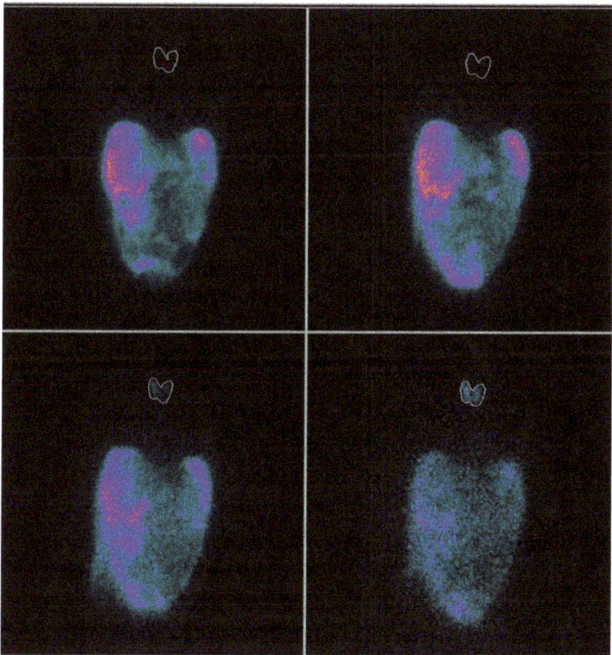

Fig. 1. Consecutive anteroposterior decay corrected scans (γ-camera) of the abdominal and thoracic area of a patient in the study by Andersson et al., 2009. The thyroid uptake, which is indicated by a region of interest in each panel, was not blocked in this patient. Images were acquired at 1.5 (top left), 5 (top right), 11.5 (bottom left), and 19.5 (bottom right) hours after infusion of ^{211}At-MX35 F(ab')2. The figure is reprinted by permission of the Society of Nuclear Medicine from Andersson H, Cederkrantz E, Bäck T, et al. Intraperitoneal α-particle radioimmunotherapy of ovarian cancer patients: pharmacokinetics and dosimetry of ^{211}At-MX35 F(ab´)2 - a phase I study. J Nucl Med 2009;50:1153-1160.

So far, the only clinical study using an α-particle emitter, ^{211}At, for treating ovarian cancer has been performed at our institution (Andersson et al., 2009). In a phase I study the pharmacokinetics and toxicity of α-RIT using ^{211}At- MX35 F(ab')2, in 9 patients with relapsed ovarian cancer was studied after 2nd or 3rd line of chemotherapy. Laparoscopy to exclude presence of macroscopic tumor growth or adhesions was performed prior to infusion with 20.1-101 MBq (0.54-2.73 mCi)/L ^{211}At-MX35 F(ab')2 via a peritoneal catheter. The study demonstrated that it is possible to achieve therapeutic absorbed doses in microscopic tumors without significant toxicity using up to 101 MBq. The potential thyroid toxicity of ^{211}At could be successfully blocked by potassium perchlorate/iodide, (unblocked thyroid, 24.7 ± 11.1 mGy/(MBq/L); blocked thyroid, 1.4 ± 1.6 mGy/(MBq/L)). Two patients have no evidence of disease at 39 and 72 months. A multicenter, phase II study is currently being planned, intended as an upfront adjuvant treatment for a patient population that has received cytoreductive surgery and chemotherapy.

6.1 Tolerability and toxicity

Generally the side effects have been mild, maximum tolerated doses (MTD) depends both on the nuclide used and the specific construct. The highest used activities can be infused using ^{131}I constructs up to 5-6 GBq have been infused using different antibodies, but due to a long half-life (8 days) the bone marrow suppression have been evident (Epenetos et al., 1987; Crippa et al., 1995; Stewart et al., 1989a, 1989b). The long half-life and gamma emission are also a concern regarding the unintentional irradiation of staff, relatives and other patients. In modelling bone marrow absorbed doses (Buchsbaum et al., 1999) using the CC49 antibody, and based on limiting the bone marrow absorbed dose to 2 Gy, the maximum possible administered activity of each of the following radionuclide was calculated: ^{188}Re: 6.2 GBq (167.6 mCi), ^{166}Ho: 4.1 GBq (110.8 mCi), ^{177}Lu: 3.9 GBq (105.4 mCi), ^{186}Re: 2.6 GBq (70.2 mCi), ^{131}I: 2.2 GBq (59.5 mCi), and ^{90}Y: 1.3 GBq (35.1 mCi). Thus, ^{188}Re was found to deliver the lowest RM absorbed dose, primarily because it had the shortest half-life, whereas ^{90}Y delivered the highest RM dose (high energy, long path-length).

For ^{90}Y a variation in MTD depending on the used antibody, from 370 MBq with B72.3 (Rosenblum et al., 1999) up to 895 MBq with CC49 (Alvarez et al., 2002) is described. Prior to the large phase III study, a MTD of 685 MBq was found (Hird et al., 1990; Maraveyas et al., 1994; Stewart et al.,1990) for ^{90}Y using the HFG1-antibody with the bone marrow as dose limiting organ. Subsequently an activity of 666 MBq was used (Nicholson et al., 1998; Verheijen et al., 2006), the most common side effects of nausea, fatigue, arthralgia, myalgia and abdominal discomfort were transient and mainly mild. The expected bone marrow toxicity was evident as thrombocytopenia with as much as 24% of the patients experiencing more than grade 3 toxicity, peeking at 6 weeks after treatment and a few cases 2,4% lasting until 6 months after treatment (Verheijen et al., 2006).

Two combined modality treatment protocols have been reported with subcutaneous IFN α2b and i.p. paclitaxel (100 mg/m^2), combined with i.p. ^{90}Y-CC49, MTD of 895 MBq, (Alvarez et al., 2002) or i.p. ^{177}Lu-CC49-RIT (Meredith et al., 2001). The addition of IFN increased hematologic toxicity such that the MTD of the combination with ^{177}Lu-CC49 was 1.5 GBq/m^2 compared to 1.7 GBq/m^2. Considering the much shorter range of the emitted β-particles from ^{177}Lu (mean range ≈ 0.2 mm) compared to those emitted from ^{90}Y (mean range ≈ 4 mm), ^{177}Lu theoretically has a higher therapeutic index than ^{90}Y for a microscopic disease, due to its ability to more specifically irradiate the tumor cells while sparing healthy tissue.

Strategies to increase the tumor activity and decrease the activity in dose limiting organs have been tested also in small clinical studies. Firstly, data have been presented using EDTA as an effective myeloprotective drug to suppress the bone uptake (Rosenblum et al., 1999). Continuous i.v. infusion of EDTA immediately before i.p. administration of up to 1,665 MBq ^{90}Y-B72.3 presented the expected dose-limiting toxicities of thrombocytopenia and neutropenia but at a higher MTD, and analysis of biopsies demonstrated that the bone and marrow content of the ^{90}Y was 15-fold lower (<0.001% ID/g) in the group receiving EDTA infusion. Secondly, the concept of pretargeted RIT based on the avidin-biotin system, was evaluated in 38 patients (Grana et al., 2004). A three-step protocol: biotinylated mAbs and avidin were i.p. injected (first and second step), and 12–18 h later ^{90}Y-biotin (either i.v. or i.p.) was injected as the third step. Sixteen were treated by i.p. injection only, whereas 22 patients received the combined treatment (i.v. + i.p.), doses ranged from 370 to 3,700 MBq of ^{90}Y-biotin. Both regimens were well tolerated, but two patients showed temporary grade III–IV hematologic toxicity. In conclusion, excellent tolerability and a good potential therapeutic role of pretargeted RIT in advanced ovarian cancer.

7. Radiation dosimetry in the clinical situation

Dosimetry is needed to optimize the amount of radiopharmaceutical that should be administered to the patient (Palm et al., 2011). This involves estimating the maximum administered radioactivity possible at which critical normal organs reach an acceptable degree of toxicity. Dosimetric calculations are mostly only needed for a few critical normal organs. Derived organ absorbed radiation doses, combined with the knowledge about tolerance absorbed doses, provide a guide for estimating the maximum tolerable activity (MTA) that should be given. This approach has been applied in the therapy with β-particle-emitting radiopharmaceuticals when tolerance absorbed doses for critical normal organs have been established. An example is the therapy with ^{177}Lu-octreotate, in which the administered activity is based on dosimetry for the kidneys (Garkavij et al., 2010). The clinical experience with β-particle emitters and estimation of tolerance absorbed doses could possibly be used to predict the outcome for the therapy with α-particle emitters. A first correction should then be made for the higher relative biological effectiveness (RBE) of α-particles. In the first clinical studies, an RBE of 5 has been applied for the estimation of equivalent absorbed doses (Andersson et al., 2009; Bruland et al., 2006; Sgouros et al., 1999). The concept of RBE and the uncertainties of its precise value for α-particles are still under debate and investigated. The weighting factors applied for the estimation of the effective absorbed dose (where a factor of 20 often is recommended by regulators for α-particle radiation) should not be used for predicting therapeutic efficacy and toxicity in patients undergoing radionuclide therapy. These weighting factors were conservatively derived for the stochastic effects and were never meant for use in estimating the deterministic effects relevant for therapy. The clinical experience using α-particles is still very limited, and no tolerance absorbed radiation doses in humans have been determined yet. The current knowledge is therefore limited to *in vitro* and *in vivo* studies. For current and planned clinical studies of α-particle–emitting radiopharmaceuticals, it is therefore very important to gain more insight into the toxic effects of α-particles and its relationship to absorbed dose for different organs. The tolerance absorbed doses found for α-particles could then gradually become established and used for the treatment planning of patients.

Besides the special challenges regarding α-particles, the establishment of pharmacokinetic data for dosimetry calculations does not differ from that of the more conventional β-particle therapies. Nuclear medicine imaging is often used for the quantification of the dosimetric calculations. Much software have been developed for the calculation of the absorbed radiation doses to organs and tumors based on serial 3D imaging and anatomical information from computed tomography (CT) or magnetic resonance imaging (MRI) (Sgouros et al., 2008). Accurate quantification of γ-camera and positron-emission tomography (PET) images and measurements of for example the radioactive blood content over time, are also becoming increasingly important for many diagnostic nuclear medicine procedures. Repeated sample measurements using, for example, a gamma-well counter can provide valuable pharmacokinetic data that allow for accurate absorbed dose calculations. Blood and urine sampling is often possible for patients undergoing therapy. Repeated sampling of peritoneal fluid has also been reported (Andersson et al., 2009). In principle, measurements or images of biopsies from organs of interest would be valuable (Bäck et al., 2010), but the increased dosimetric accuracy gained must be weighed against the discomfort such invasive procedures cause the patient. Simple, non-invasive methods using uptake probes can also provide important information on the pharmacokinetics for an individual patient. Gaze et al. have demonstrated the usefulness of such an approach for patient dosimetry following ^{131}I-MIBG treatments (Gaze et al., 2005).

Imaging using a γ-camera is commonly used for quantifying the biodistribution of therapeutic radiopharmaceuticals. A prerequisite, of course, being the presence of emitted γ-photons, characteristic X-ray, or bremsstrahlung radiation. The image quality depends on photon energy, photon yields, energy settings, and appropriate matching of collimator and photon energy. The decay chains of the α-particle emitters used hitherto in clinical studies (^{225}Ac, ^{213}Bi, ^{211}At, and ^{223}Ra) all include emissions of photons useful for γ-camera imaging. However, the spatial resolution of γ-camera images is inferior to what is needed to resolve activity distributions within organ compartments or in small tumors. Administered activity and the presence of photons are also much lower compared to the diagnostic situation, resulting in a low signal-to-noise ratio. The possibility of serial γ-camera imaging of patients receiving α-particle therapy is therefore limited for providing quantitative data for dosimetry of whole organs. Low count rates make the preferred 3D SPECT (three dimensional single photon-emission computed tomography) imaging of the radionuclide distribution very time consuming. Serial imaging might therefore be restricted to planar imaging with possibly lower accuracy for the quantification of radioactivity. Such planar images can provide useful quantitative information, and the accuracy can also be increased by using co-registration with CT images (Sjögren et al., 2002).

A focus committee of the Society of Nuclear Medicine provided a review in 1995 of the different factors affecting quantitative SPECT (Rosenthal et al., 1995). The field has developed since then, but the main factors that affect the quantification using SPECT remain the same. Many factors influence the accuracy of the quantification of PET/CT images and include: correction for attenuation, noise, image resolution, and ROI (region of interest) definitions (Alessio et al., 2010; Boellard et al., 2004; Kinahan et al., 1998). Regarding all quantifications, it can be very useful to perform phantom measurements mimicking the patient situation as good as possible. Measurements of that kind can help in selecting the parameters for imaging or probe sessions as well as providing indications of the accuracy that possibly can be obtained (He et al., 2005).

7.1 Tumor and critical organ absorbed doses

Although the maximum amount of administered activity possible is directly related to the absorbed radiation dose to the critical organs, the therapeutic efficacy is determined by the absorbed dose to the tumors. If a low tumor absorbed dose can be expected, the therapy might not be justified. The tumor absorbed dose should therefore, if at all possible, be estimated before treatment. The visualization and quantification using a γ-camera can at best give an estimate of the radiopharmaceutical uptake in the organ as a whole and in large tumors. The determination of absorbed radiation dose to sub-organ compartments or to small tumors or infiltrate cancer cells is though seldom possible.

Estimating the absorbed dose to tumors following α-particle therapy is particularly difficult. Because the targeted tumors often are too small to be detected, at best indirect methods can be used for approximating the absorbed radiation dose. Using antibody or peptide-based therapies, this approximation can for example involve *in vitro* studies on the binding kinetics to antigens or receptor sites for the relevant cancer cell type. Using radionuclides having a decay chain including α-particle-emitting daughters, studies would involve investigating the retention of daughter radionuclides on or in the vicinity of the cancer cells.

Microdosimetry based on such *in vitro* studies could then provide the basis for investigations of the probability for eradicating or stopping or retarding the growth of the tumors. The theoretical basis for such dosimetry has recently been described by Sgouros et al. (Sgouros et al., 2011).

The complexity of the studies and calculations involved for the absorbed dose is considerable, particularly when translating the results to the individual patient for an outcome prediction. This initial complexity should not though prevent formulation of a first, although perhaps rough, estimate. Such estimates, including best-guess information on tumor spread and overall tumor burden, targeting ability, and the amount of delivered radioactivity, will often provide good insight into the potential usefulness of the treatment approach.

As for radionuclide therapies using β-particle emitters, the absorbed dose to critical organs often determines the MTA. The common aim should therefore be to maximize the administered activity to near the level of toxicity for these organs, even for therapies using α-particles. Therapy planning should include calculation of expected organ absorbed doses (Gy) per administered activity (Bq) to identify the optimal amount of activity to be administered. The absorbed dose calculations can either be based on pharmacokinetic data from previous patients or preferably, data from the specific patient is used. Such data could be generated by tracer studies of the actual radiopharmaceutical or a substitute with similar pharmacokinetics. If a fractionated or repeated therapy is to be used, the generation of pharmacokinetic data from each administration should be used for re-planning the remainder. However, differences can arise in the pharmacokinetics between the therapeutic radiopharmaceutical and the tracer or between subsequent therapy sessions, and methods should therefore be established to detect such changes.

7.2 General considerations

The clinical studies using targeted α-particle therapy have their origin in previously established strategies involving β-particle emitters. It is assumed that the significantly shorter track range of the α-particles compared to β-particles provides a therapeutic advantage in that the critical normal organs to a high degree will be spared and a higher absorbed radiation dose to microscopic tumors will be reached. An illustration of this fact is ^{223}Ra therapy for example, in which the bone marrow is less irradiated compared to therapies using β-particle emitters. Radium-223 binds to the skeleton, resulting in a high absorbed dose to the bone surfaces while the absorbed radiation dose to the bone marrow remains relatively low. Consequently, the hematologic toxicity is therefore limited.

If shifting from a β- to an α-particle emitting radiopharmaceutical, the dosimetry differs not only due to the different particles emitted but also due to differences in half-lives and the biokinetics of the free radionuclide. When, for example, using ^{211}At-conjugates, ^{211}At can be set free and be taken up in the thyroid as a result of the natrium iodine symporter (NIS) receptor expressed at the thyroid cells. This process is very similar to that which occurs when iodine-based conjugates are used and iodine is set free and taken up by the NIS receptor. In both of the clinical studies using ^{211}At, blocking agents like potassium perchlorate were used to reduce the uptake in the thyroid cells. This method is well known for iodine-based therapies, and both the normal uptake of iodine in the thyroid and the blocking effect of, for example, potassium iodide are well established. Regarding ^{211}At, the blocking effect can not be considered well established, and careful monitoring is therefore necessary for any unwanted uptake in the thyroid despite the use of blocking agents.

The physical half-life of α- and β-particle emitters used should ideally be matched with the kinetics of the targeting approach. The relatively short half-lives of the α-particle emitters ^{211}At and ^{213}Bi could in general be a disadvantage therefore, but are a good match for the loco-regional therapies such as intraperitoneal. Most of the decays will occur within the intraperitoneal cavity before the substance is distributed throughout the body. To be able to achieve optimal therapeutic efficacy the maximum safe amount of activity should be administered to the patient. The determination of the MTA is typically sought for a patient population but should ideally be estimated for each individual patient as mentioned above; thus, patient-specific dosimetry is needed.

Taking a control image with an analogue is relevant for ovarian cancer. In this case, it is important to determine if the infused radiopharmaceutical can disperse throughout the peritoneal cavity and access all potential microscopic tumors on the peritoneal lining. Leakage control, i.e., determining the lymphatic flow out from the peritoneal cavity, can also be done using an analogue by monitoring the activity concentration in blood over time. Such control images helps manage bone marrow absorbed doses. Pharmacokinetic data show that the variation in absorbed dose to bone marrow among patients is around 20% (Andersson et al., 2009). If the absorbed dose to the bone marrow determines the MTA, then a tracer study could be used to estimate the patient-specific MTA. However, since the peritoneum might determine the MTA for intraperitoneal therapy, only the activity concentration in the peritoneal fluid is probably needed to establish it. In this particular situation, the same activity concentration in the injected solution for all patients can be reasonable, but it is valid only if the patients are free from ascites at the time of injection.

The phase I study on ovarian cancer has generated interest in an adjuvant-targeted α-particle therapy of earlier-stage cancer patients (Andersson et al., 2009). This population would by necessity include patients who would remain disease-free even without the adjuvant therapy. In such settings, it is relevant to include stochastic and/or long-term risks such as secondary cancers and dysfunction of the peritoneum in the justification for the therapy. In this particular case, it is advised that calculation of the equivalent doses to all relevant organs is done, including a conservative estimation of the RBE for α-particles.

8. Future perspectives

The mortality of EOC has not decreased during the past decades, despite a decline in incidence and an intensification of treatment has occurred. The majority of the patients are diagnosed at an advanced stage and most of them will therefore succumb, suffering from abdominal complications. Using present diagnostics, the screening for early stage EOC has not been successful, but efforts in finding proteins in serum indicating early EOC is a vision for future improvements in ovarian cancer survival. Additional approaches are for example the development of targeted treatments, resulting hopefully in higher efficacy and lower toxicity than present day treatments, some of which have been discussed above. Such targeted therapies could include substrate analogues, ligands, or antibodies, resulting in up-regulation of receptors or surface antigens. Antibodies may exhibit a therapeutic effect on their own or as conjugates to toxins or radionuclides. Since the clinical situation is dominated by spread and complications in the abdominal cavity, such therapeutic techniques are primarily directed intraperitoneally. A successful intraperitoneal therapy may eradicate abdominal disease and complications, however, extraperitoneal metastases may become revealed. Therefore, a combination of abdominal and systemic modalities is most likely required.

As the current available standard treatments often fail to cure a micrometastatic disease, RIT, using short ranged high efficiency α-particles emitted from for example ^{211}At or ^{213}Bi and depositing the radiation energy in close vicinity of the targeted cancer cells, is an attractive approach, possibly in combination with β-particle emitters aimed at larger tumor cell clusters. Such procedures could then be given as a boost after initial cytoreductive surgery and systemic chemotherapy, primarily intraperitoneally but possibly also intravenously by pretargeting approaches, based for example on the avidin/streptavidin-biotin system. A systemic adjunctive approach may be of particular value if the disease includes retroperitoneal vascularized metastases to the lymph nodes for example (Buchsbaum et al., 2005; Frost et al., 2010; Paganelli et al., 1993). Another important concept that could potentially improve the therapeutic index would be to use fractionated RIT, expectedly resulting in decreased normal tissue toxicity while retaining the therapeutic efficacy (Elgqvist et al., 2009b). Auger emitters could also offer an alternative to the radionuclides mentioned above, due to the emitted electrons being low energy (<< 1 keV), and therefore having a very short path length in tissue. To effectively damage the DNA the Auger emitter has to be incorporated into the DNA molecule though, a biological challenge that has to be taken into account for this type of treatment.

The potential disadvantages with a treatment given intraperitoneally are: the i.p. catheter could cause pain and discomfort for the patient, the catheter could leak (and possibly therefore decreasing the therapeutic efficacy and causing a radiation protection problem for the staff), and it could cause an infection and therefore a risk of peritonitis. In order for the i.p. treatments to be successful, especially when using radionuclides that emit short-range particles such as α-particles, loculation and/or adhesions are undesirable and could decrease the therapeutic efficacy. The potential problems of toxicity (especially bone marrow, kidney, peritoneum) and HAMA response always needs to be addressed. A number of review articles have recently been published, regarding RIT in general and RIT against intraperitoneal EOC in particular (Allen, 2004, 2008; Andersson et al., 2003; Chérel, 2006; Crippa, 1993; Gadducci et al., 2005; Gaze, 1996; Goldenberg, 2002; Goldenberg & Sharkey, 2006; Imam, 2001; Kairemo, 1996; Kassis et al., 1996; Meredith et al., 2007; Mulford et al., 2005; Muto & Kassis, 1995; Oyen et al., 2007; Sharkey & Goldenberg, 2005; Zalutsky et al., 2007).

Many different parameters could influence the intraperitoneal therapeutic outcome, some of which are: the specificity of targeting construct, the degree of antigenic expression (Moltoff et al., 1991), loss of immunoreactivity of the targeting construct, amount of unlabeled antibody, diffusion barriers for penetration of the targeting construct into cancer cell clusters, the choice of radionuclide (half-life and particle range), low specific radioactivity, and tumors located extraperitoneally. If treating a microscopic disease the choice of using β-particle emitters could be problematic due to the inability of the β-particles to deliver high enough radiation energy to the target volume, i.e. the cancer cell nuclei. That is probably the reason why the clinical studies performed so far using β-particles have failed when trying to treat microscopic diseases.

The proof-of-concept using an intraperitoneal treatment has been shown in a phase III study by the Gynecologic Oncology Group that included women undergoing initial therapy for advanced ovarian cancer (Armstrong et al., 2006), and the advantage of i.p. compared to i.v. administration for the localization of radiolabeled mAbs to microscopic peritoneal disease has been shown in some studies, both in animal models and for humans (Andersson et al., 2003; Horan Hand et al., 1989; Ward et al., 1987). Finally, in order to be able to compare and evaluate different treatment strategies the need to conduct randomized, controlled, multicenter clinical studies with large enough patient numbers, enabling statistical significance to occur, must be emphasized and aimed at.

9. References

Alessio AM, Kinahan PE, Champley KM, et al. Attenuation-emission alignment in cardiac PET/CT based on consistency conditions. *Med Phys*. 2010;37(3):1191–1200.

Allen BJ, Tian Z, Rizvi SM, et al. Preclinical studies of targeted alpha therapy for breast cancer using ^{213}Bi-labelled-plasminogen activator inhibitor type 2. *Br J Cancer*. 2003;88:944–950.

Allen BJ, Raja C, Rizvi S, et al. Targeted alpha therapy for cancer. *Phys Med Biol*. 2004;4916:3703–3712.

Allen BJ. Clinical trials of targeted alpha therapy for cancer. *Rev Recent Clin Trials*. 2008;3:185–191.

Alvarez RD, Partridge EE, Khazaeli MB, et al. Intraperitoneal radioimmunotherapy of ovarian cancer with ^{177}Lu-CC49: a phase I/II study. *Gynecol Oncol*. 1997;65:94–101.

Alvarez RD, Huh WK, Khazaeli MB, et al. A phase I study of combined modality ^{90}Y-CC49 intraperitoneal radioimmunotherapy for ovarian cancer. *Clin Cancer Res*. 2002;8:2806–2811.

Andersson H, Lindegren S, Bäck T, et al. Biokinetics of the monoclonal antibodies MOv18, OV185 and OV197 labelled with ^{125}I according to the m-MeATE method or the Iodogen method in nude mice with ovarian cancer xenografts. *Acta Oncol*. 1999;38:323–328.

Andersson H, Lindegren S, Bäck T, et al. Radioimmunotherapy of nude mice with intraperitoneally growing ovarian cancer xenograft utilizing ^{211}At-labelled monoclonal antibody MOv18. *Anticancer Res*. 2000;20:459–462.

Andersson H, Lindegren S, Bäck T, et al. The curative and palliative potential of the monoclonal antibody MOv18 labelled with ^{211}At in nude mice with intraperitoneally growing ovarian cancer xenografts - A long-term study. *Acta Oncol*. 2000;39:741–745.

Andersson H, Palm S, Lindegren S, et al. Comparison of the therapeutic efficacy of ^{211}At- and ^{131}I-labelled monoclonal antibody MOv18 in nude mice with intraperitoneal growth of human ovarian cancer. *Anticancer Res*. 2001;21:409–412.

Andersson H, Elgqvist J, Horvath G, et al. Astatine-211-labeled antibodies for treatment of disseminated ovarian cancer: an overview of results in an ovarian tumor model. *Clin Cancer Res*. 2003;9:3914–3921.

Andersson H, Cederkrantz E, Bäck T, et al. Intraperitoneal α-particle radioimmunotherapy of ovarian cancer patients: pharmacokinetics and dosimetry of ^{211}At-MX35 F(ab')2 – a phase I study. *J Nucl Med*. 2009;50:1153–1160.

Arklie J, Taylor-Papadimitriou J, Bodmer WF, et al. Differentiation antigens expressed by epithelial cells in the lactating breast are also detectable in breast cancers. *Int J Cancer*. 1981;28:23–29.

Armstrong DK, Bundy B, Wenzel L, et al. Intraperitoneal cisplatin and paclitaxel in ovarian cancer. *N Engl J Med*. 2006;354:34–43.

Baker TS, Bose SS, Caskey-Finney HM, et al. Humanisation of an anti mucin antibody for breast and ovarian cancer therapy. In: Ceriani RL, ed. *Antigen and antibody molecular engineering in breast cancer diagnosis and treatment*. New York: Plenum Press, 1994.

Benham FJ, Povey MS, and Harris H. Placental-like alkaline phosphatase in malignant and benign ovarian tumours. *Clin Chim Acta*. 1978;86:201–215.

Boellaard R, Krak NC, Hoekstra OS et al. Effects of noise, image resolution, and ROI definition on the accuracy of standard uptake values: A simulation study. *J Nucl Med*. 2004;45:1519–1527.

Boerman OC, van Niekerk CC, Makkink K, et al. Comparative immunohistochemical study of four monoclonal antibodies directed against ovarian carcinoma-associated antigens. *Int J Gyn Path*. 1991;10:15–25.

Borchardt PE, Yuan RR, Miederer M, et al. Targeted Actinium-225 in vivo generators for therapy of ovarian cancer. *Cancer Res*. 2003;63:5084–5090.

Breitz HB, Durham JS, Fisher DR, et al. Pharmacokinetics and normal organ dosimetry following intraperitoneal Rhenium-186-labeled monoclonal antibody. *J Nucl Med*. 1995;36:754–761.

Bruland ØS, Nilsson S, Fisher DR et al. High-linear energy transfer irradiation targeted to skeletal metastases by the alpha-emitter ^{223}Ra: adjuvant or alternative to conventional modalities? *Clin Cancer Res*. 2006;12(20): 6250–6257.

Buchsbaum DJ, Rogers BE, Khazaeli MB, et al. Targeting strategies for cancer radiotherapy. *Clin Cancer Res*. 1999;5:3048–3055.

Buchsbaum DJ, Khazaeli MB, Axworthy DB, et al. Intraperitoneal pretarget radioimmunotherapy with CC49 fusion protein. *Clin Cancer Res*. 2005;11:8180–8185.

Buijs WC, Tibben JG, Boerman OC, et al. Dosimetric analysis of chimeric monoclonal antibody cMOv18 IgG in ovarian carcinoma patients after intraperitoneal and intravenous administration. *Eur J Nucl Med*. 1998;25:1552–1561.

Buist MR, Kenemans P, Hollander W, et al. Kinetics and tissue distribution of the radiolabeled chimeric monoclonal antibody MOv18 IgG and F(ab´)2 fragments in ovarian cancer patients. *Cancer Res*. 1993;53:5413–5418.

Buist MR, Kenemans P, Molthoff C, et al. Tumor uptake of intravenously administered radiolabeled antibodies in ovarian carcinoma patients in relation to antigen expression and other tumor characteristics. *Int J Cancer*. 1995;64:92–98.

Burchell J, Durbin H, and Taylor-Papadimitriou J. Complexity of expression of antigenic determinants recognised by monoclonal antibodies HMFG1 and HMFG2 in normal and malignant human mammary epithelial cells. *J Immunol*. 1983;131:508–513.

Bäck T, Andersson H, Divgi CR, et al. ^{211}At radioimmunotherapy of subcutaneous human ovarian cancer xenografts: evaluation of relative biologic effectiveness of an alpha-emitter in vivo. *J Nucl Med*. 2005;46:2061–2067.

Bäck T and Jacobsson L. The alpha-camera: a quantitative digital autoradiography technique using a charge-coupled device for ex vivo high-resolution bioimaging of alpha-particles. *J Nucl Med*. 2010;51(10):1616–1623.

Campbell IG, Jones TA, Foulkes WD, et al. Folate-binding protein is a marker for ovarian cancer. *Cancer Res*. 1991;51:5329–5338.

Carter P, Presta L, Gorman CM, et al. Humanization of an anti-p185^{HER2} antibody for human cancer therapy. *Proc Natl Acad Sci*. 1992;89:4285–4289.

Chérel M, Davodeau F, Kraeber-Bodéré F, et al. Current status and perspectives in alpha radioimmunotherapy. *Q J Nucl Med Mol Imaging*. 2006;50:322–329.

Colcher D, Esteban J, Carrasquillo JA, et al. Complementation of intracavitary and intravenous administration of a monoclonal antibody (B72.3) in patients with carcinoma. *Cancer Res*. 1987;47:4218–4224.

Cordier D, Forrer F, Bruchertseifer F, et al. Targeted alpha-radionuclide therapy of functionally critically located gliomas with Bi-213-DOTA-[Thi(8),Met(O-2)(11)]-substance P: a pilot trial. *Eur J Nucl Med Mol Imaging*. 2010;37:1335–1344.

Corson DR, Mackenzie KR, and Segre E. Astatine - the element of atomic number-85. *Nature*. 1947;159:24.

Crippa F. Radioimmunotherapy of ovarian cancer. *Int J Biol Markers*. 1993;8:187–191.

Crippa F, Bolis G, Seregni E, et al. Single-dose intraperitoneal radioimmunotherapy with the murine monoclonal antibody ^{131}I MOv18: clinical results in patients with minimal residual disease of ovarian cancer. *Eur J Cancer*. 1995;31A:686–690.

Davis Q, Perkins AC, Roos JC, et al. An immunoscintigraphic evaluation of the engineered human monoclonal antibody (hCTMO1) for use in the treatment of ovarian carcinoma. *Br J Obst Gynaecol*. 1999;106:31–37.

Edwards DP, Grzyb KT, Dressler LG, et al. Monoclonal antibody identification and characterization of a M_r 43,000 membrane glycoprotein associated with human breast cancer. *Cancer Res*. 1986;46:1306–1317.

Einhorn N, Tropé C, Ridderheim M, et al. A systematic overview of radiation therapy effects in ovarian cancer. *Acta Oncol*. 2003;42:562–566.

Elgqvist J, Bernhardt P, Hultborn R, et al. Myelotoxicity and RBE of ^{211}At-conjugated monoclonal antibodies compared with ^{99m}Tc-conjugated monoclonal antibodies and ^{60}Co irradiation in nude mice. *J Nucl Med*. 2005;46:464–471.

Elgqvist J, Andersson H, Bäck T, et al. Therapeutic efficacy and tumor dose estimations in radioimmunotherapy of intraperitoneally growing OVCAR-3 cells in nude mice with ^{211}At-labeled monoclonal antibody MX35. *J Nucl Med*. 2005;46:1907–1915.

Elgqvist J, Andersson H, Bäck T, et al. Alpha-radioimmunotherapy of intraperitoneally growing OVCAR-3 tumors of variable dimensions: Outcome related to measured tumor size and mean absorbed dose. *J Nucl Med*. 2006;47:1342–1350.

Elgqvist J, Andersson H, Bäck T, et al. Fractionated radioimmunotherapy of intraperitoneally growing ovarian cancer in nude mice with ^{211}At-MX35 F(ab')2: therapeutic efficacy and myelotoxicity. *Nucl Med Biol*. 2006;33:1065–1072.

Elgqvist J, Andersson H, Bernhardt P, et al. Administered activity and metastatic cure probability during radioimmunotherapy of ovarian cancer in nude mice with ^{211}At-MX35 F(ab')2. *Int J Radiat Oncol Biol Phys*. 2006;66:1228–1237.

Elgqvist J, Andersson H, Haglund E, et al. Intraperitoneal alpha-radioimmunotherapy in mice using different specific activities. *Cancer Biother Radiopharm*. 2009;24:509–513.

Elgqvist J, Andersson H, Jensen H, et al. Repeated intraperitoneal alpha-radioimmunotherapy of ovarian cancer in mice. *J Oncol*. 2009;2010;2010:394913.

Elgqvist J, Hultborn R, Lindegren S, et al. Ovarian cancer: Background and clinical perspectives. In Targeted Radionuclide Therapy. Lippincott Williams & Wilkins, 2010, Ed. Tod Speer. Chapter 29, p 380–396. ISBN: 978-0-7818-9693-4.

Epenetos AA, Nimmon CC, Arklie J, et al. Radioimmunodiagnosis of human cancer in an animal model using labeled tumor associated monoclonal antibodies. *Br J Cancer.* 1982;46:1-8.

Epenetos AA, Munro AJ, Stewart S, et al. Antibody-guided irradiation of advanced ovarian cancer with intraperitoneally administered radiolabeled monoclonal antibodies. *J Clin Oncol.* 1987;512:1890–1899.

Epenetos AA, Hird V, Lambert H, et al. Long term survival of patients with advanced ovarian cancer treated with intraperitoneal radioimmunotherapy. *Int J Gynecol Cancer.* 2000;10:44–46.

Frost S, Jensen H, and Lindegren S. In vitro evaluation of avidin antibody pretargeting using ^{211}At-labeled and biotinylated poly-L-lysine as effector molecule. *Cancer.* 2010;116:1101–1110.

Gadducci A, Cosio S, Conte PF, et al. Consolidation and maintenance treatments for patients with advanced epithelial ovarian cancer in complete response after first-line chemotherapy: a review of the literature. *Crit Rev Oncol Hematol.* 2005;55:153–166.

Garkavij M, Nickel M, Sjögreen-Gleisner K et al. ^{177}Lu-[DOTA0,Tyr3] octreotate therapy in patients with disseminated neuroendocrine tumors: Analysis of dosimetry with impact on future therapeutic strategy. *Cancer.* 2010;116:1084–1192.

Gaze MN. The current status of targeted radiotherapy in clinical practice. *Phys Med Biol.* 1996;41:1895–903.

Gaze MN, Chang YC, Flux GD et al. Feasibility of dosimetry-based high-dose ^{131}I-meta-iodobenzylguanidine with topotecan as a radiosensitizer in children with metastatic neuroblastoma. *Cancer Biother Radiopharm.* 2005;20(2):195–199.

Gendler SJ. MUC1, the renaissance molecule. *J Mammary Gland Biol Neoplasia.* 2001;6:339–353.

Goldenberg DM. Targeted therapy of cancer with radiolabeled antibodies. *J Nucl Med.* 2002;43:693–713.

Goldenberg DM and Sharkey RM. Advances in cancer therapy with radiolabeled monoclonal antibodies. *Q J Nucl Med Mol Imaging.* 2006;50:248–264.

Goldrosen MH, Biddle WC, Pancook J, et al. Biodistribution, pharmacokinetic, and imaging studies with ^{186}Re-labeled NR-LU-10 whole antibody in LS174T colonic tumor-bearing mice. *Cancer Res.* 1990;50:7973–7878.

Grana C, Bartolomei M, Handkiewicz D, et al. Radioimmunotherapy in advanced ovarian cancer: is there a role for pre-targeting with (90)Y-biotin? *Gynecol Oncol.* 2004;93:691–698.

He B, Du Y, Song X et al. A Monte Carlo and physical phantom evaluation of quantitative In-111 SPECT. *Phys Med Biol.* 2005;50:4169–4185.

Hilkens J. Biochemistry and function of mucins in malignant disease. *Cancer Rev.* 1988;11/12:25–54.

Hird V, Stewart JS, Snook D, et al. Intraperitoneally administered ^{90}Y-labelled monoclonal antibodies as a third line of treatment in ovarian cancer. A phase 1–2 trial: problems encountered and possible solutions. *Br J Cancer Suppl.* 1990;10:48–51.

Hnatowich DJ, Chinol M, Siebecker DA, et al. Patient distribution of intraperitoneally administered Yttrium-90-labeled antibody. *J Nucl Med.* 1988;29:1428–1434.

Horan Hand P, Shrivastav S, Colcher D, et al. Pharmacokinetics of radiolabeled antibodies following intraperitoneal and intravenous administration in rodents, monkeys and humans. *Antibody Immunoconj Radiopharm.* 1989;2:241–255.

Imam SK. Advancements in cancer therapy with alpha-emitters: a review. *Int J Radiat Oncol Biol Phys.* 2001;51:271–278.

Jaaback K and Johnson N. Intraperitoneal chemotherapy for the initial management of primary epithelial ovarian cancer. *The Cochrane Library.* 2009;4:1–34.

Jacobs AJ, Fer M, Su FM, et al. A phase I trial of a rhenium 186-labeled monoclonal antibody administered intraperitoneally in ovarian carcinoma: toxicity and clinical response. *Obstet Gynecol.* 1993;82:586–593.

Johnson VG, Schlom J, Paterson AJ, et al. Analysis of a human tumor-associated glycoprotein (TAG-72) identified by monoclonal antibody B72.3. *Cancer Res.* 1986;46:850–857.

Kairemo K. Radioimmunotherapy of solid cancers. *Acta Oncol.* 1996;35:343–355.

Kassis AI, Adelstein J, and Mariani G. Radiolabeled nucleoside analogs in cancer diagnosis and therapy. *Q J Nucl Med.* 1996;40:301–319.

Kerr JA and Trotman-Dickenson AF. *Strength of chemical bonds.* 59 ed., Boca Raton: CRC Press, 1977.

Kievit E, Pinedo HM, Schlüper HM, et al. Comparison of the monoclonal antibodies 17-1A and 323/A3: the influence of the affinity on tumor uptake and efficacy of radioimmunotherapy in human ovarian cancer xenografts. *Br J Cancer.* 1996;73:457–464.

Kinahan PE, Townsend DW, Beyer T et al. Attenuation correction for a combined 3D PET/CT scanner. *Med Phys.* 1998;25(10):2046–2053.

Knör S, Sato S, Huber T, et al. Development and evaluation of peptidic ligands targeting tumour-associated urokinase plasminogen activator receptor (uPAR) for use in alpha-emitter therapy for disseminated ovarian cancer. *Eur J Nucl Med Mol Imaging.* 2008;35:53–64.

Koprowski H, Steplewski Z, Mitchell H, et al. Colorectal carcinoma antigens detected by hybridoma antibodies. *Somat Cell Genet.* 1979;5:957–972.

Kosmas C, Kalofonos HP, Hird V, et al. Monoclonal antibody targeting of ovarian carcinoma. *Oncology.* 1998;55:435–446.

Larsen RH and Bruland OS. Radiolysis of radioimmunoconjugates - Reduction in antigen-binding ability by alpha-particle adiation. *J of Label Comp Radiopharm.* 1995;36:1009–1018.

Li Y, Rizvi SM, Ranson M, et al. ^{213}Bi-PAI2 conjugate selectively induces apoptosis in PC3 metastatic prostate cancer cell line and shows anti-cancer activity in a xenograft animal model. *Br J Cancer.* 2002;86:1197–1203.

Lindegren S, Frost S, Bäck T, et al. Direct procedure for the production of ^{211}At-labeled antibodies with an {varepsilon}-lysyl-3-(trimethylstannyl)benzamide immunoconjugate. *J Nucl Med.* 2008;49:1537–1545.

Macey DJ, Meredith RF. A strategy to reduce red marrow dose for intraperitoneal radioimmunotherapy. *Clin Cancer Res.* 1999;5:3044–3047.

Mahé MA, Fumoleau P, Fabbro M, et al. A phase II study of intraperitoneal radioimmunotherapy with iodine-131-labeled monoclonal antibody OC-125 in patients with residual ovarian carcinoma. *Clin Cancer Res.* 1999;5:3249–3253.

Maraveyas A, Snook D, Hird V, et al. Pharmacokinetics and toxicity of an ^{90}Y-CITC-DTPA-HMFG1 radioimmunoconjugate for intraperitoneal radioimmunotherapy of ovarian cancer. *Cancer*. 1994;73:1067–1075.

Meredith RF, Partridge EE, Alvarez RD, et al. Intraperitoneal radioimmunotherapy of ovarian cancer with Lutetium-177-CC49. *J Nucl Med*. 1996;37:1491–1496.

Meredith RF, Alvarez RD, Partridge EE, et al. Intraperitoneal radioimmunotherapy of ovarian cancer: a phase I study. *Cancer Biother Radiopharm*. 2001;16:305–315.

Meredith RF, Buchsbaum DJ, Alvarez RD, et al. Brief overview of preclinical and clinical studies in the development of intraperitoneal radioimmunotherapy for ovarian cancer. *Clin Cancer Res*. 2007;13:5643–5645.

Miotti S, Canevari S, Ménard S, et al. Characterization of human ovarian carcinoma-associated antigens defined by novel monoclonal antibodies with tumor-restricted specificity. *Int J Cancer*. 1987;39:297–303.

Molthoff CF, Calame J, Pinedo H, et al. Human ovarian cancer xenografts in nude mice: Characterization and analysis of antigen expression. *Int J Cancer*. 1991;47:72–79.

Molthoff CF, Pinedo H, Schlüper H, et al. Influence of dose and schedule on the therapeutic efficacy of ^{131}I-labelled monoclonal antibody 139H2 in a human ovarian cancer xenograft model. *Int J Cancer*. 1992;50:474–480.

Molthoff CF, Buist MR, Kenemans P, et al. Experimental and clinical analysis of the characteristics of a chimeric monoclonal antibody, MOv18, reactive with an ovarian cancer-associated antigen. *J Nucl Med*. 1992;33:2000–2005.

Molthoff CF, Prinssen HM, Kenemans P, et al. Escalating protein doses of chimeric monoclonal antibody MOv18 immunoglobulin G in ovarian carcinoma patients: A phase I study. *Cancer*. 1997;80:2712–2720.

Mukherjee P, Madsen CS, and Ginardi AR. Mucin 1-specific immunotherapy in a mouse model of spontaneous breast cancer. *J Immunother*. 2003;26:47–62.

Mulford DA, Sheinberg DA, and Jurcic JG. The promise of targeted α-particle therapy. *J Nucl Med*. 2005;46:199–204.

Muto MG, Finkler NJ, Kassis AI, et al. Intraperitoneal radioimmunotherapy of refractory ovarian carcinoma utilizing Iodine-131-labeled monoclonal antibody OC125. *Gynaecol Oncol*. 1992;45:265–272.

Muto MG and Kassis AI. Monoclonal antibodies used in the detection and treatment of epithelial ovarian cancer. *Cancer*. 1995;15:2016–2027.

Nicholson S, Gooden CS, Hird V, et al. Radioimmunotherapy after chemotherapy compared to chemotherapy alone in the treatment of advanced ovarian cancer: a matched analysis. *Oncol Rep*. 1998;5:223–226.

Nuti M, Teramoto YA, Mariani-Costantini R, et al. A monoclonal (B72.3) defines patterns of distribution of a novel tumor-associated antigen in human mammary carcinoma cell populations. *Int J Cancer*. 1982;29:539–545.

Oei AL, Verheijen RH, Seiden MV, et al. Decreased intraperitoneal disease recurrence in epithelial ovarian cancer patients receiving intraperitoneal consolidation treatment with yttrium-90-labeled murine HMFG1 without improvement in overall survival. *Int J Cancer*. 2007;120:2710–2714.

Oyen WJ, Bodei L, Giammarile F, et al. Targeted therapy in nuclear medicine - current status and future prospects. *Ann Oncol*. 2007;18:1782–1792.

Paganelli G, Magnani P, and Fazio F. Pretargeting of carcinomas with the avidin-biotin system. *Int J Biol Markers*. 1993;8:155–159.

Palm S, Humm JL, Rundqvist R, et al. Microdosimetry of astatine-211 single-cell irradiation: role of daughter polonium-211 diffusion. *Med Phys*. 2004;31:218–225.

Palm S, Elgqvist J, and Jacobsson L. Patient-specific alpha-particle dosimetry. *Curr Radiopharm*. 2011;4(4):329–335.

Persson M, Gedda L, Lundqvist H, et al. ^{177}Lu-Pertuzumab: Experimental therapy of HER-2-expressing xenografts. *Cancer Res*. 2007;67:326–331.

Poels LG, Peters D, Van Megen Y, et al. Monoclonal antibody against human ovarian tumor-associated antigens. *J Nat Cancer Inst*. 1986;76:781–787.

Pozzi OR and Zalutsky MR. Radiopharmaceutical chemistry of targeted radiotherapeutics, Part 3: alpha-particle-induced radiolytic effects on the chemical behavior of ^{211}At. *J Nucl Med*. 2007;48:1190–1196.

Qu CF, Song EY, Li Y, et al. Preclinical study of ^{213}Bi labeled PAI2 for the control of micrometastatic pancreatic cancer. *Clin Exp Metastasis*. 2005;22:575–586.

Ranson M, Tian Z, Andronicos NM, et al. In vitro cytotoxicity of ^{213}Bi-labeled-plasminogen activator inhibitor type 2 (alpha-PAI-2) on human breast cancer cells. *Breast Cancer Res Treat*. 2002;71:149–159.

Rosenblum MG, Verschraegen CF, Murray JL, et al. Phase I study of ^{90}Y-labeled B72.3 intraperitoneal administration in patients with ovarian cancer: effect of dose and EDTA coadministration on pharmacokinetics and toxicity. *Clin Cancer Res*. 1999;5:953–961.

Rosenhein NB, Leichner PK, and Vogelsang G. Radiocolloids in the treatment of ovarian cancer. *Obstet Gynecol Surv*. 1979;34:708–720.

Rosenthal MS, Cullom J, Hawkins W, et al. Quantitative SPECT imaging: a review and recommendations by the Focus Committee of the Society of Nuclear Medicine Computer and Instrumentation Council. *J Nucl Med*. 1995;36(8):1489–1513.

Rubin SC, Kostakoglu L, Divgi C, et al. Biodistribution and intraoperative evaluation of radiolabeled monoclonal antibody MX35 in patients with epithelial ovarian cancer. *Gynecol Oncol*. 1993;51:61–66.

Schlom J, Colcher D, Suer K, et al. Tumor targeting with monoclonal antibody B72.3: experimental and clinical results. In: Goldenberg D, ed. *Cancer imaging with radiolabeled antibodies*. Boston, MA: Kluwer Academic Publishing, 1990.

Sgouros G, Ballangrud AM, Jurcic JG, et al. Pharmacokinetics and dosimetry of an alpha-particle emitter labeled antibody: ^{213}Bi-HuM195 (anti-CD33) in patients with leukemia. *J Nucl Med*. 1999;40(11):1935–1946.

Sgouros G, Frey E, Wahl R et al. Three-dimensional imaging-based radiobiological dosimetry. *Semin Nucl Med*. 2008;38(5):321–334.

Sgouros G, Hobbs R, and Song H. Modelling and dosimetry for alpha-particle therapy. *Curr Radiopharm*. 2011;4(3):261–265.

Sharkey RM and Goldenberg DM. Perspectives on cancer therapy with radiolabeled monoclonal antibodies. *J Nucl Med*. 2005;46:115–127.

Sjögreen K, Ljungberg M, and Strand SE. An activity quantification method based on registration of CT and whole-body scintillation camera images, with application to ^{131}I. *J Nucl Med*. 2002;43(7):972–982.

Song YJ, Qu CF, Rizvi SM, et al. Cytotoxicity of PAI2, C595 and Herceptin vectors labeled with the alpha-emitting radioisotope Bismuth-213 for ovarian cancer cell monolayers and clusters. *Cancer Letters*. 2006;234:176–183.

Song EY, Abbas Rizvi SM, Qu CF, et al. Pharmacokinetics and toxicity of ^{213}Bi-labeled PAI2 in preclinical targeted alpha therapy for cancer. *Cancer Biol Ther*. 2007;6:898–904.

Steffen AC, Almqvist Y, Chyan MK, et al. Biodistribution of ^{211}At labeled HER-2 binding affibody molecules in mice. *Oncol Rep*. 2006;17:1141–1147.

Steffen AC, Orlova A, Wikman M, et al. Affibody-mediated tumour targeting of HER-2 expressing xenografts in mice. *Eur J Nucl Med Mol Imaging*. 2006;33:631–638.

Stewart JS, Hird V, Sullivan M, et al. Intraperitoneal radioimmunotherapy for ovarian cancer. *Br J Obstet Gynaecol*. 1989;96:529–536.

Stewart JS, Hird V, Snook D, et al. Intraperitoneal radioimmunotherapy for ovarian cancer: pharmacokinetics, toxicity, and efficacy of ^{131}I labeled monoclonal antibodies. *Int J Radiat Oncol Biol Phys*. 1989;16:405–413.

Stewart JS, Hird V, Snook D, et al. Intraperitoneal yttrium-90-labeled monoclonal antibody in ovarian cancer. *J Clin Oncol*. 1990;8:1941–1950.

Su FM, Beaumier P, Axworthy D, et al. Pretargeted radioimmunotherapy in tumored mice using an in vivo Pb-212/Bi-212 generator. *Nucl Med Biol*. 2005;32:741–747.

Sunderland CA, Davis JO, and Stirrat GM. Immunohistology of normal and ovarian cancer tissue with monoclonal antibody to placental alkaline phosphatase. *Cancer Res*. 1984;44:4496–4502.

Thor A, Gorstein F, Ohuchi N, et al. Tumor-associated glycoprotein (TAG-72) in ovarian carcinomas defined by monoclonal antibody B72.3. *J Natl Cancer Inst*. 1986;76:995–1006.

Tolmachev V, Orlova A, Pehrson R, et al. Radionuclide therapy of HER2-positive microzenografts using a ^{177}Lu-labeled HER2-specific affibody molecule. *Cancer Res*. 2007;67:2773–2782.

Travers P and Bodmer WF. Preparation and characterisation of monoclonal antibodies against placental alkaline phosphatise and other human trophoblast-associated determinants. *Int J Cancer*. 1984;33:633–641.

Turner JH, Rose AH, Glancy RJ, et al. Orthotopic xenografts of human melanoma and colonic and ovarian carcinoma in sheep to evaluate radioimmunotherapy. *Br J Cancer*. 1998;78:486–494.

Van Zanten-Przybysz I, Molthoff CF, Roos JC, et al. Radioimmunotherapy with intravenously administered ^{131}I-labeled chimeric monoclonal antibody MOvl8 in patients with ovarian cancer. *J Nucl Med*. 2000;41:1168–1176.

Van Zanten-Przybysz I, Moltoff CF, Roos JC, et al. Influence of the route of administration on targeting of ovarian cancer with the chimeric monoclonal antibody MOv18: i.v. *VS*. i.p.. *Int J Cancer*. 2001;92:106–114.

Varia MA, Stehman FB, Bundy BN, et al. Intraperitoneal radioactive phosphorus (^{32}P) versus observation after negative second-look laparotomy for stage III ovarian carcinoma: A randomized trial of the Gynecologic Oncology Group. *J Clin Oncol*. 2003;21:2849–2855.

Varki NM, Reisfeld RA, and Walker LE. Antigens associated with a human lung adenocarcinoma defined by monoclonal antibodies. *Cancer Res*. 1984;44:681–687.

Verheijen RH, Massuger LF, Benigno BB, et al. Phase III trial of intraperitoneal therapy with yttrium-90-labeled HMFG1 murine monoclonal antibody in patients with epithelial ovarian cancer after a surgically defined complete remission. *J Clin Oncol.* 2006;24:571–578.

Visser GWM, Diemer EL, and Kaspersen FM. The nature of the astatine-protein bond. *Int J Appl Radiat Isot.* 1981;32:905–912.

Ward BG, Mather SJ, Hawkins LR, et al. Localization of radioiodine conjugated to the monoclonal antibody HMFG2 in human ovarian carcinoma: assessment of intravenous and intraperitoneal routes of administration. *Cancer Res.* 1987;47:4719-4723.

Welshinger M, Yin BWT, and Lloyd KO. Initial immunochemical characterization of MX35 ovarian cancer antigen. *Gynecol Oncol.* 1997;67:188–192.

Wilbur DS, Hadley SW, Hylarides MD, et al. Development of a stable radioiodinating reagent to label monoclonal antibodies for radiotherapy of cancer. *J Nucl Med.* 1989;30:216–226.

Wilbur DS, Chyan MK, Hamlin DK, et al. Reagents for astatination of biomolecules: comparison of the in vivo distribution and stability of some radioiodinated/astatinated benzamidyl and nido-carboranyl compounds. *Bioconjug Chem.* 2004;15:203–223.

Wilbur DS, Thakar MS, Hamlin DK, et al. Reagents for astatination of biomolecules. 4. Comparison of maleimido-closo-decaborate(2-) and meta-[^{211}At]astatobenzoate conjugates for labeling anti-CD45 antibodies with [^{211}At]astatine. *Bioconjug Chem.* 2009;20:1983–1991.

Wolf BC, D'Emilia JC, Salem RR, et al. Detection of the tumor associated glycoprotein antigen (TAG-72) in premalignant lesions of the colon. *J Natl Cancer Inst.* 1989;81:1913–1917.

Yin BW, Kiyamova R, Chua R, et al. Monoclonal antibody MX35 detects the membrane transporter NaPi2b (SLC34A2) in human carcinomas. *Cancer Immun.* 2008;8:3–11.

Yordanov AT, Garmestani K, Zhang M, et al. Preparation and in vivo evaluation of linkers for ^{211}At labeling of humanized anti-Tac. *Nucl Med Biol.* 2001;28:845–856.

Zalutsky MR and Narula AS. Astatination of proteins using an N-succinimidyl tri-normal-butylstannyl benzoate intermediate. *Appl Radiat Isot.* 1988;39:227–232.

Zalutsky MR and Vaidyanathan G. Astatine-211-labeled radiotherapeutics: An emerging approach to targeted alpha-particle radiotherapy. *Curr Pharm Des.* 2000;6:1433–1455.

Zalutsky MR, Reardon DA, Pozzi OR, et al. Targeted alpha-particle radiotherapy with ^{211}At-labeled monoclonal antibodies. *Nucl Med Biol.* 2007;34:779–785.

Zalutsky MR, Reardon DA, Akabani G, et al. Clinical experience with alpha-particle-emitting At-211: Treatment of recurrent brain tumor patients with At-211-labeled chimeric antitenascin monoclonal antibody 81C6. *J Nucl Med.* 2008;49:30–38.

Zotter S, Hageman PC, Lossnitzer A, et al. Tissue and tumour distribution of human polymorphic epithelial mucin. *Cancer Rev.* 1988;11/12:55–101.

15

Vitamin K2 as a Chemotherapeutic Agent for Treating Ovarian Cancer

K. Nakaya[1], Y. Masuda[2], T. Aiuchi[3] and H. Itabe[3]
[1]*Department of Health Pharmacy, Yokohama College of Pharmacy, Yokohama*
[2]*Department of Pharmaceutical Biology, Showa Pharmaceutical University, Machida*
[3]*School of Pharmacy, Showa University, Tokyo*
Japan

1. Introduction

Ovarian cancer is the fifth most common cancer among women and approximately 200,000 women are diagnosed as ovarian cancer every year in the world (Parkin et al., 2005). Platinum-containing chemotherapeutic agents such as cisplatin (cis-diamminedichloroplatinum II) and carboplatin have been most frequently used for the treatment of ovarian cancer. These platinum compounds specifically react with guanine residues in DNA to form interstrand and intrastrand cross-links in DNA, known as DNA-adducts. This interferes with mitosis of cancer cells and causes cell death. However, ovarian cancer cells can become resistant to cisplatin and the majority of patients develop cisplatin-resistant disease (Giaccone 2000; Hennessy et al., 2009; Kartalou & Essigmann 2001), and as a result, most ovarian cancers relapse. Paclitaxel (taxol) and two analogues of camptothecin, irinotecan and topotecan, are the drugs most commonly administered to platinum-resistant ovarian cancer patients. Paclitaxel (taxol) binds to γ-tubulin and stabilizes microtubule structure, which causes a G2/M block in the cancer cell cycle. Irinotecan, also known as CPT-11 (7-ethyl-10-[4-(1-piperidino)-1-piperidino]-carbonyloxy camptothecin) and topotecan (10-hydroxy-9-dimethylaminomethyl-(*S*)-camptothecin) inhibit topoisomerase I by resealing DNA breaks, which results in the inhibition of cancer cell growth (Bookman et al., 1998; Swisher et al., 1997). However, the survival rate for relapsed patients is low; Thus, there is an urgent need for more effective chemotherapeutic approaches for ovarian cancer treatment. We have previously reported that some ovarian cancer cell lines are remarkably sensitive to vitamin K2 (Shibayama-Imazu et al, 2003, 2006, 2008). In this review, strategies for developing chemotherapeutic agents for ovarian cancer are described and vitamin K2 is proposed as a promising chemotherapeutic agent for ovarian cancer.

2. Effect of vitamin K2 on cancer cells

Natural forms of vitamin K such as vitamin K1 (phylloquinone) and vitamin K2 (menaquinones, MK) are cofactors for the post-translational γ-carboxylation of glutamate residues in vitamin K-dependent proteins (Fig. 1). Vitamin K is mainly used as a hemostatic agent because coagulation factors VII, IX, and X, which are critical to blood coagulation, are vitamin K-dependent proteins. In addition, vitamin K2 has anti-cancer activity, whereas vitamin K1 does not. This difference arises from structural differences in the side chains attached to the parent ring of vitamin K.

2.1 Structures and fundamental properties of vitamin K

The parent ring structure of vitamin K is 2-methyl-1,4-naphthoquinone (menadione), which is also known as vitamin K3 (Fig. 1). Vitamin K3 does not occur naturally and causes oxidative stress in both normal and cancer cells and is toxic to the liver. There are few successful clinical applications of vitamin K3. Vitamin K1 has a phythyl side chain at the 3 position of vitamin K3 and is present mainly in green vegetables. Vitamin K1 is converted to vitamin K2 in animals and humans (Thijssen & Drittij-Reijnders, 1996); vitamin K2 has isoprenoid side chains of various lengths attached to the 3 position of the vitamin K3 ring structure. The different forms of vitamin K2, menaquinone-n (MK-n), are categorized according to the number of repeating isoprenoid residues in the side chain. The most common form of vitamin K2 in animals is menaquinone-4 (MK-4), which has four isoprenoid residues as its side chain. MK-4 is the most biological active form of the vitamin and is produced by intestinal bacteria. Long chain menaquinones, MK-7 to MK-10, are synthesized by bacteria and are present in fermented products such as cheese (MK-8 and MK-9) and East Asian fermented soybean products, such as natto and miso (Shearer et al., 1996; Schurgers & Vermeer, 2000).

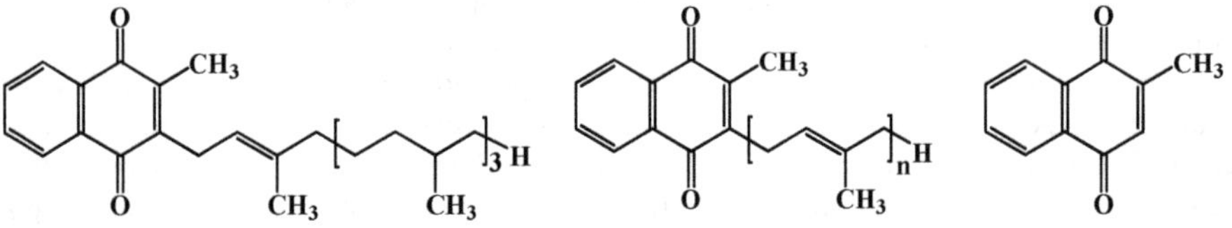

Vitamin K1 Vitamin K2 Vitamin K3

Fig. 1. Chemical Structures of vitamin K

Naturally occurring vitamin K1 contains a phytyl group, and vitamin K2 has a repeating isoprenoid group at the 3 position of the vitamin K3 menadione ring. In animals, the most common and most biologically active form of vitamin K2 is MK-4, which has four isoprenoid residues (n = 4). Unlike vitamin K1, vitamin K2 has anti-cancer activity in addition to its critical role in blood coagulation and bone metabolism. The isoprenyl side chain of vitamin K2 contributes to its unique anti-cancer activity.

2.2 Growth inhibitory activity of vitamin K2 on cancer cells

We initially demonstrated vitamin K2-induced differentiation in human leukemia cells which was unrelated to its clinical role in blood coagulation and bone metabolism (Sakai I, 1994). Inhibition of cancerous cell growth and induction of apoptosis by vitamin K2 has subsequently been observed in a variety of human cancer cell lines, including liver (Nishikawa et al., 1995; Otsuka et al., 2004), pancreatic (Shibayama-Imazu et al., 2003), ovarian (Shibayama-Imazu et al., 2003, 2006, 2008), lung (Yoshida et al., 2003; Yokoyama et al., 2005), stomach (Tokita et al., 2006), breast (Wu et al., 1993), and leukocyte (Yaguchi, 1997). The growth-inhibitory effects of vitamin K2 on various human cancer cell lines are listed in Table 1. Vitamin K2 has almost no effect on normal bone marrow cells (Miyazawa et al., 2001), and inhibition of cancerous cell growth was not observed with vitamin K1. Therefore, the side chain of vitamin K2 may be important for the anti-cancer activity of vitamin K2. The anti-cancer activity of isoprenoids is known to depend on the length of the polyprenyl alcohol side chain; polyprenoids with a geranylgeranyl group or a geranylisopropyl group have the most potent anticancer activity (Ohizumi et al., 1995). Vitamin K2 MK-4 has a geranylgeranyl side chain and is commonly used for the treatment of a variety of cancer cells. In this review, vitamin K2 MK-4 is denoted simply as vitamin K2.

Source	Cell line	IC_{50} (M)	Reference
Ovarian cancer	PA-1	5	Shibayama-Imazu et al., 2008
	TYK-nu	73	Shibayama-Imazu et al., 2008
	SK-OV-3	152	Shibayama-Imazu et al., 2008
	SW626	188	Shibayama-Imazu et al., 2008
	OVCAR3	>400	Shibayama-Imazu et al., 2008
Leukemia	U937	28	Shibayama-Imazu et al., 2003
	HL-60	150	Shibayama-Imazu et al., 2003
Liver cancer	PLC/PRF/5	>400	Shibayama-Imazu et al., 2003
	Hep2G	45	Otsuka et al., 2004
	Hep3B	112	Nishikawa et al., 1995
	HuH-7	80	Kanamori et al., 2007
Pancreatic cancer	KP-4	>400	Shibayama-Imazu et al., 2003
	MIA PaCa-2	153	Shibayama-Imazu et al., 2003
	2C6	>400	Shibayama-Imazu et al., 2003
Gastric cancer	KATO III	>400	Shibayama-Imazu et al., 2003
	NUGC-2	>400	Shibayama-Imazu et al., 2003
	MKN7	50	Tokita et al., 2006
	MKN74	25	Tokita et al., 2006
	FU97	35	Tokita et al., 2006
Lung cancer	LU-139	75	Yoshida et al., 2003

Table 1. IC_{50} values for vitamin K2 in various cancer cell lines. IC_{50} is defined as the concentration of vitamin K2 that inhibits cell growth by 50%. The values for SW626 and OVCAR3 were estimated from previously published results (Shibayama-Imazu et al., 2008). Clinical trials using vitamin K2 that were conducted successfully for leukemia and liver cancer patients are indicated by boxes.

3. Induction of apoptosis in ovarian cells by vitamin K2

Inhibition of cell growth is a good indicator of the induction of apoptosis in cancer cells by chemical agents. A comparison of the inhibition of the growth of various cancer cells by vitamin K2 showed that an ovarian cancer cell line PA-1 is the most sensitive to vitamin K2. A steroid orphan receptor TR3/Nur77, which regulates cell proliferation and apoptosis, is responsible for the induction of apoptosis in ovarian cancer PA-1 cells by vitamin K2.

3.1 Growth inhibition of ovarian cancer cells by vitamin K2

We observed that apoptosis is readily induced in some ovarian cancer cell lines by low concentrations of vitamin K2 (Shibayama-Imazu et al, 2003; 2006). Figure 2 shows that vitamin K2 is a potent inhibitor of the growth of human ovarian cancer PA-1 cells, with an IC_{50} of 5.0 $\pm$ 0.7 μM. The IC_{50} value for PA-1 cells is the lowest observed for cancer cell lines treated with vitamin K2, indicating that PA-1 cells are the most sensitive to vitamin K2 (Table 1). In contrast to PA-1 cells, SK-OV-3 cells were resistant to vitamin K2 and no significant growth inhibition was observed (Fig. 2). PA-1 and SK-OV-3 cells were used as vitamin K2-sensitive and vitamin K2-resistant cells, respectively, in order to examine the mechanism of apoptosis induction by vitamin K2.

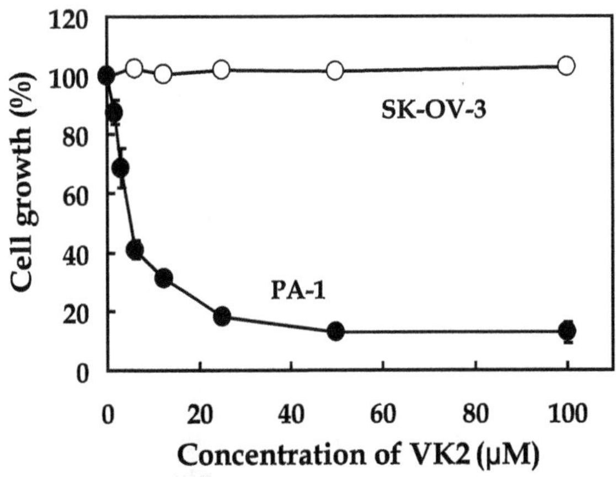

Fig. 2. Effects of vitamin K2 on the growth of human ovarian cancer PA-1 and SK-OV-3 cells. Cell proliferation was determined using the XTT assay 96 h after treatment with various concentrations of vitamin K2. Each value is represented as mean $\pm$ SD of the results from three independent experiments. Vitamin K2-sensitive PA-1(●); vitamin K2-resistant SK-OV-3 (○). [Reproduced with permission from Fig. 1 of Shibayama-Imazu et al., 2008.]

3.2 Mechanism of the induction of apoptosis by vitamin K2

The induction of apoptosis by vitamin K2 in vitamin K2-sensitive ovarian cancer PA-1 cells proceeds slowly. Fragmented nucelosomes were released into the cytosolic fraction 24 h after the start of incubation of PA-1 cells with 30 μM vitamin K2, and increased until at least 72 h after the start of incubation (Fig. 3A). After 72 h, the induction of apoptosis was evident in approximately 35% of PA-1 cells, as determined by counting apoptotic cells with condensed and fragmented nuclei stained with Hoechst 33342 (Shibayama-Imazu et al., 2008). The slow rate of apoptosis is one of the characteristic features of vitamin K2-induced apoptosis, compared to apoptosis induced by conventional anticancer agents such as camptothecin and etoposide, and by geranaylgeraniol (Masuda et al., 2000; Shibayama-Imazu et al., 2003). Mitochondria play a crucial role in the induction of apoptosis by various apoptotic agents. Cytochrome c released from mitochondria forms a complex with Apaf-1 and activates procaspase 9, which activates a downstream caspase cascade. Once the caspase cascade has been triggered, nucleases are activated to induce apoptotic chromatin condensation and DNA fragmentation. The release of cytochrome c in PA-1 cells was detected 48 h after treatment with 30 μM vitamin K2 and the release increased sharply 72 h after the treatment (Fig. 3B).

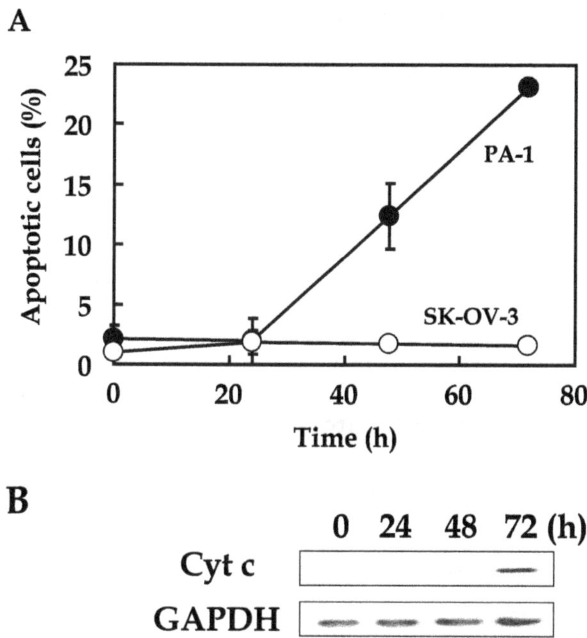

Fig. 3. Induction of apoptosis in ovarian cancer PA-1 and SK-OV-3 cells by vitamin K2. (A) Both vitamin K2-sensitive PA-1 (●) and vitamin K2-resistant SK-OV-3 (○) cells were treated with 30 μM of vitamin K2 for various times. Each value is represented as mean ± SD of the results from three independent experiments. The percentage of apoptotic cells that contained condensed and fragmented chromatin was quantified after staining with Hoechst 33342 as described previously (Shibayama-Imazu et al., 2008). (B) The panel shows immunoblotting analysis of cytochrome c released from mitochondria into the cytoplasm of PA-1 cells that had been treated with 30 μM vitamin K2 (Shibayama-Imazu et al., 2008). [Reproduced with permission from Fig. 6 of Shibayama-Imazu et al., 2008.]

3.3 Accumulation of TR3/Nur77 in mitochondria after treatment of PA-1 cells with vitamin K2

A steroid orphan receptor TR3/Nur77 is overexpressed in various cancer cells lines, including ovarian (Holmes et al., 2002), lung (Li et al., 1998), prostate (Li et al., 2000), colon (Cho et al., 2007), pancreatic (Chintharlapalli et al., 2005), bladder (Chintharlapalli et al., 2005) and stomach (Wu et al., 2002). The expression of TR3/Nur77 is rapidly induced during cancer cell apoptosis triggered by various apoptotic agents, such as phorbol ester 12-*O*-tetradecanoyl phobol-13-acetate (Li et al., 2000), etoposide (Li et al., 2000), cytosporone B (Liu et al., 2010), and the synthetic retinoid 6-[3-(1-admantyl)]-4-hydroxyphenyl]-2-naphthalene carboxylic acid (CD437, Holmes et al., 2004). TR3/Nur77 translocates from the nucleus to mitochondria in response to these apoptosis inducers, with the exception of CD437 (Li et al., 2000). TR3/Nur77 binds to Bcl-2 which switches the function of Bcl-2 from protection to the induction of cytochrome c release from the mitochondria, resulting in the induction of apoptosis (Li et al., 2000). For CD437, the levels of TR3/Nur77 in the nuclei of various pancreatic cancer cells were increased by treatment with this agent, although translocation of TR3/Nur77 from the nuclei to the mitochondria was not observed (Chintharlapalli et al., 2005).

A. TR3/Nur77 in the cell lysates

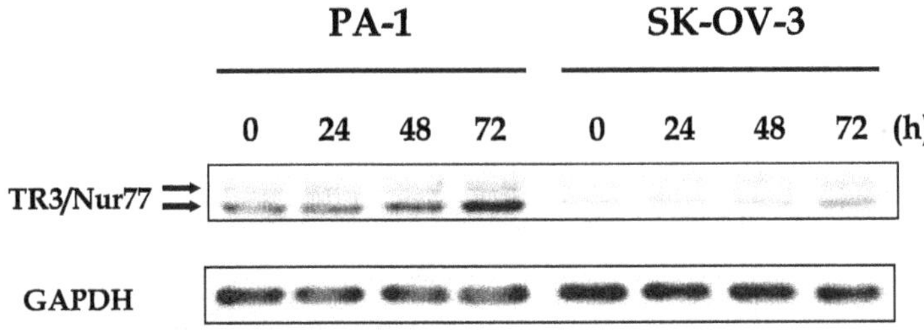

B. TR3/Nur77 in the mitochondrial fractions

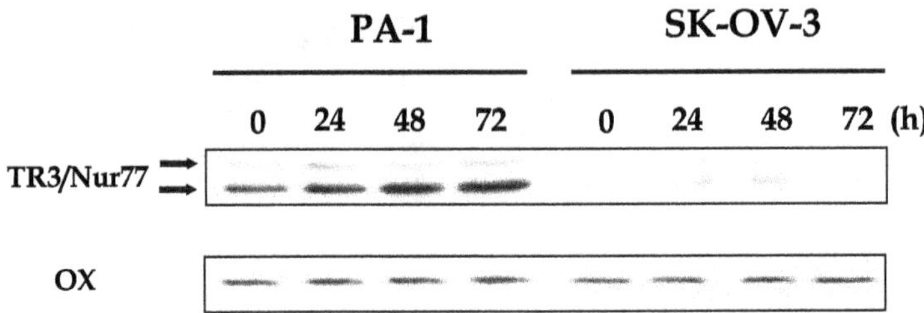

Fig. 4. Immunoblotting analysis of TR3/Nur77 in vitamin K2-sensitive PA-1 cells and vitamin K2-resistant SK-OV-3 cells. Both vitamin K2-sensitive PA-1 and vitamin K2-resistant SK-OV-3 cells were treated with 30 μM of vitamin K2 for 0 h, 24 h, 48 h, and 72 h. TR3/Nur77 in the cell lysates (A) and in the heavy mitochondrial fractions (B) were detected by immunoblotting using rabbit TR3/Nur77-specific polyclonal antibody (Shibayama-Imazu et al., 2008). Two immunostained bands were detected under our electrophoretic conditions as previously reported (Chintharlapalli et al., 2005). The more slowly migrating minor band is phosphorylated TR3/Nur77 (Pekarsky et al., 2001). The intensities of the glyceraldehyde-3-phosphate dehydrogenase (GAPDH) band and the cytochrome oxidase subunit IV (OX) band confirmed that an equal amount of cell lysate proteins and heavy mitochondrial fraction proteins, respectively, were loaded in each lane. [Reproduced with permission from Fig. 3 and Fig. 6 of Shibayama-Imazu et al., 2008.]

The level of TR3/Nur77 in vitamin K2-sensitive PA-1 cells was approximately four-fold higher than that in vitamin K2-resistant SK-OV-3 cells (Fig. 4A). The level of TR3/Nur77 in the cell lysate of PA-1 cells increased markedly in a time-dependent manner after treatment with vitamin K2. In contrast, the level of TR3/Nur77 in the cell lysate of vitamin K2-resistant SK-OV-3 cells was very low and was not significantly affected by treatment with vitamin K2. The TR3/Nur77 level in the cell lysate of SK-OV-3 cells did not reach the level observed in untreated PA-1 cells, even 72 h after the start of the treatment.

In the heavy mitochondrial fraction, which is composed mostly of mitochondria, the level of TR3/Nur77 increased sharply 48 h and 72 h after the start of the treatment of PA-1 cells with vitamin K2 (Fig. 4B). The percentage of apoptotic cells increased in parallel with the increase in TR3/Nur77 in the heavy mitochondrial fraction of PA-1 cells (Fig. 3A). In contrast, the level of TR3/Nur77 in the heavy mitochondrial fraction of vitamin K2-resistant SK-OV-3 cells was unchanged by vitamin K2 treatment (Fig. 4B). Immunofluorescence staining of PA-1 cells during vitamin K2-induced apoptosis indicates that the amounts of TR3/Nur77 present in both mitochondria and nuclei as well as in the cytosolic fraction increased after vitamin K2 treatment (Shibayama-Imazu et al., 2008). This suggests that TR3/Nur77 migrated directly from the cytoplasm to the mitochondria and no translocation from the nucleus to mitochondria occurred. It should be noted that this effect of vitamin K2 on ovarian cancer PA-1 cells is unique and different from that of apoptosis-inducing agents such as etoposide (Li et al., 2000) and cytosporone B (Liu et al., 2010) which cause translocation of TR3/Nur77 from the nuclei to the mitochondria.

4. Strategy for the improvement of chemotherapy of ovarian cancer

Combination treatments with agents that sensitize ovarian cancer cells to platinum compounds are an efficient strategy for overcoming chemoresistance acquired by ovarian cancer cells. Cancer cell survival signals can be inhibited by chemical agents, or ovarian cancer cells can be sensitized to platinum chemotherapeutic agents by preventing the repair of platinum-DNA adducts. A further method is to find chemical agents that induce apoptosis in ovarian cancer cells by a different mechanism from platinum compounds and may therefore exert synergistic apoptotic effects.

4.1 Inhibition of survival signals

The balance between cellular survival and induction of apoptosis determines the sensitivity of cancer cells to chemotherapeutic drugs. Therefore, blocking survival cascade signals or enhancing apoptosis-inducing signals enhances the sensitivity of ovarian cancer cells to chemotherapeutic agents (Vivanco & Sawyers, 2002). Topotecan, an inhibitor of topoisomerase I, inhibits Akt kinase activity in cisplatin-resistant ovarian cancer Caov-3 cells (Tsunetoh et al., 2010). The PI3K-Akt survival cascade signal in cisplatin-resistant ovarian cancer cells is inhibited by treatment with a combination of topotecan and cisplatin, which enhances the sensitivity to cisplatin *in vitro* and *in vivo* (Tsunetoh et al., 2010). The flavonoid compound, kaempherol, sensitizes ovarian cancer OVCAR-3 cells to cisplatin by down regulation of cMyc, which is involved in proliferation and is commonly activated in human cancer cells (Jung et al., 2008; Luo et al., 2010). Treatment of cisplatin resistant A2780CP ovarian cancer cells with a polyphenol, curcumin (diferulonyl methane), derived from the rhizomes of turmeric *Curcuma longa*, down regulated the expression of cMyc and pro-survival proteins such as Bcl-X_L and Mcl-1, leading to cisplatin sensitization (Yallapu, 2010). Topotecan, kaempherol, and curcumin therefore warrant further investigation as potential therapeutic agents for ovarian cancer.

4.2 Inhibition of platinum-DNA adduct repair

Inhibitors of DNA synthesis, such as gemcitabine (Touma et al., 2006), cytarabine (Swinnen et al., 2008), hydroxyurea (Raymond et al., 2001), and aphidicolin (Sargent et al., 1996), are able to inhibit the repair process of platinum-DNA adducts and have been used to increase sensitivity to chemotherapeutic platinum compounds. A phase II study using carboplatin followed by gemcitabine and paclitaxel for the treatment of ovarian cancer patients showed an improvement in therapeutic efficacy (Harries et al., 2004). However, the pulmonary toxicity observed as a side effect of this treatment still needs to be addressed.

The histone deacetylase inhibitor panobinostat, which affects the expression of various genes, showed synergistic cytotoxic effects in conjunction with conventional chemotherapeutic agents including carboplatin on ovarian cancer cell lines (Budman et al., 2010).

Arsenic trioxide inhibits UV-induced DNA repair processes (Hartwig et al., 1997), and also showed additive cytotoxic effects with cisplatin for human ovarian carcinoma cell lines *in vitro* (Uslu et al., 2000). Arsenic trioxide was successfully used for the treatment of all-trans retinoic acid resistant acute promyelocytic leukemia (Soignet et al., 1998), which suggests that it may be successful in treating cisplatin-resistant ovarian cancer patients.

4.3 Induction of apoptosis in cancer cells by activating the TR3/Nur77 gene

Indole -3-carbinol (I3C), contained in cruciferous vegetables such as broccoli, cabbage, and cauliflower, and its dimeric product 3,3′-diindolylmethane (DIM) are nontoxic, natural compounds with anticancer activities. DIM and its analogues increase the levels of TR3/Nur77 and induce apoptosis in various cancer cell lines including colon, pancreas, prostate, and breast cancer cells (Banerjee et al., 2009; Cho et al., 2007). Pancreatic cancer cells with acquired resistance to chemotherapeutic drugs, such as cisplatin, oxaliplatin, and gemcitabin, were sensitized by pretreatment with DIM (Banerjee et al., 2009). Compounds that activate the TR3/Nur77 gene and induce apoptosis in cancer cells are proposed as a new category of chemotherapeutic drugs, and include an analogue of cytosporone B (Liu et al., 2010) and 1,1-bis(3'-indolyl)-1-(*p*-substituted phenyl) methanes (C-substituted DIMs, Chintharlapalli et al., 2005). Acetylshikonin and its derivative 5,8-diacetoxyl-6-(1'-acetoxyl-4'-methyl-3'-pentenyl)-1,4-naphthaquinones (SK07) increased the level of TR3/Nur77 through posttranscriptional regulation, and induced apoptosis in various cancer cell lines including lung and cervical cancer cells (Liu et al., 2008). The positive correlation of the expression of the TR3/Nur77 subfamily member Nor-1 with survival rates of diffuse large B-cell lymphoma patients indicates the importance of TR3/Nur77 as a target for anti-cancer agents (Shipp et al., 2002). The importance of TR3-Nur77 as a therapeutic target of ovarian cancer is also demonstrated by the fact that low expression of TR3/Nur77 in tissue samples obtained from various cancer patients is significantly associated with metastasis of primary solid cancers (Ramaswamy et al., 2003).

We discovered that some ovarian cancer cell lines, such as PA-1 cells, are sensitive to vitamin K2 and apoptosis induced by stimulation of TR3/Nur77 synthesis and its accumulation in mitochondria (Fig. 5). Small interfering RNA (siRNA) directed against TR3-Nur77 (siRNA-TR3/Nur77) caused a marked decrease in the levels of TR3/Nur77 in the lysate of PA-1 cells. When ovarian cancer PA-1 cells after transfection with siRNA-TR3/Nur77 were treated with vitamin K2, the marked increase in the levels of TR3/Nur77 observed by vitamin K2 without siRNA-TR3/Nur77 was almost completely abolished (Shibayama-Imazu et al., 2008). Induction of apoptosis by vitamin K2 was also significantly inhibited by transfection of PA-1 cells with siRNA-TR3/Nur77. Furthermore, cycloheximide, an inhibitor of protein synthesis, prevented the increase in TR3/Nur77 levels, its accumulation in the mitochondria, and the induction of apoptosis in PA-1 cells caused by vitamin K2 treatment (Shibayama-Imazu et al., 2008). These results indicate that the synthesis of TR3/Nur77 and its accumulation in mitochondria are required for the induction of apoptosis in PA-1 cells by vitamin K2 and also suggest that an increase in the level of TR3/Nur77 could be the cause of sensitivity to the induction of apoptosis in PA-1 cells by vitamin K2 (Fig. 5).

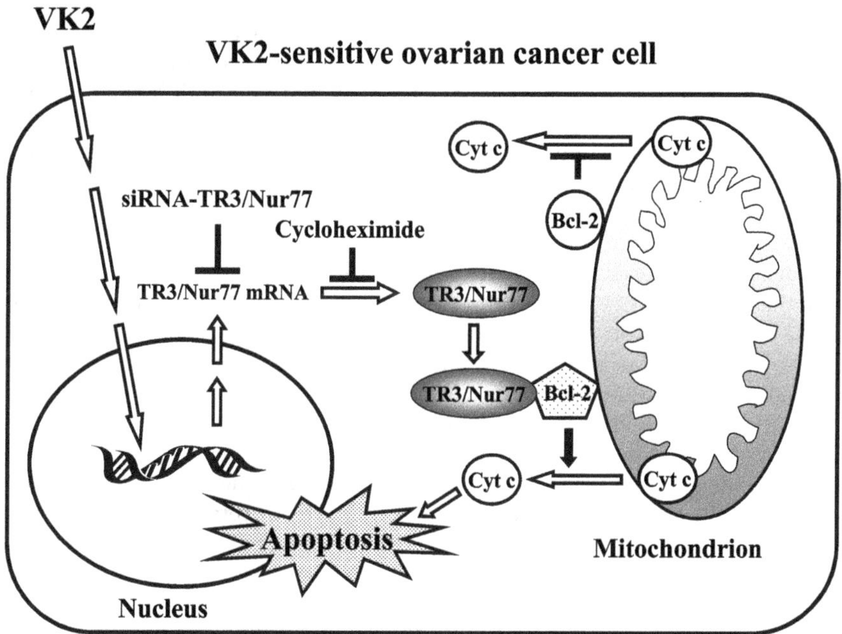

Fig. 5. A model for the induction of apoptosis in vitamin K2-sensitive ovarian cancer cells. The levels of TR3/Nur77 in vitamin K2-sensitive ovarian cancer cells are increased after treatment with vitamin K2. TR3/Nur77 synthesized in the cytoplasm migrates to the mitochondria and binds to Bcl-2, which protects the cell from apoptosis. Interaction of TR3/Nur77 with Bcl-2 induces a conformational change in Bcl-2, triggering the release of cytochrome c, which activates the caspase cascade and thus induces apoptosis. siRNA-TR3/Nur77 causes degradation of TR3/Nur77 mRNA and cycloheximide inhibits the protein synthesis of TR3/Nur77, both leading to inhibition of the induction of apoptosis by vitamin K2.

A combination of vitamin K2 and conventional chemotherapeutic agents for ovarian cancer, such as cisplatin and etoposide, which induce apoptosis by different mechanisms, might have additive or synergistic apoptotic effects on ovarian cancer cells. In addition, pretreatment with vitamin K2 or combination treatment with conventional chemotherapeutic agents could be effective for overcoming chemoresistance in ovarian cancer cells.

5. Vitamin K2 as a promising chemotherapeutic agent for ovarian cancer

Vitamin K2 induces apoptosis in blastic cells from patients with myelodysplastic syndrome (Nishimaki et al., 1999; Yaguchi et al., 1998) and has been successfully used in the clinical treatment of patients with this disorder (Miyazawa et al., 2000; Takami et al., 1999; Yaguchi et al., 1998, 1999). Oral administration of vitamin K2 with retinoic acid to a patient with relapsed acute promyelocytic leukemia resulted in complete remission (Fujita et al., 1998). In addition, oral administration of vitamin K2 also had a suppressive effect on the recurrence of hepatocellular carcinoma and improved patient survival rate (Habu et al., 2004; Mizuta et al., 2006; Tamori et al., 2007; Yoshiji et al., 2009). A recent cohort study indicates that cancer incidence and mortality were significantly decreased by dietary intake of vitamin K2 from food sources (Nimptsch et al., 2010). Vitamin K2 is also used clinically as a drug for osteoporosis in Asian countries such as Japan, Korea, and Thailand, because it also has a significant effect on bone fracture prevention (Cockayne et al., 2006; Olson, 2000; Shiraki et al., 2000). This is because calcium-binding proteins such as osteocalcin and calbindin, which are involved in calcium uptake and bone mineralization, are vitamin K-dependent proteins. A further cohort study indicated that the relative risk of coronary heart disease was also reduced by dietary intake of vitamin K2 (Geleijne et al., 2004). This may be because vitamin K-dependent proteins are associated with vascular repair processes (Benzakour & Kanthou, 2000) and the prevention of vascular calcification (Shanahan et al, 1998). No side effects from vitamin K2 therapy were observed in any of these clinical studies; even vitamin K2 dosages in excess of 40 mg/day did not cause any side effects associated with hypercoagulable states (Shiraki et al., 2000), demonstrating its excellent safety profile. However, it is unknown why some ovarian cancer cell lines are resistant to vitamin K2. It may be possible to overcome vitamin K2 resistance by using it in combination with other agents that increase the level of TR3/Nur77 in cancer cells, such as DIM, cytosporone B, and the shikonin derivative SK07. SK07 stimulates the protein synthesis of TR3/Nur77 even in cervical cancer HeLa cells, in which the basal expression level of TR3/Nur77 is low (Liu et al., 2008). Further pre-clinical and clinical evaluation of vitamin K2 is required for its use in chemotherapy for ovarian cancers.

6. Conclusion

Several ovarian cancer cell lines are sensitive to vitamin K2; the IC_{50} value of the most vitamin K2-sensitive ovarian cancer PA-1 cells is as low as 5 μM. Apoptosis is induced in PA-1 cells through the stimulation of TR3/Nur77 synthesis and its accumulation in mitochondria, which results in the release of cytochrome c and activation of the caspase cascade (Fig. 5). Because this mechanism is different from those of conventional chemotherapeutic agents for ovarian cancer such as cisplatin and etoposide, the present study demonstrates a new method for increasing the sensitivity of cisplatin resistant ovarian cancer cells to chemotherapy. Moreover, our observation suggests that the combination of vitamin K2 with cisplatin or etoposide may potentially be effective for the treatment of ovarian cancers. None of the clinical trials using high doses of vitamin K2 have recorded side effects from the treatment, and oral administration of vitamin K2 has already been successfully used for the treatment of acute promyelocytic leukemia and haepatocellular carcinoma (Table 1). We therefore propose vitamin K2 as a useful chemotherapeutic agent for ovarian cancer.

7. Acknowledgements

We are grateful for the support from Grants-in-Aid for Scientific Research from the Ministry of Education, Cultures, Sports, Science, and Technology, Japan.

8. References

Banerjee, S., Wang, Z., Kong, D. & Sarkar, FH. (2009) 3,3'-Diindolylmethane enhances chemosensitivity of multiple chemotherapeutic agents in pancreatic cancer. *Cancer Research*,Vol.69, No.13, (July 2009), pp. 5592-5600, ISSN 1538-7445

Benzakour, O. & Kanthou, C. (2000) The anticoagulant factor, protein S, is produced by cultured human vascular smooth muscle cells and its expression is up-regulated by thrombin. *Blood*. Vol.95, No.6, (March 2000), pp. 2008-2014, ISSN 0006-4971

Bookman, MA., Malmström, H., Bolis, G., Gordon, A., Lissoni, A., Krebs, JB. & Fields, SZ. (1998) Topotecan for the treatment of advanced epithelial ovarian cancer: an open-label phase II study in patients treated after prior chemotherapy that contained cisplatin or carboplatin and paclitaxel. *Journal of Clinical Oncology*, Vol.16, No.10, (October 1998), pp. 3345-3352, ISSN 0732-183X

Budman, DR., Tai, J., Calabro, A. & John, V. (2010) The histone deacetylase inhibitor panobinostat demonstrates marked synergy with conventional chemotherapeutic agents in human ovarian cancer cell lines. *Investigational New Drugs*, (May 2010), published on line: June 9, ISSN 0167-6997

Chintharlapalli, S., Burghardt, R., Papineni, S., Ramaiah, S., Yoon, K. & Safe, S. (2005) Activation of Nur77 by selected 1,1-Bis(3'-indolyl)-1-(p-substituted phenyl)methanes induces apoptosis through nuclear pathways. *The Journal of Biolical Chemistry*, Vol.280, No.26, (July 2005), pp. 24903-24914, ISSN 0021-9258

Cho, SD., Yoon, K., Chintharlapalli, S., Abdelrahim, M., Lei, P., Hamilton, S., Khan, S., Ramaiah, SK. & Safe, S. (2007) Nur77 agonists induce proapoptotic genes and responses in colon cancer cells through nuclear receptor-dependent and nuclear receptor-independent pathways. *Cancer Research*, Vol.67, No.2, (January 2007), pp. 674-683, ISSN 1538-7445

Cockayne, S., Adamson, J., Lanham-New, S., Shearer, MJ., Gilbody, S. & Torgerson, DJ. (2006) Vitamin K and the prevention of fractures: systematic review and meta-analysis of randomized controlled trials. *Archives of Internal Medicine*, Vol.166, No.12, (June 2006), pp. 1256-1261, ISSN 0003-9926

Fujita, H., Tomiyama, J. & Tanaka, T. (1998) Vitamin K2 combined with all-trans retinoic acid induced complete remission of relapsing acute promyelocytic leukemia. *British Journal of Haematology*, Vol.103, No.2, (November 1998), pp. 584-585, ISSN 0007-1048

Geleijnse, JM., Vermeer, C., Grobbee, DE., Schurgers, LJ., Knapen, MH., van der Meer, IM., Hofman, A. & Witteman, JC. (2004) Dietary intake of menaquinone is associated with a reduced risk of coronary heart disease: the Rotterdam Study. *The Journal of Nutrition*, Vol.134, No.11, (November 2004), pp. 3100-3015, ISSN 0022-3166

Giaccone, G. (2000) Clinical perspectives on platinum resistance. *Drugs*, Vol.59, Suppl. 4, pp. 9-17, ISSN 0012-6667

Habu, D., Shiomi, S., Tamori, A., Takeda, T., Tanaka, T., Kubo, S. & Nishiguchi, S. (2004) Role of vitamin K2 in the development of hepatocellular carcinoma in women with viral cirrhosis of the liver. *The Journal of the Amerian Medical Association*, Vol.292, No.3, (July 2004), pp. 358-361, ISSN 0098-7484

Harries, M., Moss, C., Perren, T., Gore, M., Hall, G., Everard, M., A'Hern, R., Gibbens, I., Jenkin, A., Shah, R., Cole, C., Pizzada, O. & Kaye, S. (2004) A phase II feasibility study of carboplatin followed by sequential weekly paclitaxel and gemcitabine as first-line treatment for ovarian cancer. *British Journal of Cancer*, Vol.91, No.4, (August 2004), pp. 627-632, ISSN 0007-0920

Hartwig, A., Groblinghoff, UD., Beyersmann, D., Natarajan, AT., Filon, R. & Mullenders, LH. (1997) Interaction of arsenic (III) with nucleotide excision repair in UV-irradiated human fibroblasts. *Carcinogenesis*, Vol.18, No.2, (February 1997), pp. 399-405, ISSN 0143-3334

Hennessy, BT., Coleman, RL. & Markman, M. (2009) Ovarian cancer. *Lancet*, Vol.374, No.9698, (October 2009), pp. 1371-1382, ISSN 0140-6736

Holmes, WF., Soprano, DR. & Soprano, KJ. (2002) Elucidation of molecular events mediating induction of apoptosis by synthetic retinoids using a CD437-resistant ovarian carcinoma cell line. *The Journal of Biological Chemistry*, Vol.277, No.47, (November 2002), pp. 45408-45419, ISSN 0021-9258

Holmes, WF., Soprano, DR &, Soprano, KJ. (2004) Synthetic retinoids as inducers of apoptosis in ovarian carcinoma cell lines. *Journal of Cellular Physiology*, Vol.199, No.3, (June 2004), pp. 317-329, ISSN 0021-9541

Jung, P., Menssen, A., Mayr, D. & Hermeking, H. (2008) AP4 encodes a c-MYC-inducible repressor of p21. *Proceedings of the Nationall Academy of Sciences of the United States of America*, Vol.105, No.39, (September 2008), pp. 15046-15051, ISSN 0027-8424

Kartalou, M. & Essigmann, JM. (2001) Mechanisms of resistance to cisplatin. *Mutation Research*, Vol.478, No. 1-2, (July 2001), pp. 23-43, ISSN 0027-5107

Li, H., Kolluri, SK., Gu, J., Dawson, MI., Cao, X., Hobbs, PD., Lin, B., Chen, G., Lu, J., Lin, F., Xie, Z., Fontana, JA., Reed, JC. & Zhang, X. (2000) Cytochrome c release and apoptosis induced by mitochondrial targeting of nuclear orphan receptor TR3. *Science*. Vol.289, No.5482, (August 2000), pp. 1159-1164, ISSN 1095-9203

Li, Y., Lin, B., Agadir, A., Liu, R., Dawson, MI., Reed, JC., Fontana, JA., Bost, F., Hobbs, PD., Zheng, Y., Chen, GQ., Shroot, B., Mercola, D. & Zhang, XK. (1998) Molecular determinants of AHPN (CD437)-induced growth arrest and apoptosis in human lung cancer cell lines. *Molecular and Cellular Biology*, Vol.18, No.8, (August 1998), pp. 4719-4731, ISSN 0270-7306

Liu, J., Zhou, W., Li, SS., Sun, Z., Lin, B., Lang, YY., He, JY., Cao, X., Yan, T., Wang, L., Lu, J., Han, YH., Cao, Zhang, XK. & Zeng, JZ. (2008) Modulation of orphan nuclear receptor Nur77-mediated apoptotic pathway by acetylshikonin and analogues. *Cancer Research*, Vol.68, No.21, (November 2008), pp. 8871-8880, ISSN 1538-7445

Liu, JJ., Zeng, HN., Zhang, LR., Zhan, YY., Chen, Y., Wang, Y., Wang, J., Xiang, SH., Liu, WJ., Wang, WJ., Chen, HZ., Shen, YM., Su, WJ., Huang, PQ., Zhang, HK. & Wu, Q. (2010) A unique pharmacophore for activation of the nuclear orphan receptor Nur77 in vivo and in vitro. *Cancer Research*, Vol.70, No.9, (May 2010), pp. 3628-3637, ISSN 1538-7445

Luo, H., Daddysman, MK., Rankin, GO., Jiang, BH. & Chen, YC. (2010) Kaempferol enhances cisplatin's effect on ovarian cancer cells through promoting apoptosis caused by down regulation of cMyc. *Cancer Cell International*, Vol. 10, (May 2010), pp. 16-25, ISSN 1475-2867

Masuda, Y., Nakaya, M., Aiuchi, T., Hashimoto, S., Nakajo, S. & Nakaya, K. (2000) The mechanism of geranylgeraniol-induced apoptosis involves activation, by a caspase-3-like protease, of a c-jun N-terminal kinase signaling cascade and differs from mechanisms of apoptosis induced by conventional chemotherapeutic drugs. *Leukemia Research*, Vol.24, No.11, (November 2000), pp. 937-950, ISSN 0145-2126

Miyazawa, K., Nishimaki, .J, Ohyashiki, K., Enomoto, S., Kuriya, S., Fukuda, R., Hotta, T., Teramura, M., Mizoguchi, H., Uchiyama, T. & Omine, M. (2000) Vitamin K2 therapy for myelodysplastic syndromes (MDS) and post-MDS acute myeloid leukemia: information through a questionnaire survey of multi-center pilot studies in Japan. *Leukemia*, Vol.14, No.6, (June 2000), pp. 1156-1157, ISSN 0887-6924

Miyazawa, K., Yaguchi, M., Funato, K., Gotoh, A., Kawanishi, Y., Nishizawa,Y., You, A. & Ohyashiki, K. (2001) Apoptosis/differentiation-inducing effects of vitamin K2 on HL-60 cells: dichotomous nature of vitamin K2 in leukemia cells. *Leukemia*, Vol.15, No.7, (July 2001), pp. 1111-1117, ISSN 0887-6924

Mizuta, T., Ozaki, I., Eguchi, Y., Yasutake, T., Kawazoe, S., Fujimoto, K. & Yamamoto, K. (2006) The effect of menatetrenone, a vitamin K2 analog, on disease recurrence and survival in patients with hepatocellular carcinoma after curative treatment: a pilot study. *Cancer*, Vol.106, No.4, (February 2006), pp. 867-872, ISSN 0008-543X

Nimptsch, K., Rohrmann, S., Kaaks, R. & Linseisen, J. (2010) Dietary vitamin K intake in relation to cancer incidence and mortality: results from the Heidelberg cohort of the European Prospective Investigation into Cancer and Nutrition (EPIC-Heidelberg). *The American Journal of Clinical Nutrition*, Vol.91, No.5, (May 2010), pp. 1348-1358, ISSN 0002-9165

Nishikawa, Y., Carr, BI., Wang, M., Kar, S., Finn, F., Dowd, P., Zheng, ZB., Kerns, J. & Naganathan S. (1995) Growth inhibition of hepatoma cells induced by vitamin K and its analogs. *The Jounal of Biological Chemistry*, Vol.270, No.47, (November 1995), pp. 28304-28310, ISSN 0021-9258

Nishimaki, J., Miyazawa, K., Yaguchi, M., Katagiri, T., Kawanishi, Y., Toyama, K., Ohyashiki, K., Hashimoto, S., Nakaya, K. & Takiguchi, T. (1999) Vitamin K2 induces apoptosis of a novel cell line established from patient with myelodysplastic syndrome in blastic transformation. *Leukemia*, Vol.13, No.9, (September 1999), pp. 1399-1405, ISSN 0887-6924

Ohizumi, H., Masuda, Y., Nakajo, S., Sakai, I., Ohsawa, S. & Nakaya, K. (1995) Geranylgeraniol is a potent inducer of apoptosis in tumor cells. *Journal of Biochemistry*, Vol.117, No.1, (January 1995), pp. 11-13, ISSN 0021-924X

Olson, RE. (2000) Osteoporosis and vitamin K intake. *The American Journal of Clinical Nutrition*, Vol.71, No.5, (May 2000), pp. 1031-1032, ISSN 0002-9165

Otsuka, M., Kato, N., Shao, RX., Hoshida, Y., Ijichi, H., Koike, Y., Taniguchi, H., Moriyama, M., Shiratori, Y., Kawabe, T. & Omata, M. (2004) Vitamin K2 inhibits the growth and invasiveness of hepatocellular carcinoma cells via protein kinase A activation. *Hepatology*, Vol.40, No.1, (July 2004), pp. 243-251, ISSN 0270-9139

Parkin, DM., Bray, F., Ferlay, J. & Pisani, P. (2005) Global Cancer Statics, 2002. *A Cancer Journal for Clinicians*, Vol.55, No. 2, (March-April 2005), pp. 74-108, ISSN 0007-9235

Pekarsky, Y., Hallas, C., Palamarchuk, A., Koval, A., Bullrich, F., Hirata, Y., Bichi, R., Letofsky, J. & Croce, CM. (2001) Akt phosphorylates and regulates the orphan nuclear receptor Nur77. *Proceedings of the National Academy of Sciences United States of America*, Vol. 98, No. 7, (March 2001), pp. 3690-3694, ISSN 0027-8424

Ramaswamy, S., Ross, KN., Lander, ES. & Golub, TR. (2003) A molecular signature of metastasis in primary solid tumors. *Nature Genetics*, Vol.33, No.1, (January 2003), pp. 49-54, ISSN 1061-4036

Raymond, E., Faivre, S., Weiss, G., McGill, J., Davidson, K., Izbicka, E., Kuhn, JG., Allred, C., Clark, GM. & Von Hoff, DD. (2001) Effects of hydroxyurea on extrachromosomal DNA in patients with advanced ovarian carcinomas. *Clinical Cancer Research*, Vol.7, No.5, (May 2001), pp. 1171-1180, ISSN 1078-0432

Sakai, I., Hashimoto, S., Yoda, M., Hida, T., Ohsawa, S., Nakajo, S. & Nakaya, K. (1994) Novel role of vitamin K2: a potent inducer of differentiation of various human myeloid leukemia cell lines. *Biochemical and Biophysical Research Communications*, Vol.205, No.2, (December 1994), pp. 1305-1310, ISSN 0006-291X

Sargent, JM., Elgie, AW., Williamson, CJ. & Taylor, CG. (1996) Aphidicolin markedly increases the platinum sensitivity of cells from primary ovarian tumours. *British Journal of Cancer*, Vol.74, No.11, (December 1996), pp. 1730-1733, ISSN 0007-0920

Shanahan, CM., Proudfoot, D., Farzaneh-Far, A. & Weissberg, PL. (1998) The role of Gla proteins in vascular calcification. *Critical Reviews in Eukaryotic Gene Expression*, Vol.8, No.3-4, (1998), pp. 357-375, ISSN 1045-4403

Shearer, MJ., Bach, A. & Kohlmeier, M. (1996) Chemistry, nutritional sources, tissue distribution and metabolism of vitamin K with special reference to bone health. *The Journal of Nutrition*, Vol.126, Suppl.4, (April 1996), pp. 1181S-1186S, ISSN 0022-3166

Schurgers, LJ. & Vermeer, C.(2000) Determination of phylloquinone and menaquinones in food. Effect of food matrix on circulating vitamin K concentrations. *Haemostasis*, Vol.30, No.6, (November-December 2000), pp. 298-307, ISSN 0301-0147

Shibayama-Imazu, T., Sakairi, S., Watanabe, A., Aiuchi, T., Nakajo, S. & Nakaya, K. (2003) Vitamin K2 selectively induced apoptosis in ovarian TYK-nu and pancreatic MIA PaCa-2 cells out of eight solid tumor cell lines through a mechanism different from geranylgeraniol. *Journal of Cancer Research and Clinical Oncology*, Vol.129, No.1, (January 2003), pp. 1-11, ISSN 0170-5216

Shibayama-Imazu, T., Sonoda, I., Sakairi, S., Aiuchi, T., Ann, WW., Nakajo, S., Itabe, H. & Nakaya, K. (2006) Production of superoxide and dissipation of mitochondrial transmembrane potential by vitamin K2 trigger apoptosis in human ovarian cancer TYK-nu cells. *Apoptosis*, Vol.11, No.9, (September 2006), pp. 1535-1543, ISSN 1360-8185

Shibayama-Imazu, T., Fujisawa, Y., Masuda, Y., Aiuchi, T., Nakajo, S., Itabe, H. & Nakaya, K. (2008) Induction of apoptosis in PA-1 ovarian cancer cells by vitamin K2 is associated with an increase in the level of TR3/Nur77 and its accumulation in mitochondria and nuclei. *Journal of Cancer Research and Clinical Oncology*, Vol.134, No.7, (January 2008), pp. 803-812, ISSN 0170-52168

Shipp, MA., Ross, KN., Tamayo, P., Weng, AP., Kutok, JL., Aguiar, RC., Gaasenbeek, M., Angelo, M., Reich, M., Pinkus, GS., Ray, TS., Koval, MA., Last, KW., Norton, A., Lister, TA., Mesirov, J., Neuber, DS., Lander, ES., Aster, JC. & Golub, TR. (2002) Diffuse large B-cell lymphoma outcome prediction by gene-expression profiling and supervised machine learning. *Nature Medicine*, Vol.8, No.1, (January 2002), pp. 68-74, ISSN 1078-8956

Shiraki, M., Shiraki, Y., Aoki, C. & Miura, M. (2000) Vitamin K2 (menatetrenone) effectively prevents fractures and sustains lumbar bone mineral density in osteoporosis. *Journsl of Bone and Mineral Research*, Vol.15, No.3, (March 2000), pp. 515-521, ISSN 0884-0431

Soignet, SL., Maslak, P., Wang, ZG., Jhanwar, S., Calleja, E., Dardashti, LJ., Corso, D., DeBlasio, A., Gabrilove, J., Scheinberg, DA., Pandolfi, PP. & Warrell, RP. Jr. (1998) Complete remission after treatment of acute promyelocytic leukemia with arsenic trioxide. *The New England Journal of Medicine*, Vol.339, No.19, (November 1998), pp. 1341-1348, ISSN 0028-4793

Swinnen, LJ., Rankin, C., Carraway, H., Albain, KS., Townsend, JJ., Budd, GT., Kish, JA., Rivkin, SE. & Blumenthal, DT. (2008) A phase II study of cisplatin preceded by a 12-h continuous infusion of concurrent hydroxyurea and cytosine arabinoside (Ara-C) for adult patients with malignant gliomas (Southwest Oncology Group S9149). *Journal of Neuro-oncology*, Vol.86, No.3, (February 2008), pp. 353-358, ISSN 0167-594X

Swisher, EM., Mutch, DG., Rader, JS., Elbendary, A. & Herzog, TJ. (1997) Topotecan in platinum- and paclitaxel-resistant ovarian cancer. *Gynecologic Oncology*. Vol.66, No.3, (September 1997), pp. 480-486, ISSN 0090-8258

Takami, A., Nakao, S., Ontachi, Y., Yamauchi, H. & Matsuda, T. (1999) Successful therapy of myelodysplastic syndrome with menatetrenone, a vitamin K2 analog. *International Journal of Hematology*, Vol.69, No.1, (January 1999), pp. 24-26, ISSN 0925-5710

Tamori, A., Habu, D., Shiomi, S., Kubo, S. & Nishiguchi, S. (2007) Potential role of vitamin K2 as a chemopreventive agent against hepatocellular carcinoma. *Hepatology Research*, Vol.37, Suppl.2, (September 2007), pp. S303-S307, ISSN 1386-6346

Thijssen, HH. & Drittij-Reijnders, MJ. (1996) Vitamin K status in human tissues: tissue-specific accumulation of phylloquinone and menaquinone-4. *British Journal of Nutrition*, Vol.75, No.1, (January 1996), pp. 121-127

Tokita, H., Tsuchida, A., Miyazawa, K., Ohyashiki, K., Katayanagi, S., Sudo, H., Enomoto, M., Takagi, Y. & Aoki, T. (2006) Vitamin K2-induced antitumor effects via cell-cycle arrest and apoptosis in gastric cancer cell lines. *International Journal of Molecular Medicine*. Vol.17, No.2, (February 2006), pp. 235-243, ISSN 1107-3756

Touma, R., Kartarius, S., Harlozinska, A., Götz, C. & Montenarh, M. (2006) Growth inhibition and apoptosis induction in ovarian cancer cells. *International Journal of Oncology*, Vol.29, No.2, (August 2006), pp. 481-488, ISSN 1019-6439

Tsunetoh, S., Terai, Y., Sasaki, H., Tanabe, A., Tanaka, Y., Sekijima, T., Fujioka, S., Kawaguchi, H., Kanemura, M., Yamashita, Y. & Ohmichi, M. (2010) Topotecan as a molecular targeting agent which blocks the Akt and VEGF cascade in platinum-resistant ovarian cancers. *Cancer Biology & Therapy*. Vol. 10, No.11, (December 2010), pp. 1137-1146, ISSN 1538-4047

Uslu, R., Sanli, UA., Sezgin, C., Karabulut, B, Terzioglu, E., Omay, SB. & Goker, E. (2000) Arsenic trioxide-mediated cytotoxicity and apoptosis in prostate and ovarian carcinoma cell lines. *Clinical Cancer Research*, Vol.6, No.12, (December 2000), pp. 4957-4964, ISSN 1078-0432

Vivanco, I. & Sawyers, CL. (2002) The phosphatidylinositol 3-Kinase AKT pathway in human cancer. *Nature Reviews. Cancer*. Vol.2, No.7, (July 2002), pp. 489-501, ISSN 1474-175X

Wu, FY., Liao, WC. & Chang, HM. (1993) Comparison of antitumor activity of vitamins K1, K2 and K3 on human tumor cells by two (MTT and SRB) cell viability assays. *Life Sciences*, Vol.52, No.22, (March 1993), pp. 1797-1804, ISSN 0024-3205

Wu, Q., Liu, S., Ye, XF., Huang, ZW. & Su, WJ. (2002) Dual roles of Nur77 in selective regulation of apoptosis and cell cycle by TPA and ATRA in gastric cancer cells. *Carcinogenesis*, Vol.23, No.10, (October 2002), pp. 1583-1592, ISSN 0143-3334

Yaguchi, M., Miyazawa, K., Katagiri, T., Nishimaki, J., Kizaki, M., Tohyama, K. & Toyama, K. (1997) Vitamin K2 and its derivatives induce apoptosis in leukemia cells and enhance the effect of all-trans retinoic acid. *Leukemia*, Vol.11, No.6, (June 1997), pp. 779-787, ISSN 0887-6924

Yaguchi, M., Miyazawa, K., Otawa, M., Katagiri, T., Nishimaki, J., Uchida, Y., Iwase, O., Gotoh, A., Kawanishi, Y. & Toyama, K. (1998) Vitamin K2 selectively induces apoptosis of blastic cells in myelodysplastic syndrome: flow cytometric detection of apoptotic cells using APO2.7 monoclonal antibody. *Leukemia*, Vol.12, No.9, (September 1998), pp. 1392-1397, ISSN 0887-6924

Yaguchi, M., Miyazawa, K., Otawa, M., Ito, Y., Kawanishi, Y. & Toyama, K. (1999) Vitamin K2 therapy for a patient with myelodysplastic syndrome. *Leukemia*, Vol.13, No.1, (January 1999), pp. 144-145, ISSN 0887-6924

Yallapu, MM., Maher, DM., Sundram, V., Bell, MC., Jaggi, M. & Chauhan, SC. (2010) Curcumin induces chemo/radio-sensitization in ovarian cancer cells and curcumin nanoparticles inhibit ovarian cancer cell growth. *Journal of Ovarian Research*, Vol.3, (April 2010), pp. 11-23, ISSN 1757-2215

Yokoyama, T., Miyazawa, K., Yoshida, T. & Ohyashiki, K. (2005) Combination of vitamin K2 plus imatinib mesylate enhances induction of apoptosis in small cell lung cancer cell lines. *International Journal of Oncology*, Vol.26, No.1, (January 2005), pp. 33-40, ISSN 1019-6439

Yoshiji, H., Noguchi, R., Toyohara, M., Ikenaka, Y., Kitade, M., Kaji, K., Yamazaki, M., Yamao, J., Mitoro, A., Sawai, M., Yoshida, M., Fujimoto, M., Tsujimoto, T., Kawaratani, H., Uemura, M. & Fukui, H. (2009) Combination of vitamin K2 and angiotensin-converting enzyme inhibitor ameliorates cumulative recurrence of hepatocellular carcinoma. *Journal of Hepatology*, Vol.51, No.2, (August 2009), pp. 315-321, ISSN 0168-8278

Yoshida, T., Miyazawa, K., Kasuga, I., Yokoyama, T., Minemura, K., Ustumi, K., Aoshima, M. & Ohyashiki, K. (2003) Apoptosis induction of vitamin K2 in lung carcinoma cell lines: the possibility of vitamin K2 therapy for lung cancer. *International Journal of Oncoogy*, Vol.23, No.3, (September 2003), pp. 627-632, ISSN 1019-6439

16

HER2 as a Therapeutic Target in Ovarian Cancer

Lukas C. Amler, Yulei Wang and Garret Hampton
Genentech Inc., South San Francisco
USA

1. Introduction

Members of the human epidermal growth factor receptor (HER) family—epidermal growth factor receptor (EGFR, HER1), HER2, HER3, and HER4—are transmembrane tyrosine kinase receptors that are important mediators of cell growth, development, and survival. Activation of the HER tyrosine kinases triggers intracellular signaling pathways, including the MAPK and PI3K-Akt pathways (Olayioye et al., 2000) (Figure 1).

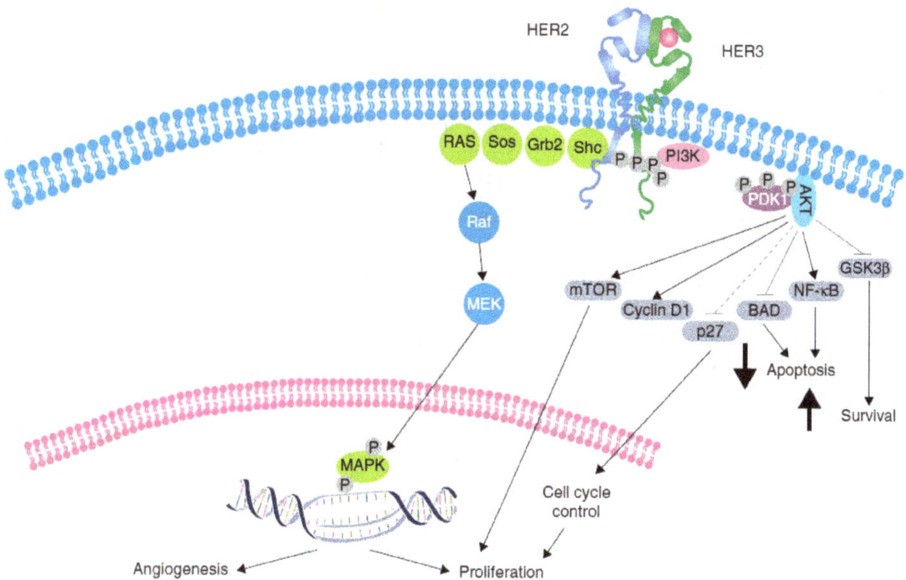

(Amler, L.C. *Expert Opinion on Biological Therapy*, 2010; Vol.10, No.9, pp.1343-1344, copyright © 2010, Informa Healthcare. Reproduced with permission of Informa Healthcare)

Fig. 1. Dimerization of HER2–HER3 initiates the PI3K and MAPK signaling pathways.

Ligand binding to HER1, 3, and 4 results in a conformational change in the extracellular domain of each protein that opens a dimerization domain and allows the receptor to form either a homo- or heterodimer with another member of the HER family (Cho & Leahy, 2002; Zhang et al., 2006). No ligand has been identified for HER2, and it exists in a conformation that is constitutively available for dimerization (Garrett et al., 2003). HER2 is therefore the preferred dimer partner of other HER family members (Graus-Porta et al., 1997). While HER2 has no known ligand, HER3 lacks intracellular tyrosine kinase activity, rendering HER2-HER3 signaling dependent on heterodimerization (Yarden & Sliwkowski, 2001). HER2-HER3 dimerization results in phosphorylation of the tyrosine kinase domain, which in turn activates intracellular signaling pathways (Zhang et al., 2006). The effect of these signaling pathways on gene transcription determines how the cell responds to the ligand activation.

HER family members can also be activated by ligand-independent mechanisms, including activation by other tyrosine kinase receptors, G-protein coupled receptors, and adhesion proteins (Siwak et al., 2010).

1.1 Role of HER2 in oncology

Members of the HER family were first associated with oncogenesis after the discovery that the sequence of the EGFR receptor was found to be very similar to that of v-*ErbB*, a transforming retroviral oncogene carried by the avian erythroblastosis virus (Downward et al., 1984). The v-*ErbB* oncogene encodes a truncated form of EGFR that can form ligand-independent dimers, thereby initiating cell signaling pathways and inducing cellular proliferation in the absence of ligand stimulation (Adelsman et al., 1996). Examination of a series of rat neuro/gliobalstomas revealed a commonly transforming gene, neu, encoding a protein serologically related to ErbB (EGFR), subsequently shown to be the HER2 oncoprotein (Coussens et al., 1985; Schechter et al., 1984).

HER2 expression is frequently dysregulated in several types of human tumors including those of the breast, head and neck, prostate, and ovary (Hynes, 1993). Of particular significance was the discovery that the HER2 protein was overexpressed, commonly by gene amplification, in about 30% of breast cancers. These studies also showed that overexpression of HER2 indicated an aggressive subtype of breast cancers with a particularly poor prognosis for the patient (Slamon et al., 1987, 1989). Overexpression of HER2 facilitates the formation of HER2 heterodimers, which trigger HER2 signaling pathways (Yarden and Sliwkowski, 2001), with excess HER2 signaling resulting in signaling cascades that promote oncogenic cell survival and proliferation (Olayioye et al., 2000; Rowinsky, 2004).

HER2 amplification /overexpression has also been reported in patients with gastric tumors where it is again linked to a poor prognosis (Jaehne et al., 1992). In addition, increased HER2 levels have been reported in some patients with salivary gland tumors (Cornolti et al., 2007) and non-small cell lung cancer (NSCLC) (Cappuzzo et al., 2006). Mutations in tumor suppressor genes may be partly responsible for the aberrant expression of HER2 in these tumors. Foe example, one tumor suppressor, *FOXP3*, normally maintains low levels of HER2 in normal cells; however, in breast cancer models the absence of *FOXP3* results in high expression of HER2 (Zuo et al., 2007).

Overexpression of HER2 is only one of several mechanisms, albeit the most frequent, by which HER2 signaling can be activated in oncogenesis. Mutations in the kinase domain of HER2 can potentially trigger signaling that is independent of ligand binding or dimerization (Anglesio et al., 2008). Ligand-dependent activation of HER2 via dimerization with other

HER family members may also play a role in HER2 oncogenesis. Of all of the different HER family dimers, the HER2-HER3 heterodimer appears to have the most potent signaling effects in cancer cells (Tzahar et al., 1996).. It appears that HER3 is crucial for mediating the dysregulated signaling in tumors overexpressing HER2 (Lee-Hoeflich et al., 2008). Cancers with HER2 amplification are frequently observed to have increased Akt activity even though HER2 cannot directly activate the PI3K-Akt pathway (Hsieh & Moasser, 2007). However, the intracellular domain of HER3 contains several binding sites for PI3K, enabling direct activation of the PI3K-Akt pathway (Figure 1), which may explain the mitogenic activity of HER2-HER3 dimers (Hsieh & Moasser, 2007). HER2 can also form a dimer with EGFR, which initiates intracellular signaling via the MAPK pathway (Campiglio et al., 1999). In summary, while HER2 amplification leading to overexpression is clearly linked to activation of HER2 in some tumor cells, activating mutations in HER2, as well as ligand-dependent activation of HER2 signaling, are also likely important mechanisms leading to HER2 oncogenesis.

2. HER2 in ovarian cancer

The HER family are important mediators of normal ovarian follicle development, and regulate the growth of ovarian epithelial cells (Conti et al., 2006). Dysregulation of HER signaling in the ovary due to overexpression of, or mutations in HER family members have been linked to the growth and proliferation of ovarian tumors.

2.1 HER2 overexpression in ovarian cancer

The proportion of ovarian cancers overexpressing HER2 is a matter of debate (Sheng & Liu, 2011). Various studies have reported that between 5% and 35% of ovarian tumors overexpress HER2 (Table 1). Some of these differences are likely to be attributable to the diagnostic technique used to measure HER2 expression. HER2 protein expression is commonly measured using immunohistochemistry (IHC), whereas *HER2* gene amplification is typically measured using hybridization techniques, such as fluorescence in situ hybridization (FISH) (Wolff et al., 2007). Recent technical improvements also enable measurement of HER2 mRNA expression levels using the quantitative real time-polymerase chain reaction (qRT-PCR) in archival samples (Muller et al., 2011).

However, the reported levels of HER2 overexpression and/or amplification may be affected by other factors including variable definitions of overexpression, small sample sizes, and variable testing conditions or assay performance (Wolff et al., 2007). It should also be noted that studies investigating only *HER2* gene amplification are likely to account for only a proportion of cancers that overexpress of the protein without amplification of the gene (Mano et al., 2004).

In a recent study of somatic copy number alterations in 489 ovarian cancer samples using multiple microarray-based platforms, 63 regions of recurrent focal amplification were identified, of which 26 regions encoded eight or fewer genes. The most common focal amplifications encoded *CCNE1*, *MYC*, and *MECOM*, each of which was highly amplified in more than 20% of tumors. By contrast, *HER2* was highly amplified in 3.1% of tumors, and a further 7% of tumors had a more moderate level of *HER2* amplification. The correlation between *HER2* copy number and mRNA expression was 0.59 (Cancer Genome Atlas Research Network, 2011).

Study	Method of assay	Pts with HER2-positive tumors, n/N (%)	Definition of 'HER2-positive'	Correlation between expression and survival[1]?	
				Yes/No	p-value
Rubin et al., 1993	IHC	36/105 (34) 12/105 (11)	2+ or 3+ membrane staining 1+ membrane staining	No†‡	NA
Meden et al., 1994	IHC	51/275 (19)	NS	Yes	p=0.001† p=0.006‡
Meden et al., 1995	IHC	48/266 (18)	NS	Yes	p=0.002† p=0.012‡
Meden et al., 1998	IHC	46/208 (22)	>5% cells had membrane staining at 100× magnification	Yes	p=0.0003†
Bookman et al., 2003	IHC	95/837 (11)	2+ or 3+ membrane staining	NA	NA
Hogdall et al., 2003	IHC	24/181 (13) 71/181 (39)	2+ or 3+ membrane staining 1+ membrane staining	Yes	p=0.003‡
Cloven et al., 2004	IHC	227/1420 (16)	≥1+ staining	NA	NA
Lassus et al., 2004[2]	IHC	66/390 (17)	2+ or 3+ membrane staining	Yes	p<0.0001†
	CISH	26/381 (7) 55/381 (14)	>5 copies of HER2 per nucleus 3–5 copies of HER2 per nucleus	Yes	p<0.0001† p<0.006‡
Kupryjanczyk et al., 2004	IHC	63/233 (27) 35/233 (15)	2+ or 3+ membrane staining 1+ membrane staining	No	NA
Nielsen et al., 2004	IHC	272/783 (35)	2+ or 3+ staining of cytoplasm or membrane	Yes/No	p=0.021†[3] p=0.76‡
Lee et al., 2005	IHC	5/102 (5)	≥1+ staining	NA	NA
Verri et al., 2005	IHC	27/194 (14) 26/194 (13)	2+ or 3+ membrane staining 1+ membrane staining	Yes/No	p=0.04† p<0.30‡
Steffensen et al., 2007[2]	IHC	18/160 (11) 39/160 (24)	2+ or 3+ membrane staining 1+ membrane staining	Yes	p=0.03†
	FISH	10/145 (7)	HER2:CEP17 ratio >2	No	p=0.39†
Tuefferd et al., 2007	IHC	41/320 (13)	2+ or 3+ membrane staining	No	p=0.6† p=0.152‡
Farley et al., 2009	FISH	9/133 (7)	HER2:CEP17 ratio >2	No	p=0.12† p=0.152‡
		12/133 (9)	HER2:nuclei ratio >4	No	p=0.42† p=0.980‡

CEP17, chromosome enumeration probe 17; CISH, chromogenic in situ hybridization; FISH; fluorescence in situ hybridization; HER2, human epidermal growth factor receptor 2; IHC, immunohistochemistry; NA, not applicable; NS, not specified; Pts, patients.

1 Overall survival of patients with HER2 positive tumors versus those with HER2 negative tumors. † Univariate analysis; ‡ Multivariate analysis.

2 Not all IHC samples were analyzable by CISH/FISH due to DNA degradation.

3 Patients with HER2 positive tumors had increased survival versus those with HER2 negative tumors.

Table 1. Expression level of HER2 in ovarian tumors in studies with >100 patients.

The HER2 mRNA level in samples taken from ovarian tumors of patients who were enrolled in a clinical trial studying platinum-sensitive disease (Kaye et al., 2008) showed a dichotomous distribution of HER2 mRNA expression (Figure 2A) similar to that observed in tumor samples from a study of patients with breast cancer (Figure 2B) (Burris et al., 2011). The prevalence of mRNA overexpression in the ovarian cancer samples was approximately 5% (Yulei Wang & Lukas Amler, unpublished data).

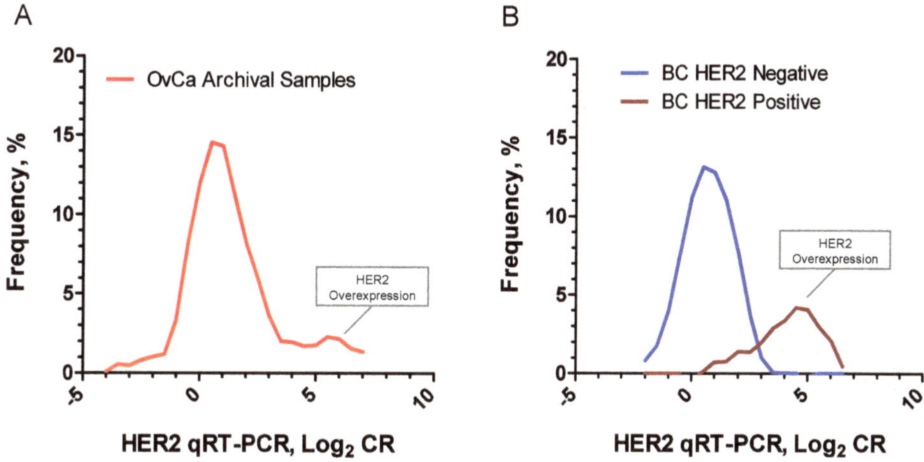

Fig. 2. Distribution of HER2 mRNA expression levels in (A) ovarian cancer and (B) breast cancer (Yulei Wang & Lukas Amler, unpublished data).

Samples from ovarian tumors were randomly chosen from archived samples collected during a clinical trial (Kaye et al., 2008). Samples from breast tumors were also collected during a clinical trial (Burris et al., 2011) but had known HER2 status (75% were HER2 negative, 25% were HER2 positive by IHC). HER2 mRNA levels in both data sets were determined by qRT-PCR (method as published in Makhija et al., 2010).

The CR of HER2:G6PDH expression was plotted as a histogram, and a smooth curve was fitted over the histogram. The ovarian cancer samples show a bimodal distribution of HER2 expression, with a small peak indicating the population of tumors that overexpress HER2 mRNA.

(BC, breast cancer; CR, concentration ratio; HER2, human epidermal growth factor receptor 2; G6PDH, glucose-6-phosphate dehydrogenase; IHC, immunohistochemistry; qRT-PCR, quantitative real time-polymerase chain reaction).

Steffenson et al. also used qRT-PCR to measure HER2 mRNA expression in 99 ovarian tumors and found that the tumor tissue had an average 5.7-fold higher level of HER2 mRNA compared with normal ovarian tissue. IHC showed HER2 overexpression (2+/3+ staining) in 11% (11/99) of tumors with a further 33% (33/99) of tumors showing 1+ staining. In contrast, all samples from normal ovarian tissue (n=23) were shown to be negative for HER2 staining (Steffensen et al., 2008).

Several studies have shown that overexpression of HER2 in ovarian tumors is an independent predictor of shorter progression-free survival and/or overall survival after multivariate analysis. However, this has not been supported by other studies (Table 1) (Serrano-Olvera et al., 2006). This discrepancy may indicate that while HER2 overexpression is of prognostic value in some groups of patients, this is not true for all patients in whom other biomarkers may be more significant. Assay quality, execution, and interpretation of data, as discussed above, may also explain differences in the observed levels of HER2 expression and its prognostic value.

2.2 Activation of HER2 in ovarian cancer

HER2 amplification and/or overexpression occurs in relatively few patients with ovarian cancer, although "normal" expression of HER2 measured by IHC 1+ staining is relatively common (Table 1). Other mechanisms, such as mutations in *HER2* or ligand-dependent activation of HER2, may play a role in HER2 oncogenesis.

Mutations in the *HER2* kinase domain are indeed found in ovarian tumors (Table 2), and the pattern of these in-frame insertions and missense mutations is similar to activating mutations found in other kinases, strongly suggesting that these mutations activate the HER2 kinase. For example, mutations in *HER2* are adjacent to or overlap with the analogous structural region of EGFR in-frame deletions that are associated with some lung tumors (Stephens et al., 2004). One study found that 6% of serous borderline ovarian tumors of low malignant potential (LMP) expressed a mutated version of HER2. LMP ovarian tumors also have a high rate of *KRAS* (18%) and *BRAF* (48%) mutations indicating that constitutive activation of the RAS-MAPK pathway may be one of the key mechanisms in the development of this type of ovarian tumor (Anglesio et al., 2008).

Nucleotide change	Amino acid change	Frequency n/N (%)	Tumor subtype	Reference
c.2325_2326 12 bp insertion	p.A775_G776 insert YVMA	1/84 (1)	Serous borderline tumors	Anglesio et al., 2008
c.2322_2323 12 bp insertion	p.M774_A775 insert AYVM	2/84 (2)	Serous borderline tumors	
c.2324_2325 12 bp insertion	p.A775_G776 insert YVMA	2/84 (2)	Serous borderline tumors	
12 bp insertion between c.2313 and c.2324	NK	2/21 (10)	Serous borderline tumors	Nakayama et al., 2006
c.2315_2316 12 bp insertion	p.A772_G773 insert YVMA	1/188 (0.5)	Serous carcinoma	Lassus et al., 2006
c.2327 G>T	p.G776V	1/6 (17)	Ovarian cell lines	Ikediobi et al., 2006
c.2570 A>G	p.N857S	1/27 (4)	Serous carcinoma	Stephens et al., 2004
c.2539 C>G	p.I767M	1/58 (2)	Serous carcinoma	Kan et al., 2010

bp, base pairs; NK, not known.

Table 2. *HER2* mutations in ovarian tumors and cell lines.

Ligand-dependent signaling via HER2-HER3 or HER2-EGFR dimers may also be important in ovarian cancer (Amler, 2010; Campiglio et al., 1999; Lewis et al., 1996). To investigate this hypothesis, Gordon et al. measured activated phosphorylated (p)HER2 by enzyme-linked immunosorbent assay and *HER2* gene amplification by FISH in 20 fresh ovarian tumor biopsies. They found that while only two tumors had *HER2* gene amplification (10%), pHER2 was detected in 45% of tumors (Gordon et al., 2006), indicating that activation of HER2 signaling probably occurs independently of gene amplification.

2.3 Biomarkers to identify HER2 activated or dependent ovarian tumors

Cumulative evidence over the past decade has demonstrated that in most cases, tumors from the same anatomic site of origin can be sub-classified into distinct molecular subsets driven by different underlying biological mechanisms and with distinct prognoses. This is best exemplified in breast cancer, where at least four distinct subtypes have been identified (Onitilo et al., 2009). Biomarkers that can differentiate between these distinct biological subsets of tumors can be used to predict the prognosis of a patient and potentially identify those who will derive the most benefit from targeted therapies (Carden et al., 2009). In breast cancer, such relevant biomarkers include measuring the expression of estrogen receptor α and the progesterone receptor to identify patients who would be sensitive to hormonal therapies, and HER2 to identify patients who would benefit from treatment with HER2-targeted therapies (Labuhn et al., 2006). Likewise, biomarkers are also used to determine the best course of treatment in a variety of other cancers. For example, patients with NSCLC or colorectal cancer (CRC) are screened for mutations in *EGFR* and *KRAS*, respectively, to determine whether they would benefit from EGFR inhibitors (Catenacci et al., 2011; Domingo et al., 2010). Mutations in both of these oncogenes are likely representative of distinct biological subsets of disease. For example, patients whose tumors harbor EGFR mutations are typically non-smokers, often female and of Asian ethnicity, and generally have a better prognosis than non-EGFR mutant NSCLC (Coate et al., 2009).

The identification of patients with ovarian tumors that express either high levels of HER2, HER2 with activating mutations, or biomarkers that indicate activated HER2 signaling, such as pHER2, could enable the patients who would derive the greatest therapeutic benefit to receive HER2-targeted therapies. Measuring the expression status of genes regulated by HER2 signaling could also identify tumors with activated HER2 signaling.

The importance of HER2-HER3 heterodimers in the HER2 signaling pathway has led to the investigation of HER3 as a prognostic biomarker in ovarian cancer (Amler, 2010). In one study of patients with ovarian cancer, those with high (≥ median; n=62) expression of HER3 protein had significantly decreased survival compared with those with low (< median; n=54) expression levels (1.80 versus 3.31 years; p=0.0034) following surgery and chemotherapy. In multivariate analysis, high HER3 expression significantly increased the risk of mortality compared with low HER3 expression (p=0.018) (Tanner et al., 2006). In contrast, patients with ovarian cancer receiving gemcitabine who had low HER3 mRNA expression (< median; n=35) had a significantly decreased progression-free survival (p=0.0002) and overall survival (p=0.003) than patients with high HER3 (≥ median; n= 24) mRNA levels. These data suggest that HER3 may be a prognostic biomarker in ovarian cancer (Makhija et al., 2010).

Interestingly, two separate studies have demonstrated that HER3 mRNA and protein levels in ovarian cancer cell lines were reduced on addition of heregulin, a ligand for HER3 (Makhija et al., 2010; Nagumo et al., 2009). The modulation of HER3 mRNA levels was found to be inversely proportional to activation of the downstream signaling molecules Akt and ERK1/2, critical components of the PI3K–Akt pathway (Nagumo et al., 2009). This suggests that low HER3 mRNA levels in HER2-positive tumors are associated with a high level of HER2–HER3 signaling. Overall these results point to a negative feedback loop that responds to the activation of HER3 by downregulation of HER3 mRNA expression (Makhija et al., 2010; Nagumo et al., 2009), and suggests that HER3 protein or mRNA levels may be a useful prognostic biomarker in patients with ovarian cancer.

3. HER2 as a drug target in human cancer

3.1 Clinical evidence for HER2 as a drug target in solid tumors

Trastuzumab (Herceptin) is a monoclonal antibody that binds to HER2 in the juxtamembrane region of the extracellular domain (Cho et al., 2003). Trastuzumab is licensed for use as a first-line treatment in combination with other chemotherapeutic agents in patients with HER2-positive breast cancer or gastric cancer in the USA and Europe. It has also been licensed for use as a single agent in patients with breast cancer who have not responded to previous chemotherapy (Genentech Inc., 2011). A trial of trastuzumab in combination with other chemotherapies in 3351 patients with breast cancer demonstrated significant improvements in disease-free survival ($p<0.0001$) and overall survival ($p=0.015$) compared with patients receiving chemotherapeutic agents alone (Romond et al., 2005). Patients who received trastuzumab after chemotherapy also exhibited a significant improvement in disease-free survival compared with those who did not ($p<0.0001$) (Piccart-Gebhart et al., 2005). In a Phase III trial of 584 patients with gastric cancer, the addition of trastuzumab to other chemotherapeutic agents significantly improved survival versus chemotherapy alone ($p=0.0046$) (Bang et al., 2010).

Lapatinib (Tyverb/Tykerb) is a small molecule inhibitor that targets the tyrosine kinase domain of HER2 and EGFR, thereby inhibiting downstream signaling from both receptors. In a Phase III trial, lapatinib increased the time to disease progression from 4.4 months in patients on capecitabine monotherapy ($n=161$) to 8.4 months in patients on a combination of the two drugs ($n=163$; $p<0.001$) (Geyer et al., 2006). The addition of lapatinib to letrozole also significantly reduced the risk of disease progression versus letrozole monotherapy ($p=0.019$) in 219 patients with HER2-positive breast tumors (Johnston et al., 2009). Following these trials, lapatinib was licensed for use in combination with letrozole as a first-line treatment for HER2-positive breast cancer, and in combination with capecitabine as a second-line treatment for breast cancer in the USA and Europe (GlaxoSmithKline, 2011).

A third agent targeting the HER2 signaling pathway, pertuzumab, is another monoclonal antibody that binds to the extracellular domain of HER2 and inhibits HER2 dimerization. The clinical development of pertuzumab is most advanced in breast cancer. In a Phase II trial of 66 patients with HER2-positive advanced breast cancer whose disease had progressed while on trastuzumab monotherapy, pertuzumab in combination with trastuzumab resulted in a complete response for 6% of patients. An additional 18% of patients had a partial response to therapy and 26% achieved stable disease for ≥6 months. Overall, 50% of patients benefited from the pertuzumab–trastuzumab combination (Baselga et al., 2010). Pertuzumab is currently undergoing several clinical trials for the treatment of HER2-positive breast cancer in combination with various other agents including trastuzumab (clinicaltrials.gov; Baselga & Swain, 2010).

Other HER2-targeted therapies in development for cancer are shown in Table 3.

HER2-targeting agent	Mechanism of action	Clinical stage	Cancer type	Clinicaltrials.gov identifier
Neratinib	TKI Dual HER2/EGFR inhibitor	Phase III	Breast	NCT00878709 NCT00915018
Afatinib	TKI Dual HER2/EGFR inhibitor	Phase III	Breast NSCLC	NCT01125566 NCT01121393
		Phase II	CRC Prostate Glioma Head and neck	NCT01152437 NCT01320280 NCT00727506 NCT00514943
		Phase I	Advanced solid tumors	NCT01206816
Varlitinib	TKI Triple HER2/EGFR/ HER4 inhibitor	Phase I/II	Advanced solid tumors	NCT00862524
MGAH22	HER2 mAb	Phase I	NSCLC Prostate Bladder Ovarian Breast	NCT01195935 NCT01148849

CRC, colorectal cancer; EGFR, epidermal growth factor receptor; HER2/4, human epidermal growth factor receptor 2/4; mAb, monoclonal antibody; NSCLC, non-small cell lung cancer; TKI, tyrosine kinase inhibitor.

Table 3. HER2-targeted therapies in clinical testing for the treatment of cancer (data from clinicaltrials.gov).

3.2 Preclinical evidence for HER2 as a target in ovarian cancer

Trastuzumab, pertuzumab, and lapatinib have all been studied in cell and animal models of ovarian cancer, demonstrating the potential use of these therapies to treat patients.

For example, in SKOV3 cells, a cell line derived from the ascites of an ovarian adenocarcinoma, trastuzumab has been shown to reduce pHER2 and pAkt levels, indicating that trastuzumab reduced the activation of HER2 signaling pathways (Larbouret et al., 2007). Moreover, both trastuzumab and lapatinib have been shown to reduce the ability of SKOV3 cells to form spheres in a dose-dependent manner, suggesting that both agents have an effect on the growth or viability of ovarian cancer cells (Magnifico et al., 2009). Pertuzumab and trastuzumab have been shown to reduce HER2-EGFR dimerization in SKOV3 cells by 24% and 44%, respectively, while lapatinib had little effect on dimerization (Gaborit et al., 2011). Finally, trastuzumab was shown to reduce tumor progression of SKOV3 xenografts in mice (Larbouret et al., 2007; Magnifico et al., 2009).

A number of studies have also investigated the effect of HER2 inhibitors on ligand-dependent signaling. Pertuzumab has been shown to reverse ligand-stimulated growth by inhibiting the phosphorylation of HER2 and subsequent activation of downstream signaling pathways (Mullen et al., 2007). Makhija et al. showed that HER3 mRNA expression was reduced by ligand stimulation in six of the eight ovarian cell lines tested. This effect was reversed by the addition of pertuzumab, small interfering RNAs (siRNAs) targeting the HER2 transcript, or inhibition of PI3K activity using a small molecule inhibitor. In contrast, siRNAs targeting the EGFR transcript, or a MEK inhibitor were not able to suppress ligand stimulation, indicating that pertuzumab inhibits HER2–HER3 signaling (Makhija et al., 2010). In a separate study, down-regulation of HER3 mRNA by heregulin-dependent activation of HER3 was reversed by pertuzumab. These authors also demonstrated that a change in HER3 mRNA levels was accompanied by changes in Akt and ERK signaling (Nagumo et al., 2009).

Other preclinical studies have suggested that levels of the HER2 extracellular domain may be a biomarker of response or resistance to some therapies used to treat ovarian cancer (Vazquez-Martin et al., 2011).

3.3 Clinical evidence for HER2 as a target in ovarian cancer

Trastuzumab, pertuzumab and lapatinib have also been studied in a number of clinical trials of ovarian cancer (Table 4).

Drug	Combination	No. pts	Clinical stage	Reference
Trastuzumab	Monotherapy	41	Phase II	Bookman et al., 2003
Lapatinib	Carboplatin	11	Phase I	Kimball et al., 2008
	Carboplatin and paclitaxel	21	Phase I/II	Rivkin et al., 2008
	Topotecan	18	Phase II	Weroha et al., 2011
Pertuzumab	Monotherapy	117	Phase II	Gordon et al., 2006
	Carboplatin with gemcitabine or paclitaxel	84		Kaye et al., 2008
	Gemcitabine	130		Makhija et al., 2010

Table 4. A summary of completed clinical trials of trastuzumab, lapatinib, and pertuzumab in HER2-positive ovarian cancer.

3.3.1 Trastuzumab

In HER2-positive ovarian cancer (2+/3+ staining by IHC), a Phase II trial of trastuzumab in 41 patients demonstrated an overall response rate of 7% (3 patients). One patient had a complete response to trastuzumab, and two patients had partial responses to treatment, while a further 16 patients (39%) achieved stable disease (Bookman et al., 2003). There are no reports of further development of trastuzumab for the treatment of ovarian cancer.

3.3.2 Lapatinib

Although studies of lapatinib for the treatment of ovarian cancer are at a relatively early stage, available evidence suggests that lapatinib may be effective in some patients with ovarian cancer. Of 11 patients with platinum-sensitive ovarian cancer receiving lapatinib plus carboplatin in a Phase Ib trial, three (27%) had a partial response to treatment and a further three patients achieved stable disease (Kimball et al., 2008). Rivkin et al. reported preliminary results from a Phase I/II study of lapatinib in combination with carboplatin and paclitaxel in 21 patients with ovarian cancer. Complete responses were observed in 21% of patients, with a further 29% of patients experiencing a partial response and 29% achieving stable disease (Rivkin et al., 2008). Lapatinib has also been studied in ovarian cancer in combination with topotecan. Results from this Phase II trial with 18 patients showed that four patients (22%) experienced clinical benefit from the combination (one partial response and three patients who achieved stable disease) (Weroha et al., 2011). In terms of further development, a Phase I trial is underway of lapatinib in combination with paclitaxel in patients with advanced solid tumors including ovarian tumors (clinicaltrials.gov identifier NCT00313599).

3.3.3 Pertuzumab

Pertuzumab has been more extensively studied in patients with ovarian cancer than other HER2-targeted agents. Studies have included trials of pertuzumab monotherapy as well as trials of pertuzumab in combination with other agents (Langdon et al., 2010). In a Phase II trial of pertuzumab alone, a partial response was observed in 4% of patients with a further 7% achieving stable disease for ≥6 months. Interestingly, patients with tumors that had a detectable level of HER2 phosphorylation (eight out of 28 tumors tested), had longer progression-free survival following pertuzumab treatment than those who did not express pHER2 (20.9 vs 5.8 weeks), although this difference was not statistically significant (p=0.14) (Gordon et al., 2006). These results, while very preliminary, suggest that pHER2 may indicate active HER2 signaling in these tumors and thus benefit from HER2 targeted therapy.

In trials of pertuzumab in combination with carboplatin, gemcitabine, or paclitaxel, patients with platinum-sensitive ovarian cancer achieved a 64% response rate compared with 52% for patients receiving chemotherapy alone (Kaye et al., 2008; Langdon et al., 2010). Pertuzumab has also been tested in combination with gemcitabine versus gemcitabine alone in 130 patients with ovarian cancer. A partial response was observed in 14% of patients receiving the combination therapy versus 5% receiving gemcitabine alone (Makhija et al., 2010).

Exploratory biomarker analyses in the Makhija and Kaye studies demonstrated that patients with ovarian tumors that express a low level of HER3 mRNA have a better response to pertuzumab than those with higher HER3 mRNA levels. Makhija et al. observed that patients with low (< median) HER3 mRNA levels receiving pertuzumab and gemcitabine demonstrated better response rates than those receiving gemcitabine alone (p=0.0002) (Makhija et al., 2010). Kaye et al. reported that in patients with tumors expressing a low level of HER3 mRNA who had a treatment-free interval of 6-12 months, those receiving pertuzumab had a longer progression-free survival time compared with those who received chemotherapy alone; however, this difference was not statistically significant (hazard ratio 0.55; p=0.16) (Amler, 2010; Kaye et al., 2008).

3.4 Summary

Preclinical data demonstrate that HER2 inhibitors reduce tumor cell signaling via HER2 in ovarian cancer cells and tumor models. In the clinic, a subset of patients with HER2-positive ovarian tumors responds to HER2-targeted treatment. Studies by Makhija et al. and Kaye et al. suggest that measuring the HER3 mRNA level may help to identify a subset of patients with ligand-dependent activation of HER2 signaling pathways who may benefit from treatment with a combination of pertuzumab and chemotherapy.

4. The future of the HER family as targets in oncology

Clinical validation of HER2 as a relevant target in ovarian cancer opens up several possibilities for therapeutic development in this area. These include the use of HER family antibody conjugates, bispecific antibodies, and novel targeted combinations, all of which are likely to require advanced and clinically integrated biomarker strategies to identify appropriate patient subsets for treatment.

HER2 antibodies can be conjugated with other anticancer drugs or radioactive entities to target chemotherapy and radiotherapy to cancerous cells that express HER2. Radiolabeled trastuzumab and pertuzumab have both been shown to delay tumor progression in mice with SKOV3 xenografts (Palm et al., 2007; Persson et al., 2007) and reduce the growth of SKOV3 cells in vitro (Heyerdahl et al., 2011), while trastuzumab–platinum (II) conjugates have been shown to increase SKOV3 cell death in vitro (Gao et al., 2008). Trastuzumab-DM1 (T-DM1) conjugates enable the targeted delivery of the antimicrotubule agent DM1 to cancer cells overexpressing HER2. In a single-arm Phase II study of T-DM1 therapy, a response rate of 26% was observed in 112 patients with HER2-positive metastatic breast cancer (Burris et al., 2011).

The bispecific, trifunctional antibody ertumaxomab, targets HER2 expressed on cancer cells and CD3 on T cells, and binds to Fcγ type I/III receptors via its Fc portion. In this way, ertumaxomab brings HER2-expressing cells into close contact with T cells and macrophages, facilitating antibody-dependent cellular cytotoxicity (ADCC) (Kiewe et al., 2006). In vitro studies have also demonstrated that ertumaxomab is able to kill cell lines with low HER2 expression derived from breast, lung, and colorectal cancers, whereas trastuzumab had no cytotoxic effect in these cells (Jager et al., 2009). In a Phase I trial of ertumaxomab in patients with HER2-positive metastatic breast cancer, five of 15 patients experienced an antitumor response (Kiewe et al., 2006).

Tumor cells commonly develop resistance to single-agent targeted therapies, thus combinations of agents that target different mechanisms of cell proliferation and survival often improve response compared with monotherapy alone. For example, the combination of trastuzumab with chA21 significantly reduced tumor size in mice with SKOV3 xenografts compared with antibody monotherapy ($p<0.05$) (A. Zhang et al., 2010). Similar results were observed with pertuzumab–trastuzumab combinations (Faratian et al., 2011) that have shown promise in the clinic (see Section 3.1) (Baselga et al., 2010). However, early clinical results for lapatinib and trastuzumab are not as promising. In a clinical trial of 282 patients with breast cancer, the combination of 1000 mg lapatinib with trastuzumab did not improve progression-free survival compared with 1500 mg lapatinib alone (16.3 versus 12.3 weeks; $p=0.18$) (Wu et al., 2011). Clinical trials of trastuzumab combined with pertuzumab (Baselga & Swain, 2010) and T-DM1 combined with pertuzumab (clinicaltrials.gov identifier NCT01120184) are ongoing in breast cancer.

Therapies targeting HER2 can also be combined with EGFR inhibitors in order to block multiple signaling pathways. Addition of matuzumab, an EGFR inhibitor, to trastuzumab was shown to reduce tumor progression in mice with SKOV3 xenografts to a greater extent than either antibody alone (Larbouret et al., 2007). The combination of trastuzumab or pertuzumab with another EGFR inhibitor, cetuximab, significantly inhibited cell growth in OVCAR-3 and IGROV-1 cells, although this effect was not observed in SKOV3 cells, possibly because of high basal levels of pERK and pAkt (Bijman et al., 2009). A combination of cetuximab and trastuzumab has also been shown to inhibit HER2–EGFR dimerization in SKOV3 cells, and this effect was shown to improve median survival and the percentage of tumor-free animals in a mouse model of ovarian cancer (Gaborit et al., 2011).

To date, clinical trials of anti-HER2/EGFR combinations have only been performed in non-ovarian cancer. Trastuzumab has been studies in breast cancer in combination with the EGFR inhibitors, gefitinib (Arteaga et al., 2008) and erlotinib (Britten et al., 2009). However, the trial of trastuzumab with erlotinib was terminated early, and the study with gefitinib showed increased toxicity with no apparent increase in the expected clinical benefit with trastuzumab monotherapy. Currently, there is one ongoing Phase I trial of trastuzumab with cetuximab in breast cancer (clinicaltrials.gov identifier NCT00367250). Trials are also underway to evaluate pertuzumab in combination with erlotinib or cetuximab in several types of cancer (clinicaltrials.gov identifiers NCT00947167, NCT01108458, NCT00855894, NCT00551421) and patients with CRC are being recruited for a trial of lapatinib in combination with cetuximab (clinicaltrials.gov identifier NCT01184482).

Combining agents that target HER2 with inhibitors of downstream signaling pathway components, such as PI3K, mTOR, or MEK, may also lead to increased clinical activity. A preclinical study investigating the PI3K inhibitor PKI-587 demonstrated tumor regression in xenograft models of breast cancer, which was enhanced when PKI-587 was combined with the dual HER2/EGFR tyrosine kinase inhibitor neratinib or a MEK inhibitor, PD0325901 (Mallon et al., 2011). A number of clinical trials are underway in breast cancer to investigate the efficacy of combining trastuzumab with PI3K inhibitors, including BKM120 (clinicaltrials.gov identifier NCT01132664) and XL-147 (clinicaltrials.gov identifier NCT01042925), as well as the combination of neratinib and temsirolimus, an allosteric mTOR inhibitor (clinicaltrials.gov identifier NCT01111825).

Preclinical and early clinical data suggest that targeting HER3 directly may also be therapeutically relevant in several types of cancer, including ovarian. The HER3 monoclonal antibody MM-121 has been shown to inhibit ovarian tumor growth in vivo (Sheng et al., 2010) and in vitro studies of another antibody, MM-111, have demonstrated that it inhibits cell growth alone and in combination with lapatinib (Oyama et al., 2010) and trastuzumab (Huhalov et al., 2010). A Phase I trial of U3-1287 in 31 patients with solid tumors, including one patient with ovarian cancer, showed that 26% of patients achieved stable disease for ≥70 days (Berlin et al., 2011). These antibodies are undergoing early-stage clinical testing in combination with other agents including HER2 and EGFR inhibitors (clinicaltrials.gov). MEHD7945A a dual-specific antibody targeting HER3 and EGFR has also shown in vivo activity in an ovarian xenograft model suggesting a potential benefit of combined inhibition of ErbB members (Schaefer et al., 2011).

4.1 The future use of biomarkers in ovarian cancer

Preclinical and clinical data suggest that amplification and overexpression of HER2 protein or mRNA, while infrequent, clearly exists in some ovarian tumors. Treatment with trastuzumab or a HER2 antibody-drug conjugate could be a potential option for these patients. Rare mutations in the *HER2* gene may be of particular relevance in ovarian LMP tumors where mutations in the *BRAF* and *KRAS* oncogenes are also common (see Section 2.2) (Anglesio et al., 2008). LMP tumors are usually treated successfully with surgery; however treatment options are limited in patients who relapse following surgery as this tumor type does not respond well to currently available chemotherapy. Further clinical evaluation with agents that inhibit HER2 signaling, such as lapatinib or trastuzumab, are warranted to determine the benefit of these agents to patients with progressed LMP lesions.

Based on the available data, it appears that ligand-dependent activation of HER2 signaling could be a more important mechanism for HER2 oncogenesis in ovarian cancer. Expression of pHER2 or HER3 may also be biomarkers that could identify tumors with oncogenic ligand-dependent HER2-activation. Further studies with inhibitors of HER2 dimerization, such as pertuzumab, will be useful in assessing their clinical potential in patients with ligand-dependent activation of the pathway.

5. Conclusion

Targeting HER2 with trastuzumab and lapatinib has proven successful in treating HER2-positive breast cancer. Other molecules, such as pertuzumab, are in advanced clinical development for the treatment of this indication, further validating the clinical relevance and importance of this target. In contrast to breast cancer, in which HER2 is overexpressed in up to 30% of cases, a much lower proportion of ovarian tumors show activation of HER2 by this mechanism. Nonetheless, trials of HER2-targeted agents in patients identified with HER2-positive ovarian tumors have shown improved progression-free survival and overall survival in a small proportion of patients.

Importantly, there are patients with ovarian tumors with no evidence of HER2 amplification or overexpression, but in whom HER2-targted therapeutics appear to be beneficial. In these patients, activating mutations in *HER2* or high levels of ligand-dependent activation of HER2/HER3 signaling may play a more important role in mediating HER2 oncogenesis. Identifying these patients through the use of novel biomarkers, such as assessment of HER3 mRNA levels, could significantly improve the clinical benefit of HER2-targeted therapies in this setting.

In conclusion, the use of targeted HER2 therapies in ovarian cancer warrants further investigation, particularly with regard to the development and validation of appropriate diagnostic tests.

6. Acknowledgement

Support for third-party writing assistance for this manuscript was provided by Genentech Inc.

7. References

Adelsman, M.A., Huntley, B.K. & Maihle, N.J. (1996). Ligand-independent dimerization of oncogenic v-*erbB* products involves covalent interactions. *Journal of Virology,* Vol.70, No.4, pp. 2533–2544

Amler, L.C. (2010). HER3 mRNA as a predictive biomarker in anticancer therapy. *Expert Opinion on Biological Therapy,* Vol.10, No.9, pp. 1343–1355

Anglesio, M.S., Arnold, J.M., George, J., Tinker, A.V., Tothill, R., Waddell, N., Simms, L., Locandro, B., Fereday, S., Traficante, N., Russell, P., Sharma, R., Birrer, M.J., deFazio, A., Chenevix-Trench, G. & Bowtell, D.D. (2008). Mutation of ERBB2 provides a novel alternative mechanism for the ubiquitous activation of RAS-MAPK in ovarian serous low malignant potential tumors. *Molecular Cancer Research,* Vol.6, No.11, pp. 1678–1690

Arteaga, C.L., O'Neill, A., Moulder, S.L., Pins, M., Sparano, J.A., Sledge, G.W. & Davidson, N.E. (2008). A phase I-II study of combined blockade of the ErbB receptor network with trastuzumab and gefitinib in patients with HER2 (ErbB2)-overexpressing metastatic breast cancer. *Clinical Cancer Research,* Vol.14, No.19, pp. 6277–6283

Bang, Y.J., van Cutsem, E., Feyereislova, A., Chung, H.C., Shen, L., Sawaki, A., Lordick, F., Ohtsu, A., Omuro, Y., Satoh, T., Aprile, G., Kulikov, E., Hill, J., Lehle, M., Ruschoff, J. & Kang, Y.K. (2010). Trastuzumab in combination with chemotherapy versus chemotherapy alone for treatment of HER2-positive advanced gastric or gastro-oesophageal junction cancer (ToGA): a phase 3, open-label, randomised controlled trial. *Lancet,* Vol.376, No.9742, pp. 687–697

Baselga, J., Gelmon, K.A., Verma, S., Wardley, A., Conte, P., Miles, D., Bianchi, G., Cortes, J., McNally, V.A., Ross, G.A., Fumoleau, P. & Gianni, L. (2010). Phase II trial of pertuzumab and trastuzumab in patients with human epidermal growth factor receptor 2-positive metastatic breast cancer that had progressed during prior trastuzumab therapy. *Journal of Clinical Oncology,* Vol.28, No.7, pp. 1138–1144

Baselga, J. & Swain, S.M. (2010). CLEOPATRA: a phase III evaluation of pertuzumab and trastuzumab for HER2-positive metastatic breast cancer. *Clinical Breast Cancer,* Vol.10, No.6, pp. 489–491

Berlin, J., Keedy, V.L., Janne, P.A., Yee, L., Rizvi, A., Jin, X., Copigneaux, C., Hettmann, T., Beaupre, D.M. & LoRusso, P. (2011). A first-in-human phase I study of U3-1287 (AMG 888), a HER3 inhibitor, in patients (pts) with advanced solid tumors. *Journal of Clinical Oncology,* Vol.29 (Suppl.), Abstract 3026

Bijman, M.N., van Berkel, M.P., Kok, M., Janmaat, M.L. & Boven, E. (2009). Inhibition of functional HER family members increases the sensitivity to docetaxel in human ovarian cancer cell lines. *Anticancer Drugs,* Vol.20, No.6, pp. 450–460

Bookman, M.A., Darcy, K.M., Clarke-Pearson, D., Boothby, R.A. & Horowitz, I.R. (2003). Evaluation of monoclonal humanized anti-HER2 antibody, trastuzumab, in patients with recurrent or refractory ovarian or primary peritoneal carcinoma with overexpression of HER2: A Phase II trial of the Gynecologic Oncology Group. *Journal of Clinical Oncology,* Vol.21, No.2, pp. 283–290

Britten, C.D., Finn, R.S., Bosserman, L.D., Wong, S.G., Press, M.F., Malik, M., Lum, B.L. & Slamon, D.J. (2009). A phase I/II trial of trastuzumab plus erlotinib in metastatic HER2-positive breast cancer: a dual ErbB targeted approach. *Clinical Breast Cancer,* Vol.9, No.1, pp. 16–22

Burris, H.A., Rugo, H.S., Vukelja, S.J., Vogel, C.L., Borson, R.A., Limentani, S., Tan-Chiu, E., Krop, I.E., Michaelson, R.A., Girish, S., Amler, L., Zheng, M., Chu, Y.W., Klencke, B. & O'Shaughnessy, J.A. (2011). Phase II study of the antibody drug conjugate trastuzumab-DM1 for the treatment of human epidermal growth factor receptor 2

(HER2)-positive breast cancer after prior HER2-directed therapy. *Journal of Clinical Oncology,* Vol.29, No.4, pp. 398–405

Campiglio, M., Ali, S., Knyazev, P.G. & Ullrich, A. (1999). Characteristics of EGFR family-mediated HRG signals in human ovarian cancer. *Journal of Cellular Biochemistry,* Vol.73, No.4, pp. 522-532

Cancer Genome Atlas Research Network. (2011). Integrated genomic analyses of ovarian carcinoma. *Nature,* Vol.474, No.7353, pp. 609–615

Cappuzzo, F., Bemis, L. & Varella-Garcia, M. (2006). HER2 mutation and response to trastuzumab therapy in non-small-cell lung cancer. *New England Journal of Medicine,* Vol.354, No.24, pp. 2619–2621

Carden, C.P., Banerji, U., Kaye, S.B., Workman, P. & De Bono, J.S. (2009). From darkness to light with biomarkers in early clinical trials of cancer drugs. *Clinical Pharmacology and Therapeutics,* Vol.85, No.2, pp. 131–133

Catenacci, D.V., Kozloff, M., Kindler, H.L. & Polite, B. (2011). Personalized colon cancer care in 2010. *Seminars in Oncology,* Vol.38, No.2, pp. 284–308

Cho, H.S. & Leahy, D.J. (2002). Structure of the extracellular region of HER3 reveals an interdomain tether. *Science,* Vol.297, No.5585, pp. 1330–1333

Cho, H.S., Mason, K., Ramyar, K.X., Stanley, A.M., Gabelli, S.B., Denney, D.W., Jr & Leahy, D.J. (2003). Structure of the extracellular region of HER2 alone and in complex with the Herceptin Fab. *Nature,* Vol.421, No.6924, pp. 756–760

Cloven, N.G., Kyshtoobayeva, A., Burger, R.A., Yu, I.R. & Fruehauf, J.P. (2004). In vitro chemoresistance and biomarker profiles are unique for histologic subtypes of epithelial ovarian cancer. *Gynecologic Oncology,* Vol.92, No.1, pp. 160–166

Coate, L.E., John, T., Tsao, M. & Shepherd, F.A. (2009). Molecular predictive and prognostic markers in non-small-cell lung cancer. *Lancet Oncology,* Vol.10, pp. 1001–1010

Conti, M., Hsieh, M., Park, J.Y. & Su, Y.Q. (2006). Role of the epidermal growth factor network in ovarian follicles. *Molecular Endocrinology,* Vol.20, No.4, pp. 715–723

Cornolti, G., Ungari, M., Morassi, M.L., Facchetti, F., Rossi, E., Lombardi, D. & Nicolai, P. (2007). Amplification and overexpression of HER2/neu gene and HER2/neu protein in salivary duct carcinoma of the parotid gland. *Archives of Otolaryngology-Head & Neck Surgery,* Vol.133, No.10, pp. 1031–1036

Coussens, L., Yang-Feng, T.L., Liao, Y.C., Chen, E., Gray, A., McGrath, J., Seeburg, P.H., Libermann, T.A., Schlessinger, J. & Francke, U. (1985). Tyrosine kinase receptor with extensive homology to EGF receptor shares chromosomal location with neu oncogene. *Science,* Vol.230, No.4730, pp. 1132–1139

Domingo, G., Perez, C.A., Velez, M., Cudris, J., Raez, L.E. & Santos, E.S. (2010). EGF receptor in lung cancer: a successful story of targeted therapy. *Expert Review of Anticancer Therapy,* Vol.10, No.10, pp. 1577–1587

Downward, J., Yarden, Y., Mayes, E., Scrace, G., Totty, N., Stockwell, P., Ullrich, A., Schlessinger, J. & Waterfield, M.D. (1984). Close similarity of epidermal growth factor receptor and v-erb-B oncogene protein sequences. *Nature,* Vol.307, No.5951, pp. 521–527

Faratian, D., Zweemer, A., Nagumo, Y., Sims, A.H., Muir, M., Dodds, M., Mullen, P., Um, I., Kay, C., Hasmann, M., Harrison, D.J. & Langdon, S.P. (2011). Trastuzumab and pertuzumab produce changes in morphology and estrogen receptor signaling in ovarian cancer xenografts revealing new treatment strategies. *Clinical Cancer Research,* Vol.17, No.13, pp. 4451-4461

Farley, J., Fuchiuji, S., Darcy, K.M., Tian, C., Hoskins, W.J., McGuire, W.P., Hanjani, P., Warshal, D., Greer, B.E., Belinson, J. & Birrer, M.J. (2009). Associations between ERBB2 amplification and progression-free survival and overall survival in advanced stage, suboptimally-resected epithelial ovarian cancers: a Gynecologic Oncology Group Study. *Gynecologic Oncology,* Vol.113, No.3, pp. 341-347

Gaborit, N., Larbouret, C., Vallaghe, J., Peyrusson, F., Bascoul-Mollevi, C., Crapez, E., Azria, D., Chardes, T., Poul, M.A., Mathis, G., Bazin, H. & Pelegrin, A. (2011). Time-resolved fluorescence resonance energy transfer (TR-FRET) to analyze the disruption of EGFR/HER2 dimers: a new method to evaluate the efficiency of targeted therapy using monoclonal antibodies. *Journal of Biological Chemistry,* Vol.286, No.13, pp. 11337-11345

Gao, J., Liu, Y.G., Liu, R. & Zingaro, R.A. (2008). Herceptin-platinum(II) binding complexes: novel cancer-cell-specific agents. *ChemMedChem,* Vol.3, No.6, pp. 954-962

Garrett, T.P., McKern, N.M., Lou, M., Elleman, T.C., Adams, T.E., Lovrecz, G.O., Kofler, M., Jorissen, R.N., Nice, E.C., Burgess, A.W. & Ward, C.W. (2003). The crystal structure of a truncated ErbB2 ectodomain reveals an active conformation, poised to interact with other ErbB receptors. *Molecular Cell,* Vol.11, No.2, pp. 495-505

Genentech Inc. (2011). *Trastuzumab prescribing information,* Accessed June 1, 2011, Available from: http://www.accessdata.fda.gov/scripts/cder/drugsatfda/

Geyer, C.E., Forster, J., Lindquist, D., Chan, S., Romieu, C.G., Pienkowski, T., Jagiello-Gruszfeld, A., Crown, J., Chan, A., Kaufman, B., Skarlos, D., Campone, M., Davidson, N., Berger, M., Oliva, C., Rubin, S.D., Stein, S. & Cameron, D. (2006). Lapatinib plus capecitabine for HER2-positive advanced breast cancer. *New England Journal of Medicine,* Vol.355, No.26, pp. 2733-2743

GlaxoSmithKline. (2011). *Lapatinib prescribing information,* Accessed June 1, 2011, Available from: http://www.accessdata.fda.gov/scripts/cder/drugsatfda/

Gordon, M.S., Matei, D., Aghajanian, C., Matulonis, U.A., Brewer, M., Fleming, G.F., Hainsworth, J.D., Garcia, A.A., Pegram, M.D., Schilder, R.J., Cohn, D.E., Roman, L., Derynck, M.K., Ng, K., Lyons, B., Allison, D.E., Eberhard, D.A., Pham, T.Q., Dere, R.C. & Karlan, B.Y. (2006). Clinical activity of pertuzumab (rhuMAb 2C4), a HER dimerization inhibitor, in advanced ovarian cancer: potential predictive relationship with tumor HER2 activation status. *Journal of Clinical Oncology,* Vol.24, No.26, pp. 4324-4332

Graus-Porta, D., Beerli, R.R., Daly, J.M. & Hynes, N.E. (1997). ErbB-2, the preferred heterodimerization partner of all ErbB receptors, is a mediator of lateral signaling. *EMBO Journal,* Vol.16, No.7, pp. 1647-1655

Heyerdahl, H., Krogh, C., Borrebaek, J., Larsen, A. & Dahle, J. (2011). Treatment of HER2-expressing breast cancer and ovarian cancer cells with alpha particle-emitting 227Th-trastuzumab. *International Journal of Radiation Oncology, Biology, Physics,* Vol.79, No.2, pp. 563-570

Hogdall, E.V., Christensen, L., Kjaer, S.K., Blaakaer, J., Bock, J.E., Glud, E., Norgaard-Pedersen, B. & Hogdall, C.K. (2003). Distribution of HER-2 overexpression in ovarian carcinoma tissue and its prognostic value in patients with ovarian carcinoma: from the Danish MALOVA Ovarian Cancer Study. *Cancer,* Vol.98, No.1, pp. 66–73

Hsieh, A.C. & Moasser, M.M. (2007). Targeting HER proteins in cancer therapy and the role of the non-target HER3. *British Journal of Cancer,* Vol.97, No.4, pp. 453–457

Huhalov, A., Adams, S., Paragas, V., Oyama, S., Overland, R., Luus, L., Gibbons, F., Zhang, B., Nhuyen, S., Nielson, U.B., Niyikiza, C., McDonagh, C.F. & Kudla, A.J. (2010). MM-1111, an ErbB2/ErbB3 bispecific antibody with potent activity in ErbB2-overexpressing cells, positively combines with trastuzumab to inhibit growth of breast cancer cells driven by the ErbB2/ErbB3 oncogenic unit. *Proceedings of 101st Annual Meeting of the American Association for Cancer Research,* Washington, DC, April 17-21, 2010

Hynes, N.E. (1993). Amplification and overexpression of the *erbB-2* gene in human tumors: Its involvement in tumor development, significance as a prognostic factor, and potential as a target for cancer therapy. *Seminars in Cancer Biology,* Vol.4, No.1, pp. 19–26

Ikediobi, O.N., Davies, H., Bignell, G., Edkins, S., Stevens, C., O'Meara, S., Santarius, T., Avis, T., Barthorpe, S., Brackenbury, L., Buck, G., Butler, A., Clements, J., Cole, J., Dicks, E., Forbes, S., Gray, K., Halliday, K., Harrison, R., Hills, K., Hinton, J., Hunter, C., Jenkinson, A., Jones, D., Kosmidou, V., Lugg, R., Menzies, A., Mironenko, T., Parker, A., Perry, J., Raine, K., Richardson, D., Shepherd, R., Small, A., Smith, R., Solomon, H., Stephens, P., Teague, J., Tofts, C., Varian, J., Webb, T., West, S., Widaa, S., Yates, A., Reinhold, W., Weinstein, J.N., Stratton, M.R., Futreal, P.A. & Wooster, R. (2006). Mutation analysis of 24 known cancer genes in the NCI-60 cell line set. *Molecular Cancer Therapeutics,* Vol.5, No.11, pp. 2606–2612

Jaehne, J., Urmacher, C., Thaler, H.T., Friedlander-Klar, H., Cordon-Cardo, C. & Meyer, H.J. (1992). Expression of *Her2/neu* oncogene product p185 in correlation to clinicopathological and prognostic factors of gastric carcinoma. *Journal of Cancer Research and Clinical Oncology,* Vol.118, No.6, pp. 474–479

Jager, M., Schoberth, A., Ruf, P., Hess, J. & Lindhofer, H. (2009). The trifunctional antibody ertumaxomab destroys tumor cells that express low levels of human epidermal growth factor receptor 2. *Cancer Research,* Vol.69, No.10, pp. 4270–4276

Johnston, S., Pippen, J., Jr, Pivot, X., Lichinitser, M., Sadeghi, S., Dieras, V., Gomez, H.L., Romieu, G., Manikhas, A., Kennedy, M.J., Press, M.F., Maltzman, J., Florance, A., O'Rourke, L., Oliva, C., Stein, S. & Pegram, M. (2009). Lapatinib combined with letrozole versus letrozole and placebo as first-line therapy for postmenopausal hormone receptor-positive metastatic breast cancer. *Journal of Clinical Oncology,* Vol.27, No.33, pp. 5538–5546

Kan, Z., Jaiswal, B.S., Stinson, J., Janakiraman, V., Bhatt, D., Stern, H.M., Yue, P., Haverty, P.M., Bourgon, R., Zheng, J., Moorhead, M., Chaudhuri, S., Tomsho, L.P., Peters, B.A., Pujara, K., Cordes, S., Davis, D.P., Carlton, V.E., Yuan, W., Li, L., Wang, W., Eigenbrot, C., Kaminker, J.S., Eberhard, D.A., Waring, P., Schuster, S.C., Modrusan, Z., Zhang, Z., Stokoe, D., de Sauvage, F.J., Faham, M. & Seshagiri, S. (2010). Diverse somatic mutation patterns and pathway alterations in human cancers. *Nature,* Vol.466, No.7308, pp. 869–873

Kaye, S.B., Poole, C.J., Bidzinski, M., Gianni, L., Gorbunova, V., Novikova, E., Strauss, A., McNally, V.A., Ross, G. & Vergote, I. (2008). A randomised phase II study evaluating the combination of carboplatin-based chemotherapy with pertuzumab (P) versus carboplatin-based therapy alone in patients with relapsed, platinum-sensitive ovarian cancer. *Journal of Clinical Oncology,* Vol.26 (Suppl. 15S), Abstract 5520

Kiewe, P., Hasmuller, S., Kahlert, S., Heinrigs, M., Rack, B., Marme, A., Korfel, A., Jager, M., Lindhofer, H., Sommer, H., Thiel, E. & Untch, M. (2006). Phase I trial of the trifunctional anti-HER2 x anti-CD3 antibody ertumaxomab in metastatic breast cancer. *Clinical Cancer Research,* Vol.12, No.10, pp. 3085–3091

Kimball, K.J., Numnum, T.M., Kirby, T.O., Zamboni, W.C., Estes, J.M., Barnes, M.N., Matei, D.E., Koch, K.M. & Alvarez, R.D. (2008). A phase I study of lapatinib in combination with carboplatin in women with platinum sensitive recurrent ovarian carcinoma. *Gynecologic Oncology,* Vol.111, No.1, pp. 95–101

Kupryjanczyk, J., Madry, R., Plisiecka-Halasa, J., Bar, J., Kraszewska, E., Ziolkowska, I., Timorek, A., Stelmachow, J., Emerich, J., Jedryka, M., Pluzanska, A., Rzepka-Gorska, I., Urbanski, K., Zielinski, J. & Markowska, J. (2004). TP53 status determines clinical significance of ERBB2 expression in ovarian cancer. *British Journal of Cancer,* Vol.91, No.11, pp. 1916–1923

Labuhn, M., Vuaroqueaux, V., Fina, F., Schaller, A., Nanni-Metellus, I., Kung, W., Eppenberger-Castori, S., Martin, P.M. & Eppenberger, U. (2006). Simultaneous quantitative detection of relevant biomarkers in breast cancer by quantitative real-time PCR. *International Journal of Biological Markers,* Vol.21, No.1, pp. 30–39

Langdon, S.P., Faratian, D., Nagumo, Y., Mullen, P. & Harrison, D.J. (2010). Pertuzumab for the treatment of ovarian cancer. *Expert Opinion on Biological Therapy,* Vol.10, No.7, pp. 1113–1120

Larbouret, C., Robert, B., Navarro-Teulon, I., Thezenas, S., Ladjemi, M.Z., Morisseau, S., Campigna, E., Bibeau, F., Mach, J.P., Pelegrin, A. & Azria, D. (2007). In vivo therapeutic synergism of anti-epidermal growth factor receptor and anti-HER2 monoclonal antibodies against pancreatic carcinomas. *Clinical Cancer Research,* Vol.13, No.11, pp. 3356–3362

Lassus, H., Leminen, A., Vayrynen, A., Cheng, G., Gustafsson, J.A., Isola, J. & Butzow, R. (2004). ERBB2 amplification is superior to protein expression status in predicting patient outcome in serous ovarian carcinoma. *Gynecologic Oncology,* Vol.92, No.1, pp. 31–39

Lassus, H., Sihto, H., Leminen, A., Joensuu, H., Isola, J., Nupponen, N.N. & Butzow, R. (2006). Gene amplification, mutation, and protein expression of EGFR and mutations of ERBB2 in serous ovarian carcinoma. *Journal of Molecular Medicine,* Vol.84, No.8, pp. 671–681

Lee, C.H., Huntsman, D.G., Cheang, M.C., Parker, R.L., Brown, L., Hoskins, P., Miller, D. & Gilks, C.B. (2005). Assessment of Her-1, Her-2, and Her-3 expression and Her-2 amplification in advanced stage ovarian carcinoma. *International Journal Gynecological Pathology,* Vol.24, No.2, pp. 147–152

Lee-Hoeflich, S.T., Crocker, L., Yao, E., Pham, T., Munroe, X., Hoeflich, K.P., Sliwkowski, M.X. & Stern, H.M. (2008). A central role for HER3 in *HER2*-amplified breast cancer: implications for targeted therapy. *Cancer Research,* Vol.68, No.14, pp. 5878–5887

Lewis, G.D., Lofgren, J.A., McMurtrey, A.E., Nuijens, A., Fendly, B.M., Bauer, K.D. & Sliwkowski, M.X. (1996). Growth regulation of human breast and ovarian tumor cells by heregulin: Evidence for the requirement of ErbB2 as a critical component in mediating heregulin responsiveness. *Cancer Research,* Vol.56, No.6, pp. 1457–1465

Magnifico, A., Albano, L., Campaner, S., Delia, D., Castiglioni, F., Gasparini, P., Sozzi, G., Fontanella, E., Menard, S. & Tagliabue, E. (2009). Tumor-initiating cells of HER2-positive carcinoma cell lines express the highest oncoprotein levels and are sensitive to trastuzumab. *Clinical Cancer Research,* Vol.15, No.6, pp. 2010–2021

Makhija, S., Amler, L.C., Glenn, D., Ueland, F.R., Gold, M.A., Dizon, D.S., Paton, V., Lin, C.Y., Januario, T., Ng, K., Strauss, A., Kelsey, S., Sliwkowski, M.X. & Matulonis, U. (2010). Clinical activity of gemcitabine plus pertuzumab in platinum-resistant ovarian cancer, fallopian tube cancer, or primary peritoneal cancer. *Journal of Clinical Oncology,* Vol.28, No.7, pp. 1215–1223

Mallon, R., Feldberg, L.R., Lucas, J., Chaudhary, I., Dehnhardt, C., Santos, E.D., Chen, Z., Dos, S.O., Ayral-Kaloustian, S., Venkatesan, A. & Hollander, I. (2011). Antitumor Efficacy of PKI-587, a highly potent dual PI3K/mTOR kinase inhibitor. *Clinical Cancer Research,* Vol.17, No.10, pp. 3193–3203

Mano, M.S., Awada, A., Di Leo, A., Durbecq, V., Paesmans, M., Cardoso, F., Larsimont, D. & Piccart, M. (2004). Rates of topoisomerase II-alpha and HER-2 gene amplification and expression in epithelial ovarian carcinoma. *Gynecologic Oncology,* Vol.92, No.3, pp. 887–895

Meden, H., Marx, D., Rath, W., Kron, M., Fattahi-Meibodi, A., Hinney, B., Kuhn, W. & Schauer, A. (1994). Overexpression of the oncogene c-*erb B2* in primary ovarian cancer: evaluation of the prognostic value in a Cox proportional hazards multiple regression. *International Journal Gynecological Pathology,* Vol.13, No.1, pp. 45–53

Meden, H., Marx, D., Raab, T., Kron, M., Schauer, A. & Kuhn, W. (1995). EGF-R and overexpression of the oncogene c-*erbB-2* in ovarian cancer: immunohistochemical findings and prognostic value. *Journal of Obstetrics and Gynaecology,* Vol.21, No.2, pp. 167–178

Meden, H., Marx, D., Roegglen, T., Schauer, A. & Kuhn, W. (1998). Overexpression of the oncogene c-*erbB-2* (*HER2/neu*) and response to chemotherapy in patients with ovarian cancer. *International Journal of Gynecological Pathology,* Vol.17, No.1, pp. 61–65

Mullen, P., Cameron, D.A., Hasmann, M., Smyth, J.F. & Langdon, S.P. (2007). Sensitivity to pertuzumab (2C4) in ovarian cancer models: cross-talk with estrogen receptor signaling. *Molecular Cancer Therapeutics,* Vol.6, No.1, pp. 93–100

Muller, B.M., Kronenwett, R., Hennig, G., Euting, H., Weber, K., Bohmann, K., Weichert, W., Altmann, G., Roth, C., Winzer, K.J., Kristiansen, G., Petry, C., Dietel, M. & Denkert, C. (2011). Quantitative determination of estrogen receptor, progesterone receptor, and HER2 mRNA in formalin-fixed paraffin-embedded tissue—a new option for predictive biomarker assessment in breast cancer. *Diagnostic Molecular Pathology,* Vol.20, No.1, pp. 1–10

Nagumo, Y., Faratian, D., Mullen, P., Harrison, D.J., Hasmann, M. & Langdon, S.P. (2009). Modulation of HER3 is a marker of dynamic cell signaling in ovarian cancer: implications for pertuzumab sensitivity. *Molecular Cancer Research,* Vol.7, No.9, pp. 1563–1571

Nakayama, K., Nakayama, N., Kurman, R.J., Cope, L., Pohl, G., Samuels, Y., Velculescu, V.E., Wang, T.L. & Shih, I. (2006). Sequence mutations and amplification of PIK3CA and AKT2 genes in purified ovarian serous neoplasms. *Cancer Biology and Therapy,* Vol.5, No.7, pp. 779–785

Nielsen, J.S., Jakobsen, E., Holund, B., Bertelsen, K. & Jakobsen, A. (2004). Prognostic significance of p53, Her-2, and EGFR overexpression in borderline and epithelial ovarian cancer. *International Journal of Gynecological Cancer,* Vol.14, No.6, pp. 1086–1096

Olayioye, M.A., Neve, R.M., Lane, H.A. & Hynes, N.E. (2000). The ErbB signaling network: receptor heterodimerization in development and cancer. *EMBO Journal,* Vol.19, No.13, pp. 3159–3167

Onitilo, A.A., Engel, J.M., Greenlee, R.T. & Mukesh, B.N. (2009). Breast cancer subtypes based on ER/PR and Her2 expression: comparison of clinicopathologic features and survival. *Clinical Medicine and Research,* Vol.7, No.1/2, pp. 4–13

Oyama, S.K., Paragas, V., Adams, S., Luus, L., Huhalov, A., Kudla, A.J., Overland, R., Nielsen, U.B., Niyikiza, C., McDonagh, C.F. & MacBeath, G. (2010). MM-111, an ErbB2/ErbB3 bispecific antibody, effectively combines with lapatinib to inhibit growth of ErbB2-overexpresing tumor cells. *101st Annual Meeting of the American Association for Cancer Research,* Washington, DC, April 17–21, 2010

Palm, S., Back, T., Claesson, I., Danielsson, A., Elgqvist, J., Frost, S., Hultborn, R., Jensen, H., Lindegren, S. & Jacobsson, L. (2007). Therapeutic efficacy of astatine-211-labeled trastuzumab on radioresistant SKOV-3 tumors in nude mice. *International Journal of Radiation Oncology Biology Physics,* Vol.69, No.2, pp. 572–579

Persson, M., Gedda, L., Lundqvist, H., Tolmachev, V., Nordgren, H., Malmström, P.U. & Carlsson, J. (2007). [^{177}Lu]Pertuzumab: experimental therapy of HER-2-expressing xenografts. *Cancer Research,* Vol.67, No.1, pp. 326–331

Piccart-Gebhart, M.J., Procter, M., Leyland-Jones, B., Goldhirsch, A., Untch, M., Smith, I., Gianni, L., Baselga, J., Bell, R., Jackisch, C., Cameron, D., Dowsett, M., Barrios, C.H., Steger, G., Huang, C.S., Andersson, M., Inbar, M., Lichinister, M., Láng, I., Nitz, U., Iwata, H., Thomssen, C., Lohrisch, C., Suter, T.M., Rüschoff, J., Sütö, T., Greatorex, V., Ward, C., Straehle, C., McFadden, E., Dolci, M.S. & Gelber, R.D. (2005). Trastuzumab after adjuvant chemotherapy in HER2-positive breast cancer. *New England Journal of Medicine,* Vol.353, No.16, pp. 1659–1672

Rivkin, S.E., Muller, C., Iriarte, D., Arthur, J., Canoy, A. & Reid, H. (2008). Phase I/II lapatinib plus carboplatin and paclitaxel in stage III or IV relapsed ovarian cancer patients. *Journal of Clinical Oncology,* Vol.26 (Suppl.), Abstract 5556

Romond, E.H., Perez, E.A., Bryant, J., Suman, V.J., Geyer, C.E., Davidson, N.E., Tan-Chiu, E., Martino, S., Paik, S., Kaufman, P.A., Swain, S.M., Pisansky, T.M., Fehrenbacher, L., Kutteh, L.A., Vogel, V.G., Visscher, D.W., Yothers, G., Jenkins, R.B., Brown, A.M., Dakhil, S.R., Mamounas, E.P., Lingle, W.L., Klein, P.M., Ingle, J.N. & Wolmark, N. (2005). Trastuzumab plus adjuvant chemotherapy for operable HER2-positive breast cancer. *New England Journal of Medicine,* Vol.353, No.16, pp. 1673–1684

Rowinsky, E.K. (2004). The erbB family: targets for therapeutic development against cancer and therapeutic strategies using monoclonal antibodies and tyrosine kinase inhibitors. *Annual Review of Medicine,* Vol.55, pp. 433–457

Rubin, S.C., Finstad, C.L., Wong, G.Y., Almadrones, L., Plante, M. & Lloyd, K.O. (1993). Prognostic significance of HER-2/neu expression in advanced epithelial ovarian cancer: a multivariate analysis. *American Journal of Obstetric Gynecology*, Vol.168, No.1 Pt.1, pp. 162–169

Schaefer et al. (2011). A Two-in One Antibody Against HER3 and EGFR has Superior Inhbitory Activity Compared to Monospecific Antibodies. Under revision.

Schechter, A.L., Stern, D.F., Vaidyanathan, L., Decker, S.J., Drebin, J.A., Greene, M.I. & Weinberg, R.A. (1984). The *neu* oncogene: an *erb-B*-related gene encoding a 185,000-Mr tumour antigen. *Nature*, Vol.312, No.5994, pp. 513–516

Serrano-Olvera, A., Duenas-Gonzalez, A., Gallardo-Rincon, D., Candelaria, M. & Garza-Salazar, J. (2006). Prognostic, predictive and therapeutic implications of HER2 in invasive epithelial ovarian cancer. *Cancer Treatment Reviews*, Vol.32, No.3, pp. 180–190

Sheng, Q., Liu, X., Fleming, E., Yuan, K., Piao, H., Chen, J., Moustafa, Z., Thomas, R.K., Greulich, H., Schinzel, A., Zaghlul, S., Batt, D., Ettenberg, S., Meyerson, M., Schoeberl, B., Kung, A.L., Hahn, W.C., Drapkin, R., Livingston, D.M. & Liu, J.F. (2010). An activated ErbB3/NRG1 autocrine loop supports in vivo proliferation in ovarian cancer cells. *Cancer Cell*, Vol.17, No.3, pp. 298–310

Sheng, Q. & Liu, J. (2011). The therapeutic potential of targeting the EGFR family in epithelial ovarian cancer. *British Journal of Cancer*, Vol.104, No.8, pp. 1241–1245

Siwak, D.R., Carey, M., Hennessy, B.T., Nguyen, C.T., McGahren Murray, M.J., Nolden, L. & Mills, G.B. (2010). Targeting the epidermal growth factor receptor in epithelial ovarian cancer: current knowledge and future challenges. *Journal of Oncology*, Vol.2010, Article ID 568938

Slamon, D.J., Clark, G.M., Wong, S.G., Levin, W.J., Ullrich, A. & McGuire, W.L. (1987). Human breast cancer: correlation of relapse and survival with amplification of the *HER-2/neu* oncogene. *Science*, Vol.234, No.4785, pp. 177–182

Slamon, D.J., Godolphin, W., Jones, L.A., Holt, J.A., Wong, S.G., Keith, D.E., Levin, W.J., Stuart, S.G., Udove, J. & Ullrich, A. (1989). Studies of the *HER-2/neu* proto-oncogene in human breast and ovarian cancer. *Science*, Vol.244, No.4905, pp. 707–712

Steffensen, K.D., Waldstrom, M., Jeppesen, U., Jakobsen, E., Brandslund, I. & Jakobsen, A. (2007). The prognostic importance of cyclooxygenase 2 and HER2 expression in epithelial ovarian cancer. *International Journal of Gynecological Cancer*, Vol.17, No.4, pp. 798–807

Steffensen, K.D., Waldstrom, M., Andersen, R.F., Olsen, D.A., Jeppesen, U., Knudsen, H.J., Brandslund, I. & Jakobsen, A. (2008). Protein levels and gene expressions of the epidermal growth factor receptors, HER1, HER2, HER3 and HER4 in benign and malignant ovarian tumors. *International Journal of Oncology*, Vol.33, No.1, pp. 195–204

Stephens, P., Hunter, C., Bignell, G., Edkins, S., Davies, H., Teague, J., Stevens, C., O'Meara, S., Smith, R., Parker, A., Barthorpe, A., Blow, M., Brackenbury, L., Butler, A., Clarke, O., Cole, J., Dicks, E., Dike, A., Drozd, A., Edwards, K., Forbes, S., Foster, R., Gray, K., Greenman, C., Halliday, K., Hills, K., Kosmidou, V., Lugg, R., Menzies, A., Perry, J., Petty, R., Raine, K., Ratford, L., Shepherd, R., Small, A., Stephens, Y., Tofts, C., Varian, J., West, S., Widaa, S., Yates, A., Brasseur, F., Cooper, C.S.,

Flanagan, A.M., Knowles, M., Leung, S.Y., Louis, D.N., Looijenga, L.H., Malkowicz, B., Pierotti, M.A., Teh, B., Chenevix-Trench, G., Weber, B.L., Yuen, S.T., Harris, G., Goldstraw, P., Nicholson, A.G., Futreal, P.A., Wooster, R. & Stratton, M.R. (2004). Lung cancer: intragenic ERBB2 kinase mutations in tumours. *Nature,* Vol.431, No.7008, pp. 525-526

Tanner, B., Hasenclever, D., Stern, K., Schormann, W., Bezler, M., Hermes, M., Brulport, M., Bauer, A., Schiffer, I.B., Gebhard, S., Schmidt, M., Steiner, E., Sehouli, J., Edelmann, J., Lãuter, J., Lessig, R., Krishnamurthi, K., Ullrich, A. & Hengstler, J.G. (2006). ErbB-3 predicts survival in ovarian cancer. *Journal of Clinical Oncology,* Vol.24, No.26, pp. 4317-4323

Tuefferd, M., Couturier, J., Penault-Llorca, F., Vincent-Salomon, A., Broet, P., Guastalla, J.P., Allouache, D., Combe, M., Weber, B., Pujade-Lauraine, E. & Camilleri-Broet, S. (2007). HER2 status in ovarian carcinomas: a multicenter GINECO study of 320 patients. *PLoS One,* Vol.2, No.11, pp. e1138

Tzahar, E., Waterman, H., Chen, X., Levkowitz, G., Karunagaran, D., Lavi, S., Ratzkin, B.J. & Yarden, Y. (1996). A hierarchical network of interreceptor interactions determines signal transduction by Neu differentiation factor/neuregulin and epidermal growth factor. *Molecular Cell Biology,* Vol.16, No.10, pp. 5276-5287

Vazquez-Martin, A., Oliveras-Ferraros, C., Cufi, S., del Barco, S., Martin-Castillo, B. & Menendez, J.A. (2011). Lapatinib, a dual HER1/HER2 tyrosine kinase inhibitor, augments basal cleavage of HER2 extracellular domain (ECD) to inhibit HER2-driven cancer cell growth. *Journal of Cell Physiology,* Vol.226, No.1, pp. 52-57

Verri, E., Guglielmini, P., Puntoni, M., Perdelli, L., Papadia, A., Lorenzi, P., Rubagotti, A., Ragni, N. & Boccardo, F. (2005). HER2/neu oncoprotein overexpression in epithelial ovarian cancer: evaluation of its prevalence and prognostic significance. Clinical study. *Oncology,* Vol.68, No.2-3, pp. 154-161

Weroha, S.J., Oberg, A.L., Ziegler, K.L., Dakhilm, S.R., Rowland, K.M., Hartmann, L.C., Moore, D.F., Jr, Keeney, G.L., Peethambaram, P.P. & Haluska, P. (2011). Phase II trial of lapatinib and topotecan (LapTop) in patients with platinum-refractory/resistant ovarian and primary peritoneal carcinoma. *Gynecologic Oncology,* Vol.122, No.1, pp. 116-120

Wolff, A.C., Hammond, M.E., Schwartz, J.N., Hagerty, K.L., Allred, D.C., Cote, R.J., Dowsett, M., Fitzgibbons, P.L., Hanna, W.M., Langer, A., McShane, L.M., Paik, S., Pegram, M.D., Perez, E.A., Press, M.F., Rhodes, A., Sturgeon, C., Taube, S.E., Tubbs, R., Vance, G.H., van de Vijver, M., Wheeler, T.M. & Hayes, D.F. (2007). American Society of Clinical Oncology/College of American Pathologists guideline recommendations for human epidermal growth factor receptor 2 testing in breast cancer. *Journal of Clinical Oncology,* Vol.25, No.1, pp. 118-145

Wu, Y., Amonkar, M.M., Sherrill, B.H., O'Shaughnessy, J., Ellis, C., Baselga, J., Blackwell, K.L. & Burstein, H.J. (2011). Impact of lapatinib plus trastuzumab versus single-agent lapatinib on quality of life of patients with trastuzumab-refractory HER2+ metastatic breast cancer. *Annals of Oncology,* March 15, 2011, Epub ahead of print

Yarden, Y., Sliwkowski, M.X. (2001). Untangling the ErbB signalling network. *Nature Reviews. Molecular Cell Biology,* Vol.2, No.2, pp. 127-137

Zhang, A., Shen, G., Zhao, T., Zhang, G., Liu, J., Song, L., Wei, W., Bing, L., Wu, Z. & Wu, Q. (2010). Augmented inhibition of angiogenesis by combination of HER2 antibody chA21 and trastuzumab in human ovarian carcinoma xenograft. *Journal of Ovarian Research,* Vol.3, pp. 20-27

Zhang, X., Gureasko, J., Shen, K., Cole, P.A. & Kuriyan, J. (2006). An allosteric mechanism for activation of the kinase domain of epidermal growth factor receptor. *Cell,* Vol.125, No.6, pp. 1137–1149

Zuo, T., Wang, L., Morrison, C., Chang, X., Zhang, H., Li, W., Liu, Y., Wang, Y., Liu, X., Chan, M.W., Liu, J.Q., Love, R., Liu, C.G., Godfrey, V., Shen, R., Huang, T.H., Yang, T., Park, B.K., Wang, C.Y., Zheng, P. & Liu, Y. (2007). *FOXP3* is an X-linked breast cancer suppressor gene and an important repressor of the *HER-2/ErbB2* oncogene. *Cell,* Vol.129, No.7, pp. 1275–1286

17

Second-Line Chemotherapy for Platinum- and Taxane-Resistant Epithelial Ovarian Cancer: Pegylated Liposomal Doxorubicin (PLD), Irinotecan, and Combination Therapies at Lower Doses

Toru Sugiyama
Obstetrics and Gynecology, Iwate Medical University School of Medicine, Morioka City Japan

1. Introduction

Epithelial ovarian cancer is sensitive to chemotherapy and approximately 75% of patients achieve complete clinical remission after the initial treatment. However, most develop a recurrence which results in death after a chronic course. Therefore, most patients are candidates for second-line chemotherapy, including approximately 20% among of these patients with platinum- and taxane-resistant disease. Patients with platinum-and taxane-resistant disease have poor outcomes, and most would like to prolong their survival with relieved symptoms and the best possible quality of life (QOL). The effects of several drugs which are being used for these purposes are similar, but it is usually difficult to relieve recurrent disease with one drug. Monotherapy has been generally chosen for having the most favorable toxicity profile in patients with platinum- and taxane-resistant disease. However, it is not clear whether this strategy is optimal with the various novel anticancer drugs and targeted agents under development. In this article, pegylated liposomal doxorubicin (PLD), which is used worldwide, and irinotecan, the predominant agent in Japan for the treatment of platinum- and taxane-resistant ovarian cancer, are evaluated for their effects and toxicity in monotherapy and in combination at lower doses with other drugs.

2. Objectives

Platinum- and taxane-resistant epithelial ovarian cancer is not curable; therefore, patients give fully informed consent and are treated to maintain their QOL. The initial treatment aims to cure cancer while the second-line chemotherapy seeks palliation as the primary goal. To be specific, the aim is to balance toxicity and the beneficial effects, and considering the toxicities after the initial treatment and patient's desires, more convenient and less toxic agents should be chosen. Second-line chemotherapy is intended to prevent deterioration of cancer lesions and to relieve symptoms.

3. Principle for choosing therapy

In the treatment of recurrent ovarian cancer, the issues to consider are the treatment-free interval (TFI), toxicity continuously observed from the initial treatment, recurrent tumor diameter and increased CA125. The TFI is the most important for selecting regimens, and the longer the TFI, the higher the response rate (Figure 1).[1,2] In selecting regimens, when the TFI is 6 months or longer, the tumor is considered to be sensitive to chemotherapy. In contrast, when the TFI is less than 6 months, the tumor is considered to be resistant to chemotherapy. For patients with a platinum- and taxane- resistant disease, a drug without cross-resistance to paclitaxel and carboplatin must be selected. On the other hand, recommended therapies for tumors sensitive to drugs, based on the results of randomized controlled trials and meta-analyses, are carboplatin- combination therapy with or without a targeted agent. However, 6-12 months of TFI is considered to be a gray zone (platinum-resistant factor remains; partially sensitive) and more careful consideration should be needed in choosing regimens.

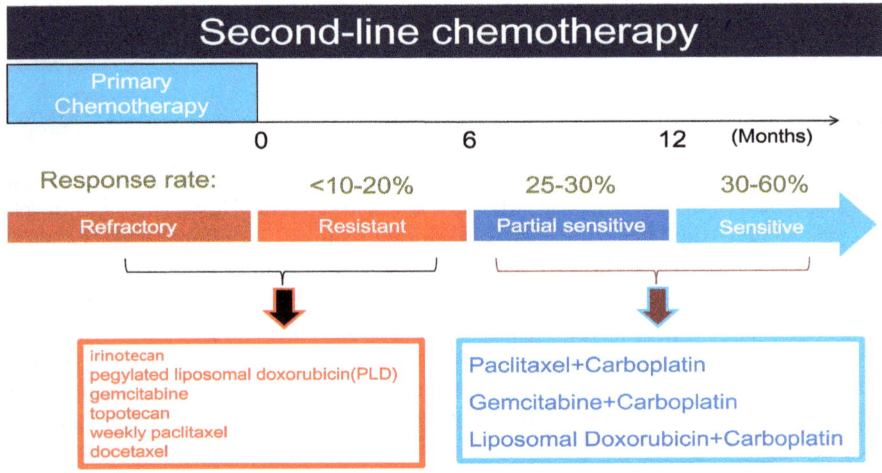

Fig. 1. Principle for choosing therapy.

Pegylated liposomal doxorubicin (PLD), topotecan, and weekly paclitaxel are the drugs approved by the Food and Drug Administration (FDA), and gemcitabine (GEM), oral etoposide, and docetaxel can also be used. In Japan, weekly irinotecan is frequently used. The effects of drugs on patients with platinum- and taxane-resistant disease are similar and no drug can complete the treatment in most patients. Based on the performance status (PS) and toxicity persisting from the initial treatment and the bone-marrow function of an individual patient, drugs to be administered should be presented to the patient. PLD is safer for heavily pretreated patients than topotecan and GEM due to mild bone-marrow toxicity, however, nonhematotoxity such as hand-foot syndrome (HFS), stomatitis and mucositis frequently develop, patient's desire is considered, finally, the drugs are selected.[3] However, it is usually difficult to completely relieve cancer with one drug with high efficacy and low toxicity, and the drugs are therefore changed as required while assessing the effect and toxicity.

4. Effects and toxicities

4.1 Effects

The response rate of anticancer drugs in platinum-resistant ovarian cancer ranges from 12% to 32%, and the survival (median) is around 8-10 months. The effect of anticancer drugs is generally evaluated by the change in tumor diameter; i.e., if the tumor diameter increases, outcomes are judged to be progressive disease (PD) and the treatment is discontinued or changed, and if the tumor diameter decreases, the treatment is evaluated to be effective and continued if no toxicity-related problem occurs. However, it was shown in several studies that such direct evaluation results of tumor diameter do not always correlate with survival time. We investigated the relationship between the drug-induced change in tumor diameter and survival, albeit in a small-size population, and showed that there was no difference in the survival time between the patients with complete response (CR) or partial response (PR) and those with stable disease (SD), and that only patients with PD showed particularly poor outcomes (the IGCS Symposium, Edinburgh, 2004). Cesano et al. showed similar results. [4] Rose et al. recently analyzed outcomes of patients with platinum-resistant ovarian ovarian cancer who were enrolled in 11 GOG phase II clinical trials (1996-2004) and compared the survival time between the CR/PR, SD and PD groups (Figure 2). [5] The results showed no difference between the CR/PR and the SD groups while the overall survival (OS) in the PD group was significantly poorer than that in the CR/PR/SD group ($p<0.001$). Given these corroborating results, it is important to evaluate the effect of treatment by the total percent of responders and patients with SD who have no increase in tumor size (disease control rate) in treatments of patients with platinum-resistant disease. This percent is expressed as the clinical benefit. Consequently, it is considered that patients with platinum- and taxane-resistant ovarian cancer who have tumors evaluable as SD as well as CR/PR are given effective treatment when patients have no toxicity problems and can maintain their QOL.

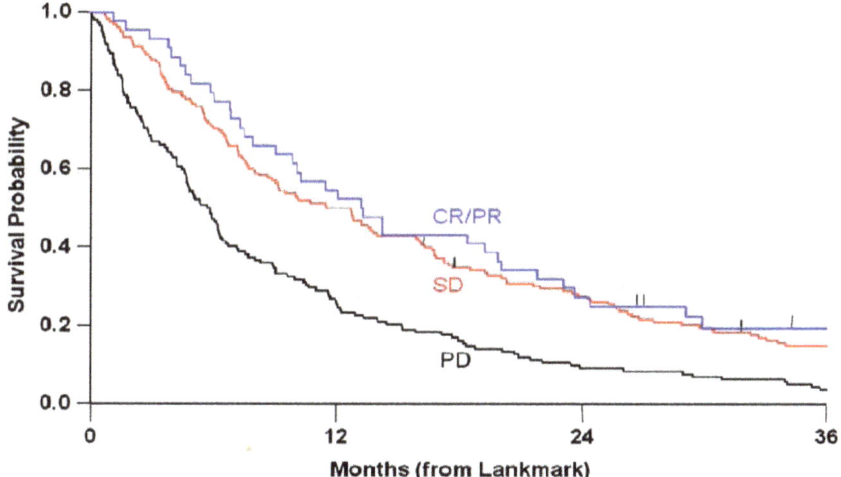

Fig. 2. Survival by tumor response status (landmark analysis)

4.2 Toxicity

The toxicity depends on agents but generally tends to increase with the frequency of chemotherapy. Therefore, in the treatment of platinum- and taxane- resistant ovarian cancer, much attention should be given to the occurrence of toxicities. Topotecan, GEM, docetaxel are highly hemotoxic, and patients using PLD, irinotecan, or weekly paclitaxel should be monitored for non-hemotoxic events that reduce the QOL. There is concern about HFS occurring in treatment with PLD, diarrhea with irinotecan, and peripheral neuropathy and arthralgia during weekly paclitaxel therapy. When a patient is treated with irinotecan, diarrhea is frequently induced, therefore, informed consent for determination of UGT1A1 polymorphism should be obtained from the patient and the assay is carried out as needed.[6,7)]

5. Pgylated liposomal doxorubicin (PLD)

PLD was approved in 1999 by the FDA and in 2000 by the European Medicines Evaluation Agency as treatment for chemorefractory and chemoresistant epithelial ovarian cancer and has been used as the first option for patients with chemorefractory and chemoresistant epithelial ovarian cancer over the world.

5.1 Efficacy

The results of phase II/III studies of PLD showed response rates to platinum-resistant disease ranging from 8.7% to 31.4%, SD rates from 18.2% to 51.3% and a high clinical benefit around 60%, and no difference in the efficacy between 50 and 40 mg/m^2 of PLD. A phase II study has recently been completed in Japan and the response rate for recurrent platinum-resistant ovarian cancer was 21.0%, the SD rate was 40.3% and the clinical benefit was 61.3%, which was similar to those in the studies in Europe and the United States.[8-15)]

5.2 Safety

The data in Europe and the United States show that PLD is accompanied by a low incidence and low severity of hematotoxicities such as neutropenia. The incidence of neutropenia of grade 3/4 ranges from 10% to 20%, and granulocyte colony stimulating factor (G-CSF) drugs are seldom needed. The incidence of thrombopenia is lower. On the other hand, PLD is accompanied by high incidences of subjective non-hematotoxities including HFS and stomatitis at FDA-approved doses and schedules. HFS and stomatitis developed in approximately 40% of patients; however, HFS of grade 2 or higher were found in 19.8% to 31.5% of patients treated with PLD at a dose of 50 mg/m^2 and 2.8% to 15.5% (less than half as frequently) at doses of 40 mg/m^2 and less. Stomatitis of grade 2 or higher developed in 14% to 38% or more of patients treated with PLD at a dose of 50 mg/m^2 and in 8.0% of those treated with 40 mg/m^2.[8-15)] We showed the efficacy of cooling the wrists and ankles during infusion to prevent HFS (ESMO, Milan, 2010). We are currently conducting a clinical trial of stomatitis prevention.

Based on the review of previous studies, no difference in the efficacy between 50 and 40 mg/m^2 of PLD, therefore, a dose of 40 mg/m^2 is preferable for patients with platinum-resistant disease to reduce adverse events. To scientifically confirm the dosage, the Japanese Gynecologic Oncology Group (JGOG) has started a randomized comparative study of 50 and 40 mg/m^2 of PLD in patients with platinum-and taxane- resistant ovarian cancer (TFI < 6 months).

5.3 Japanese-specific toxicity

The incidences and severity of PLD-induced toxicity in the Japanese population are different from those in European and the United States populations. In a Phase II trial in Japan, the incidence of HFS was 78% (Grade 2 or more: 51%) and that of neutropenia of grade 3 or more was 68%, suggesting the necessity of toxicity monitoring and treatment.[16)]

5.4 Comparison with other drugs in Phase III trials

- Topotecan: The response rate of topotecan was around 14% in patients with platinum- and taxane-resistant ovarian cancer. In a phase III comparative study with paclitaxel, the response rate of topotecan was 13.3% in the platinum-resistant ovarian cancer group, better than paclitaxel's rate of 6.7%.[17)] The time to progression in the topotecan group was significantly better than that in the paclitaxel group; consequently, topotecan was confirmed to have at least an equivalent effect to paclitaxel. In comparison with PLD, topotecan had a tendency of being more effective in terms of the progression free survival (PFS) and overall survival (OS) in the platinum-resistant ovarian cancer group; on the other hand, PLD was significantly more effective than topotecan in the platinum-sensitive ovarian cancer group (Table 1).[18)]

	Progression-free survival (median, week)		Overall survival (median, week)	
Gordon et al. (2001)				
Platinum-sensitive				
PLD (n=109)	28.9	*P=0.037*	108	*p=0.008*
topotecan (n=111)	23.3		71	
Platinum-resistant				
PLD (n=130)	9.1	*p=0.733*	36	*p=0.455*
topotecan (n=124)	13.6		41	
Mutch et al. (2007)				
Platinum-resistant				
PLD (n=96)	3.1*	*p=0.870*	13.5*	*p=0.997*
gemcitabine (n=99)	3.6*		12.7*	
Ferrandina et al. (2008)**				
PLD (n=75)	16**	*p=0.411*	56**	*p=0.048*
gemcitabine (n=77)	20**		51**	

*** months**
****Patients with treatment-free interval < 12 months**

Gordon AN et al Gynecol Oncol 2004;95: 1-8
Mutch DG et al J Clin Oncol 2007;25: 2811-2818
Ferrandina G et al J Clin Oncol 2008;26: 890-896

Table 1. Survival of Randomized studies.

- Gemcitabine: The response rate at doses of 800-1,000 mg/m^2/week and the schedule of days 1, 8 and 15 and one-week withdrawal was 13-14% in the platinum-resistant ovarian cancer group. Mutch et al. conducted a phase III comparative study with gemcitabine (GEM) that showed no significant differences in PFS and OS between PLD and GEM. [14] Ferrandina et al. reported no differences in PFS between PLD and GEM in relapsed patients with a treatment-free interval (TFI) of 12 months or less, but a significant efficacy in OS with PLD compared to GEM (Table 1). [15] From the results of the above phase III studies, PLD was considered to have similar efficacy as other novel drugs on platinum-resistant disease; however, it was more effective at improving the survival rate in patients with recurrent ovarian cancer, including platinum-sensitive cancer, than other drugs.

- Difference in toxicity: The results of phase III comparative studies with topotecan or GEM confirmed that HFS and stomatitis significantly developed in patients treated with 50 mg/m^2 of PLD while the incidence of HFS was slightly higher in patients treated with 40 mg/m^2 of PLD compared with those treated with GEM and no difference was found in the incidence of stomatitis between PLD and GEM. On the other hand, PLD induced hematotoxicity less than topotecan and gemcitabine. Although neutropenia of grade 3 or more developed in 10% to 20% of patients treated with 50 mg/m^2 of PLD, febrile neutropenia was rarely found. The incidence of thrombocytopenia was further less. [13-15]

5.5 Combination with other drugs

In multidrug therapy, toxicity is often increased by the combination of multiple drugs at doses recommended for monotherapy. In contrast to initial chemotherapy, which aims to cure cancer, second-line chemotherapy aims to combine drugs at lower doses, considering the toxicity based on the results of phase I clinical studies. In particular, drugs with non-hematotoxicity such as PLD should be used in accordance with the above consideration. [3] In fact, in phase II clinical trials, the incidence and severity of PLD-specific non-hematotoxicities (HFS, stomatitis) were reduced without loss of efficacy when PLD was administered at lower doses in combination with GEM, topotecan, vinorelbine, and oxaliplatin.

In vitro data suggested a potential synergistic interaction between PLD and GEM. [19] Combination chemotherapy of PLD and GEM achieved good response rates ranging from 22% to 33%, however, the clinical benefit was between 28% and 61%, which was similar to PLD monotherapy. [20-23] As for hematotoxicity, neutropenia of grade 3/4 was slightly higher and HFS of grade 2/3 was slightly less. The combination of PLD and GEM is an active and acceptably tolerated option in the treatment of patients with platinum-resistant ovarian cancer (Table 2). The combination at the dosages chosen seems suitable for this patient population. Synergism between PLD and topotecan was demonstrated in platinum-resistant disease. [24] A median total response rate of 28% and clinical benefit of 72% were demonstrated, with a median TTP of 30+weeks in the combination of PLD and topotecan for platinum-resistant disease (Table 3).[25] These data compare favorably to the data of both the drugs administered as single agent. In comparison of two studies of combination chemotherapy of PLD and oxaliplatin, the response rates for platinum-resistant disease were 28.6% and 38.5% and the clinical benefit was 71.4% and 76.9%, suggesting the higher efficacy compared with PLD monotherapy. [26,27] Furthermore, the response rates for platinum-sensitive disease were 66.7% and 81.5% and the clinical benefit was 82.8% and 100%, showing the efficacy similar or more to other platinum combination chemotherapy (Table 3). The incidence of HFS was low and no marked increase in hematotoxicity was found, consequently, it was considered to be controllable. Consequently, PLD, with its low hematotoxicity but specific non-hematotoxicities, is recommended for use not as a monotherapy but in low-doses combinations for improved patient QOL.

Author (year)	No. of pts with pl-resist.	Dose/ Schedule	RR(%)	Clinical benefit(%)	Response duration(wk)	Toxicity(%) G3/4neutro	Toxicity(%) PPE
Agostino[1] (2003)	38	P: 30mg/m²(d1) G: 1000mg/m²(d1,8) q3wk	25.0	61.1	18.0	35.6	25.7 (G2/3)
Ferrandina[2] (2005)Q3wk	66	P: 30mg/m²(d1) G: 1000mg/m²(d1,8) q3wk	21.6	53.6	20.5	28.8	14.4 (G3)
Skarlos[3] (2005)	37	P: 25mg/m² (d1) G: 650mg/m² (d1,8) q4wk	22.0	27.5	2.7*	18.9	5.4 (G2/3)
Petru[4] (2006)	31	P: 30mg/m² (d1) G: 650mg/m² (d1,8) q4wks	33.0	46.7	3.0**	26.0	16.0 (G2/3)

* time to failure (month)
** month
Pl-resist: platinum resistant or refractory
RR: response rate, G: grade, neutro: neutropenia
PPE: palmar-plantar erythrodysesthesia

1. BJC 2003;89: 1180-1184
2. Gynecol Oncol 2005;98: 267-273
3. AntiCancer Res 2005; 25: 3103-3108
4. Gynecol Oncol 2006;102: 226-229

Table 2. Phase II studies of PLD + GEM inpatients with platinum-resistant disease.

Author (year)	No. of pts	Dose/ Schedule	RR(%)	Clinical benefit(%)	Response duration (wk)	Toxicity(%) G3/4neutro	Toxicity(%) PPE
Verhar-Langeris[1] (2006)	27*	P: 30mg/m²(d1) T: 1mg/m²/d(d1-5) q3wk	28.0*	72.0*	NR	70.4	3.7 (G3)
Katsaros[2] (2005)	32	P: 30mg/m2(d1) V: 30mg/m2(d1) q3wk	43.3	70.0	NR	12.5	6.3 (G3/4)
Nicoletto[3] (2005)	43	P: 30-35mg/m² (d1) O: 70mg/m² (d1) q4wk	66.7** (28.6*)	82.8** (71.4*)	NR	9.3	4.7(G2)
Recchia[4] (2007)	40	P: 40mg/m² over 2days O: 120mg/m² over 2days q3wks	81.5** (38.5*)	100** (76.9*)	NR	37.5	10.0 (G2)

*patients with platinum-resistant
** patients with platinum-sensitive
T: topotecan, V: vinorelbine, O: oxaliplatin,
RR: response rate, G: grade, neutro: neutropenia
PPE: palmar-plantar erythrodysesthesia

1. Int J Gynecol Cancer 2006;16:65-70
2. Ann Oncol 2005;16:300-306
3. Gynecol Oncol 2006;100:318-323
4. Gynecol Oncol 2007;106: 164-169

Table 3. Phase II studies of PLD-combination in platinum- and taxane-pretreated patients.

6. Irinotecan

Irinotecan has achieved a response rate of 23.6% in recurrent ovarian cancer. 28) Irinotecan/cisplatin combination chemotherapy has shown a response rate of 33% in platinum-resistant ovarian cancer, 29) and 76% when used as the initial regimen for epithelial ovarian cancer. [30] Regarding dose-limiting toxicity, although neutropenia and diarrhea were observed, diarrhea was thought to cause no remarkable problems in the combination regimen examined. Based on these results, irinitecan is considered to be useful drug in chemotherapy for ovarian cancer. There were two phase II studies of single agent of irinotecan for platinum- and taxane-resistant ovarian cancer. Matsumoto et al. treated 28 patients with platinum- and taxane-resistant or refractory ovarian cancer with irinotecan (irinotecan 100mg/m2, days 1,8,15, every 4 weeks), and they observed a response rate of 28.5% with a SD rate of 32.1%, and the clinical benefit was obtained in 60.7% of the patients. [31] Grade3 or 4 neutropenia and diarrhea were shown in 17.9% and 10.7% of the patients, respectively. They concluded that the weekly dosing schedule of irinotecan seems to be effective and safe salvage chemotherapy regimen for platinum- and taxane-resisitant or refractory epithelial ovarian cancer. There are few studies of irinotecan, commonly used in Japan for second-line chemotherapy, from Europe and the United States. Bodurka et al. conducted a clinical trial of irinotecan at a dose of 300 mg/m^2 every 3 weeks in 31 platinum-resistant and platinum-refractory patients. [32] The response rate was 17% and lower than that Matsumoto et al. reported; however, irinotecan had at least an equivalent effect to topotecan and GEM. Furthermore, 14 (48%) patients had stable disease (SD) and 65% showed a clinical benefit, which was similar to the result of Matsumoto et al. There are no data directly comparing irinotecan and topotecan, which have similar active mechanism; however, in a comparison between the results of a phase II study in Japanese patients with recurrent ovarian cancer (topotecan: 1.2 mg/m^2, days 1-5, every 3 weeks), [33] the results of Matsumoto et al. (irinotecan: 100 mg/m^2, days 1, 8 and 15, every 4 weeks), [31] and the results of Bodurka et al. (irinotecan: 300 mg/m^2, every 3 weeks), [32] toxicities markedly differed. The incidences of hematotoxicity of grade 3 or more were higher in the topotecan group; i.e., the incidence of neutropenia of grade 3 or more was 95.8% in the topotecan group, but 17.9% and 35.5% in the irinotecan groups of Matsumoto et al. and Bodurka et al., respectively. Furthermore, thrombopenia occurred in 97% of the topotecan group, but rarely in the irinotecan groups (0% and 6.5% in studies of Matsumoto et al. and Bodurka et al., respectively). Diarrhea frequently occurred in the irinotecan groups with ≥grade 3 incidences of 10.7% and 32.3% in Matsumoto et al. and Bodurka et al., respectively. On the other hand, the incidence in the topotecan group was low (7.1%). As shown above, in treatment with topotecan and irinotecan for patients with recurrent ovarian cancer, hematotoxicity and diarrhea should be monitored, respectively.

6.1 Combination with cisplatin

The synergism between irinotecan and cisplatin, [34] the different mechanism of action between the two drugs, [35] some lack of cross-resistance, [36] and the relative absence of overlapping principal toxicities support the rationale behind considering combination therapy with these agents. Minagwa et al. reported that in cisplatin-resistant Hela cells cisplatin showed a collateral sensitivity to SN-38, an active metabolite of irinotecan. [37] Furthermore, isobologram analysis indicated synergistic interaction of cisplatin and SN-38 for cisplatin-resistant Hela cells. Based on the results of a phase I study, our group conducted a phase II study with irinotecan and cisplatin. [29] Twenty-five patients with recurrent ovarian cancer who had previously undergone platinum-based combination chemotherapy received this treatment consisting of 50 or 60mg/m2 of irinotecan on days 1, 8, and 15, and 50 or 60mg/m2 of cisplatin on day1 every 4 weeks administrated intravenously. The overall response rate was 40%. Even when the analysis was limited to 21 platinum-resistant cases, the response rate was 33.3% with a stable disease (SD) rate of 38.1%, and the clinical benefit was obtained in 15/21 (71.4%) patients (Table 4). Neutropenia occurred in 54.5% of cycles and 64% of patients. Although diarrhea was observed in 31.8% of the courses, there were only a few severe cases (3.0%), and this condition could be managed with the administration of loperamide and/or Kanpo medicine along with adequate hydration. Irinotecan/cisplatin represented a useful doublet regimen for platinum-resistant disease because high clinical benefit was shown, and irinotecan may induce relatively mild hematologic toxicity, particularly, thrombocytopenia, compared with topotecan. Neutropenia was reserved by short-term G-CSF. Although diarrhea frequently occurs during irinitecan monotherapy, it is no longer thought to be a serious toxicity in combination chemotherapy due to irinotecan dose reduction.

Author	No. of pts	Dose/ Schedule	RR(%)	Clinical Benefit (mo)	Time to Progression (mo)	G3/4Toxicity(%)/per patients Neutropenia	Diarrhea
Irinotecan/ Cisplatin							
Sugiyama (1998)	21	P: 50 or 60mg/m²(d1) I : 50 or 60mg/m²(d1,8,15) q4wk	33.3	71.4	6.0	64.0	4.0
Irinotecan/ Oral etoposide							
Nishio (2007)	27	I: 70mg/m²(d1,15) E: 50mg/day (d1-21) q4wk	44.4	85.1	9.0	59.3	7.4
Shoji (2010))	31	I: 70mg/m²(d1,8) E: 50mg/day (d1-21) q4wk	41.9	77.4	7.0 (SD 11.0)	52.4	4.8

*month
SD: stable disease

1. Cancer Lett 1998;128: 211-218
2. Gynecol Oncol 2007;106: 342-347
3. Int J Gynecol Cancer 2010

Table 4. Phase II studies of irinotecan-combinations in patients with platinum-resistant disease.

6.2 Combination with oral etoposide

Etoposide, a topoisomerase-II inhibitor, has high antitumor activity against various animal and human malignancies. The efficacy of etoposide may be regimen-dependent, since prolonged oral administration has yielded better results than intravenous administration. The largest study to date, performed by the Gynecologic Oncology Group (GOG), reported a response rate of 8.3%.[38] Rose et al. gave oral etoposide (50mg/kg of body weight) from days 1 to 21 every 4 weeks to 41 patients with platinum-resistant or 25 patients with platinum-/taxane-resistant ovarian cancer and obtained response rates of 26.8% and 32%, respectively.[39]

DNA topoisomerase-I and -II are nuclear enzymes that participate in various genetic processes, including transcription, replication, recombination and chromosome segregation at mitosis. [40] These two DNA topoisomerases are functionally related and act in concert. Both seem to be essential for maintaining cell viability throughout the cell cycle. Topoisomerase-I treatment induces an increase in the S-phase cell population with an increase in topoisomerase-II mRNA expression. Thus, topoisomerase-I can modulate topoisomerase-II levels to enhance the effect of topoisomerase-II inhibitors. [41,42] Therefore, combined use of topoisomerase-I and-II targeting agents could theoretically inhibit both DNA and RNA synthesis completely, resulting in synergistic cytotoxicity.

We undertook a pilot study and a phase II study to evaluate the antitumor efficacy and toxicity of a combination of irinotecan and oral etoposide in women with platinum- and taxane-resistant ovarian cancer. [43,44] In both studies, irinotecan was administered in an intravenous dose of 60 or 70mg/m^2 as a 90-min infusion on days 1 and 15 of a 28-day cycle, and etoposide was administered in an oral dose of 50mg/body on days 1 to 21. The two studies showed very similar results for efficacy (according to the RECIST and CA125 criteria) and toxicity (Table 4). A pilot study of irinotecan and oral etoposide in platinum- and taxane-resistant ovarian cancer reported an overall response rate of 44.4% in 12/27cases, and the median duration of response was 11 months. [43] Adding 11 patients with SD, a high clinical benefit was shown in 23/27 cases (85.1%). The median time to progression and the median survival in the study group as a whole was 9 months and 17 months, respectively. The major toxicity was neutropenia (grade 3/4, 59%), but was managed easily by administration of short-term G-CSF. Febrile neutropenia was observed in only one patient. Diarrhea was infrequent and mild. The other study was conducted in the northern area of Japan (Tohoku Gynecologic Cancer Unit).[44] Forty-two patients with recurrent epithelial ovarian cancer who had previously undergone platinum-based combination chemotherapy were registered in this study, and the overall response rate was 50.0%. Even when the analysis was limited to 31 platinum-resistant cases, a response rate of 41.9% and clinical benefit of 77.4% were achieved. As for toxicity, grade 3/4 neutropenia was observed in 22 patients (52.4%) and febrile neutropenia in 3 patients (7.1%). Grade 3/4 diarrhea occurred in only two patients (4.8%). Acute myeloid leukemia (AML) developed as a secondary malignancy in one patient in each study. Topoisomerase-II-related AML, initially noted as a therapy-related complication of childhood leukemia, is characterized by the lack of a myelodysplastic phase, no dysplastic change in diagnostic bone marrow specimens, balanced chromosomal translocations involving 11q23, and variable chemosensitivity. This leukemia is characteristically related to the cumulative dose of etoposide and has a shorter latency period (median, 24 to 30 months) than the AML associated with alkylating agent therapy. In general, a total dose of etoposide of more than 6g may be associated with an increased risk of developing leukemia. The total dose of etoposide received by the two patients who had AML in the two studies was 10.5g and 14.2g, respectively. We strongly recommended that this regimen not be given for more than 6 cycles, even if the response or stable disease is sustained. These results of the two studies justify further studies of irinotecan plus oral etoposide in patients with platinum- and taxane-resistant epithelial ovarian cancer.

7. Conclusions

In the treatment of platinum- and taxane- resistant recurrent ovarian cancer, monotherapy is recommended from the perspective of toxicity. However, monotherapy of PLD and irinotecan, which have specific non-hematotoxicities, increases the incidence and severity of

HFS, stomatitis and diarrhea, resulting in a decreased patient QOL. We investigated whether combination therapy of these drugs with other drugs would exploit their advantages at lower doses. The results of studies of combination therapy of PLD or irinotecan showed lower incidences of the non-hematotoxicities specific to these drugs at the same time good patient QOL was maintained; furthermore, a good clinical benefit was shown without loss of the effect in comparison with that of monotherapy. In conclusion, we propose the use of combination therapy using PLD or irinotecan in the treatment of platinum- and taxane- resistant recurrent ovarian cancer.

8. Summary

In the treatment of platinum- and taxane-resistant recurrent cancer, monotherapy is recommended as the standard treatment from the perspective of toxicity. However, pegylated liposomal doxorubicin (PLD) and irinotecan have specific non-hematotoxicities that impair the quality of life (QOL) of patients; therefore, combination therapy at lower doses may provide better clinical benefit than monotherapy, especially as it can be maintained for a longer time because the lowering of the doses decreases the specific toxicities.

9. References

[1] Blackledge G, Lawton F, Redman C, et al. Response of patients in phase II studies of chemotherapy in ovarian cancer: Implications for patients treatment and the design of phase II trilas. Br J Cancer 1989;59: 650-3

[2] Markman M, Reichman B, Hakes T, et al. Response to second-line cisplatin-based intraperitoneal therapy in ovarian cancer: Influence of a prior response to intravenous cisplatin. J Clin Oncol 1991;9:1801-5

[3] Sugiyama T and Kumagai S. Pegylated liposomal doxorubicin for advanced ovarian cancer in women who are refractory to both platinum- and paclitaxel-based chemotherapy regimens. Clinical Medicine: Therapeutics 2009;1:1227-1236.

[4] Cesano A, Lane SR, Poulin R, Ross G, Fields S. Stabilization of disease as a useful predictor of survival following second-line chemotherapy in small cell lung cancer and ovarian cancer. Int J Oncol 1999;15: 1233-1238.

[5] Rose P, Tian C, Bookman MA. Assessment of tumor response as a surrogate endpoint of survival in recurrent/platinum-resistant ovarian carcinoma: a Gynecologic Oncology Group study. Gynecol Oncol 2010;117: 324-329.

[6] Ando Y, Saka H, Ando M, et al. Polymorphisms of UDP-glucuronosyltransferase I in Gilbert's syndrome. Cancer Res 2000;60: 6921-6926.

[7] Takano M, Kato M, Yoshikawa T, et al. Clinical significance of UDP-glucuronosyltransferase 1A1*6 for toxicities of combination chemotherapy with irinotecan and cisplatin in gynecologic cancers. Oncology 2009;76: 315-321.

[8] Muggia FM, Hainsworth JD, Jeffers S, Miller P, Groshen S, Tan M, Roman L, Uziely B, Muderspach L, Garcia A, Burnett A, Greco FA, Morrow CP, Paradiso LJ, Liang Li-J. Phase II study of liposomal doxorubicin in refractory ovarian cancer: antitumor activity and toxicity modification by liposomal encapsulation. J Clin Oncol 1997;15: 987-993.

[9] Gordon AN, Granai CO, Rose PG, Hainsworth J, Lopez A, Weissman C, Rosales R, Sharpington T. Phase II study of liposomal doxorubicin in platinum- and paclitaxel-refractory epithelial ovarian cancer. J Clin Oncol 2000;18:3093-3100.

[10] Markman M, Kennedy A, Webster K, Peterson G, Kulp B, Belinson J. Phase 2 trial of liposomal doxorubicin (40 mg/m2) in platinum/paclitaxel-refractory ovarian and fallopian tube cancers and primary carcinoma of the peritoneum. Gynecol Oncol 2000;78: 369-372.

[11] Wilailak S, Linasmita V. A study of pegylated liposomal doxorubicin in platinum-refractory epithelial ovarian cancer. Oncology 2004;67: 183-186.

[12] Chou HH, Wang KL, Chen CA, Wei LH, Lai CH, Hsieh CY, Yang YC, Twu NF, Chang TC, Yen MS. Pegylated liposomal doxorubicin (Lipo-Dox) for platinum-resistant or refractory epithelila ovarian carcinoma: a Taiwanese gynecologic oncology group study with long-term follow-up. Gynecol Oncol 2006;101: 423-428.

[13] Gordon AN, Fleagle JT, Guthrie D, Parkin DE, Gore ME, Lacave AJ. Recurrent epithelial ovarian carcinoma: a randomized phase III study of pegylated liposomal doxorubicin versus topotecan. J Clin Oncol 2001;19: 3312-3322.

[14] Mutch DG, Orlando M, Goss T, Teneriello MG, Gordon AN, McMeekin SD, Wang Y, Scribner Jr DR, Marciniack M, Naumann RW, Secord AA. Randomized phase III trial of gemcitabine compared with pegylated liposomal doxorubicin in patients with platinum-resistant ovarian cancer. J Clin Oncol 2007;25: 2811-2818.

[15] Ferrandina G, Ludovisi M, Lorusso D, Pignata S, Breda E, Savarese A, Del Medico P, Scaltriti L, Katsaros D, Priolo D, Scambia G. Phase III trial of gemcitabine compared with pegylated liposomal doxorubicin in progressive or recurrent ovarian cancer. J Clin Oncol 2008;26: 890-896.

[16] Katsumata N, Fujiwara Y, Kamura T, Nakanishi T, Hatae M, Aoki D, Tanaka K, Tsuda H, Kamiura S, Takehara K, Sugiyama T, Kigawa J, Fujiwara K, Ochiai K, Ishida R, Inagaki M, Noda K. Phase II clinical trial of pegylated liposomal doxorubicin (JNS002) in Japanese patients with mullerian carcinoma (epithelial ovarian carcinoma, primary carcinoma of fallopian tube, peritoneal carcinoma) having a therapeutic history of platinum-based chemotherapy: a phase II study of the Japanese Gynecologic Oncology Group. Jpn J Clin Oncol 2008;38: 777-785.

[17] Ten Bokkel Huinink W, Gore M, Carmichael J, et al. Topotecan versus paclitaxel for the treatment of recurrent epithelial ovarian cancer. J Clin Oncol 1997;15: 2183-2193.

[18] Gordon AN, Tonda M, Sun S, Rackoff W, on behalf of the Doxil Study 30-49 investigators.Long-term survival advantage for women treated with pegylated liposomal doxorubicin compared with topotecan in a phase 3 randomized study of recurrent and refractory epithelial ovarian cancer. Gynecol Oncol 2004;95: 1-8.

[19] Chow KU, Ries J, Weidmann E, Pourebrahim F, Napieralski S, Stieler M, Boehrer S, Rummel MJ, Stein J, Hoelzer D, Mitrou PS. Induction of apoptosis using 2′,2′difluorodeoxycytidine (gemcitabine) in combination with antimetabolites or anthracyclines on malignant lymphatic and myeloid cells. Antagonism or synergism depends on incubation schedule and origin of neoplastic cells. Ann Hematol 2000;79: 485-492.

[20] D'Agostino G, Ferrandia G, Ludovisi M, Testa A, Lorusso D, Gbaguidi N, Breda E, Mancuso S, Scambia G. Phase II study of liposomal doxorubicin and gemcitabine in the salvage treatment of ovarian cancer. Br J Cancer 2003;89: 1180-1184.

[21] Ferrandina G, Paris I, Ludovisi M, D'Agostino G, Testa A, Lorusso D, Zanghi M, Pisconti S, Pezzella G, Adamo V, Breda E, Scambia G. Gemcitabine and liposomal doxorubicin in the salvage treatment of ovarian cancer: updated results and long-term survival. Gynecol Oncol 2005;98: 267-273.

[22] Skarlos DV, Kalofonos HP, Fountzilas G, Dimopoulos MA, Pavlidis N, Razis E, Economopoulos T, Pectasides D, Gogas H, Kosmidis P, Bafaloukos D, Klouvas G, Kyratzis G, Aravantinos G. Gemcitabine plus pegylated liposomal doxorubicin in patients with advanced epithelial ovarian cancer resistant/refractory to platinum and/or taxanes. A HeCOG phase II study. Anticancer Res 2005; 25: 3103-3108.

[23] Petru E, Angleitner-Boubenizek L, Reinthaller A, Deibl M, Zeimet AG, Volgger B, Stempfl A, Marth C. Combined PEG liposomal doxorubicin and gemcitabine are active and have acceptable toxicity in patients with platinum-refractory and -resistant ovarian cancer after previous platinum-taxane therapy: a phase II Austrian AGO study. Gynecol Oncol 2006;102: 226-229.

[24] Jonsson E, Friborg H, Nygren P, Larsson R. Synergistic interactions of combinations of topotecan with standard drugs in primary cultures of human tumor cells from patients. Eur J Clin Pharmacol 1998;54: 509-514.

[25] Verhaar-Langereis M, Karakus A, van Eijkeren M, Voest E, Witteveen E. Phase II study of the combination of pegylated liposomal doxorubicin and topotecan in platinum-resistant ovarian cancer. Int J Gynecol Cancer 2006;16: 65-70.

[26] Nicoletto MO, Falci C, Pianalto D, Artioli G, Azzoni P, De Masi G, Ferrazzi E, Perin A, Donach M, Zoli W. Phase II study of pegylated liposomal doxorubicin and oxaliplatin in relapsed advanced ovarian cancer. Gynecol Oncol 2006;100: 318-323.

[27] Recchia F, Saggio G, Amiconi G, Di Blasio A, Cesta A, Candeloro G, Carta G, Necozione S, Mantovani G, Rea S. A multicenter phase II study of pegylated liposomal doxorubicin and oxaliplatin in recurrent ovarian cancer. Gynecol Oncol 2007;106: 164-169.

[28] Takeuchi S, Dobashi K, Fujimoto S, et al. A late phase II study of CPT-11 on uterine cervical cancer and ovarian cancer. Research Groups of CPT-11 in Gynecologic Cancers. Jpn J Cancer Chemother 1991;18: 1861-1869.

[29] Sugiyama T, Yakushiji M, Nishida T, et al. Irinotecan (CPT-11) combined with cisplatin in patients with refractory or recurrent ovarian cancer. Cancer Lett 1998;128: 211-218.

[30] Sugiyama T, Yakushiji M, Kamura T, et al. Irinotecan (CPT-11) and cisplatin as first-line chemotherapy for advanced ovarian cancer. Oncology 2002;63: 16-22.

[31] Matsumoto K, Katsumata N, Yamanaka Y, Yonemori K, Kohno T, Shimizu C, et al. The safety and efficacy the weekly dosing of irinotecan for platinum and taxanes-resistant ovarian cancer. Gynecol Oncol 2006;100: 412-416.

[32] Bodurka DC, Levenback C, Wolf JK Gano J, Wharton JT, Kavanagh JJ, et al. Phase II trial of irinotecan in patients with metastatic epithelial ovarian or peritoneal cancer. J Clin Oncol 2003;21: 291-297.

[33] Aoki D, Katsumata N, Nakanishi T, et al. A phase II clinical trial of topotecan in Japanese patients with relapsed ovarian carcinoma. Jpn J Clin Oncol 2010;

[34] Kudoh S, Takada M, Masuda N, et al. Enhanced anti-tumor efficacy of a combination of CPT-11, a new derivative of camptothecin, and cisplatin against lung tumor xenografts. Jpn J Cancer Res 1993;84: 203-207.

[35] Kunimoto T, Nitta K, Tanaka T, et al. Antitumor activity of 7-ethyl-10-[4-(1-piperidino)-1-piperidino]carbonyloxy-camptothecin, a novel water-soluble derivative of camptothecin, against murine tumors. Cancer Res 1987;47: 5944-5947.

[36] Tsuruo T, Matsuzaki T, Matsushita M et al. Antitimor effect of CPT-11, a new derivative of camptothecin, against pleiotropic drug-resistant tumors in vitro and in vivo. Cancer Chemother Pharmacol 1988;21: 71-74.

[37] Minagawa Y, Kigawa J, Ishihara H, Itamochi H, Terakawa N. Synergistic enhancement of cisplatin cytotoxicity by SN-38, an active metabolite of CPT-11, for cisplatin-resistant HeLa cells. Jpn J Cancer Res. 1994; 85: 966-971.

[38] Slayton RE, Creasman WT, Petty W, et al. Phase II trial of VP-16-213 in the treatment of advanced squamous cell carcinoma of the cervix and adenocarcinoma of the ovary. A Gynecologic Oncology Group study. Cancer Treat Rep 1979;63: 2089-2092.

[39] Rose PG, Blessing JA, Mayer AR, Homesley HD. Prolonged oral etoposide as second-line therapy for platinum-resistant and platinum-sensituve ovarian carcinoma: a Gynecologic Oncology Group study. J Clin Oncol 1998;16: 405-410.

[40] Wang JC. DNA topoisomerases. Annu Rev Biochem 1985;54: 665-697.

[41] Kim R, Hirabayashi N, Nishiyama M, et al. Experimental studies on biochemical modulation targeting topoisomerase I and II in human tumor xenografts in nude mice. Int J Cancer 1992;50: 760-766.

[42] Masumoto N, Nakano S, Esaki T, et al. Sequence-dependent modulation of anticancer drug activities by 7-ethyl-10-hydroxycamptothecin in an HST-1 human squamous carcinoma cell line. Anticancer Res 1995;14: 405-409.

[43] Nishio S, Sugiyama T, Souji T, et al. Pilot study evaluationg the efficacy and toxicity of irinotecan plus oral etoposide for platinum- and taxane-resistant epithelial ovarian cancer. Gynecol Oncol 2007;106: 342-347.

[44] Shoji T, Takatori E, Omi H, et al. Phase II clinical study of the combination chemotherapy regimen of irinotacan plus oral etoposide for the treatment of recurrent ovarian cancer (Tohoku Gynecologic Cancer Unit 101 Group study). Int J Gynecol Cancer 2010;21:44-50.

Permissions

The contributors of this book come from diverse backgrounds, making this book a truly international effort. This book will bring forth new frontiers with its revolutionizing research information and detailed analysis of the nascent developments around the world.

We would like to thank Samir A. Farghaly, MD, PhD, for lending his expertise to make the book truly unique. He has played a crucial role in the development of this book. Without his invaluable contribution this book wouldn't have been possible. He has made vital efforts to compile up to date information on the varied aspects of this subject to make this book a valuable addition to the collection of many professionals and students.

This book was conceptualized with the vision of imparting up-to-date information and advanced data in this field. To ensure the same, a matchless editorial board was set up. Every individual on the board went through rigorous rounds of assessment to prove their worth. After which they invested a large part of their time researching and compiling the most relevant data for our readers. Conferences and sessions were held from time to time between the editorial board and the contributing authors to present the data in the most comprehensible form. The editorial team has worked tirelessly to provide valuable and valid information to help people across the globe.

Every chapter published in this book has been scrutinized by our experts. Their significance has been extensively debated. The topics covered herein carry significant findings which will fuel the growth of the discipline. They may even be implemented as practical applications or may be referred to as a beginning point for another development.

The editorial board has been involved in producing this book since its inception. They have spent rigorous hours researching and exploring the diverse topics which have resulted in the successful publishing of this book. They have passed on their knowledge of decades through this book. To expedite this challenging task, the publisher supported the team at every step. A small team of assistant editors was also appointed to further simplify the editing procedure and attain best results for the readers.

Our editorial team has been hand-picked from every corner of the world. Their multi-ethnicity adds dynamic inputs to the discussions which result in innovative outcomes. These outcomes are then further discussed with the researchers and contributors who give their valuable feedback and opinion regarding the same. The feedback is then collaborated with the researches and they are edited in a comprehensive manner to aid the understanding of the subject.

Apart from the editorial board, the designing team has also invested a significant amount of their time in understanding the subject and creating the most relevant covers. They scrutinized every image to scout for the most suitable representation of the subject and create an appropriate cover for the book.

The publishing team has been involved in this book since its early stages. They were actively engaged in every process, be it collecting the data, connecting with the contributors or procuring relevant information. The team has been an ardent support to the editorial, designing and production team. Their endless efforts to recruit the best for this project, has resulted in the accomplishment of this book. They are a veteran in the field of academics and their pool of knowledge is as vast as their experience in printing. Their expertise and guidance has proved useful at every step. Their uncompromising quality standards have made this book an exceptional effort. Their encouragement from time to time has been an inspiration for everyone.

The publisher and the editorial board hope that this book will prove to be a valuable piece of knowledge for researchers, students, practitioners and scholars across the globe.

List of Contributors

Sherri L. Stewart
Division of Cancer Prevention and Control, Centers for Disease Control and Prevention, USA

Duangmani Thanapprapasr and Sarikapan Wilailak
Department of Obstetrics and Gynecology, Faculty of Medicine, Ramathibodi Hospital, Mahidol University, Thailand

Gina M. Mantia-Smaldone and Nathalie Scholler
Penn Ovarian Cancer Research Center, University of Pennsylvania, Philadelphia, USA

Susanna Syriac
Roswell Park Cancer Institute, Department of Pathology, Division of Surgical Oncologic Pathology Buffalo, USA

Faith Ough
University of Southern California, Department of Pathology, Division of Cytopathology, Los Angeles, USA

Paulette Mhawech-Fauceglia
University of Southern California, Department of Pathology, Division of Gynecologic Oncologic Pathology, Los Angeles, USA

Gennaro Cormio, Maddalena Falagario and Luigi E. Selvaggi
University of Bari, Italy

Dan Ancuşa, Octavian Neagoe, Răzvan Ilina, Adrian Carabineanu, Corina Şerban and Marius Craina
University of Medicine and Pharmacy „Victor Babeş" Timişoara, Romania

Yi Pan
Department of Neurology & Psychiatry, Saint Louis University, USA

Antonios-Apostolos K. Tentes
Didimotichon General Hospital, Greece

Nicolaos Courcoutsakis and Panos Prasopoulos
Alexandroupolis University Hospital, Greece

Constantine Gennatas
Areteion Hospital, University of Athens, Greece

Samir A. Farghaly
The Joan and Sanford I. Weill/ The Graduate School of Medical Sciences and The New York Presbyterian Hospital -Weill Cornell Medical Center, Cornell University, New York, NY, USA

Carlos M. Telleria and Alicia A. Goyeneche
Division of Basic Biomedical Sciences, Sanford School of Medicine, The University of South Dakota, Vermillion, South Dakota, USA

Juliane Farthmann and Annette Hasenburg
University Hospital, Dept. of Gynecology, Freiburg, Germany

Wei-Chu Chie
Institute of Epidemiology and Preventive Medicine, College of Public Health, National Taiwan University, Taiwan

Elfriede Greimel
Department of Obstetrics and Gynaecology, Medical University Graz, Graz, Austria

J. Elgqvist and P. Albertsson
Department of Oncology, Sahlgrenska Academy, University of Gothenburg, Sweden

S. Lindegren
Department of Radiation Physics, Sahlgrenska Academy, University of Gothenburg, Sweden

K. Nakaya
Department of Health Pharmacy, Yokohama College of Pharmacy, Yokohama

Y. Masuda
Department of Pharmaceutical Biology, Showa Pharmaceutical University, Machida, Japan

T. Aiuchi and H. Itabe
School of Pharmacy, Showa University, Tokyo, Japan

Toru Sugiyama
Obstetrics and Gynecology, Iwate Medical University, School of Medicine, Morioka City, Japan